Cosmeceutical Science in Clinical Practice

Cosmeceuticals – skin care products that fall between a cosmetic and a pharmaceutical, with active ingredients that counter skin aging and promote skin rejuvenation – are an invaluable adjunct to the cosmetic dermatologist or plastic surgeon performing minimally invasive aesthetic procedures. This guide from expert researchers and practitioners explains how best to integrate the potential of cosmeceutical products into the best international clinical practice, with new chapters to cover the very latest developments in this area.

Series in Cosmetic and Laser Therapy

About the Series

The world of cosmetic and aesthetic medicine and surgery has grown greatly in size and complexity over recent years, and the series in *Cosmetic and Laser Therapy* keeps readers up to date with the latest clinical therapies to improve and rejuvenate the appearance of skin, hair, and nails. Published in association with the *Journal of Cosmetic and Laser Therapy*, each volume in the series is prepared separately and typically focuses on a topical theme. Volumes are published on an occasional basis, according to the emergence of new developments.

Handbook of Cosmetic Skin Care, Second Edition
Avi Shai, Howard I. Maibach, Robert Baran

Cosmetic Bootcamp Primer: Comprehensive Aesthetic Management
Kenneth Beer, Mary P. Lupo, Vic A. Narurkar

Illustrated Manual of Injectable Fillers: A Technical Guide to the Volumetric Approach to Whole Body Rejuvenation, First Edition
Neil S. Sadick, Paul J. Carniol, Deborshi Roy, Luitgard Wiest

Comprehensive Aesthetic Rejuvenation: A Regional Approach
Jenny Kim, Gary Lask, Andrew Nelson

Textbook of Chemical Peels: Superficial, Medium, and Deep Peels in Cosmetic Practice, Second Edition
Philippe Deprez

Textbook of Cosmetic Dermatology, Fifth Edition
Robert Baran, Howard I. Maibach

Disorders of Fat and Cellulite: Advances in Diagnosis and Treatment
David J. Goldberg, Alexander L. Berlin

Botulinum Toxins in Clinical Aesthetic Practice 3E, Volume One: Clinical Adaptations
Anthony V. Benedetto

Botulinum Toxins in Clinical Aesthetic Practice 3E, Volume Two: Functional Anatomy and Injection Techniques
Anthony V. Benedetto

Aesthetic Rejuvenation Challenges and Solutions: A World Perspective
Paul J. Carniol, Gary D. Monheit

Illustrated Manual of Injectable Fillers, Second Edition
Neil S. Sadick

Adapting Dermal Fillers in Clinical Practice
Yates Yen-Yu Chao, Sebastian Cotofana

Cosmeceutical Science in Clinical Practice, Second Edition
Neil S. Sadick, Mary P. Lupo, Zoe Diana Draelos

For more information about this series please visit: https://www.crcpress.com/Series-in-Cosmetic-and-Laser-Therapy/book-series/CRCCOSLASTHE

Cosmeceutical Science in Clinical Practice

Second Edition

Edited by

Neil S. Sadick MD, FAAD, FAACS, FACP, FACPh

Weill Medical College of Cornell University and
Sadick Dermatology and Aesthetic Surgery
New York, New York, USA

Mary P. Lupo MD, FAAD

Tulane University Medical Center and Lupo Center for Aesthetic and
General Dermatology
New Orleans, Louisiana, USA

Zoe Diana Draelos MD, FAAD

Duke University School of Medicine Durham, North Carolina, USA
Dermatology Consulting Services, High Point, North Carolina, USA

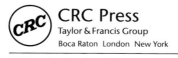

CRC Press
Taylor & Francis Group
Boca Raton London New York

CRC Press is an imprint of the
Taylor & Francis Group, an **informa** business

Cover image: © Shutterstock

Second edition published 2023
by CRC Press
6000 Broken Sound Parkway NW, Suite 300, Boca Raton, FL 33487-2742

and by CRC Press
4 Park Square, Milton Park, Abingdon, Oxon, OX14 4RN

CRC Press is an imprint of Taylor & Francis Group, LLC

© 2023 Taylor & Francis Group, LLC

ISBN: 9781138055506 (hbk)
ISBN: 9781032485058 (pbk)
ISBN: 9781315165905 (ebk)

DOI: 10.1201/9781315165905

Typeset in Times
by KnowledgeWorks Global Ltd.

Contents

Contributors

Fadwa Ahmed
The Warren Alpert Medical School of Brown
    University
Providence, Rhode Island

Macrene Alexiades
Yale University School of Medicine
New Haven, Connecticut

Andrew F. Alexis
Weill Cornell Medicine
New York, New York

Susan Bard
Vive Dermatology
Brooklyn, New York

Diane S. Berson
Weill-Cornell Medical School
New York, New York

Ronda Farah
University of Minnesota Medical School
Minneapolis, Minnesota

Laurel Naversen Geraghty
Dermatology & Laser Associates of Medford
Medford, Oregon

Jasmine Gibson
The Warren Alpert Medical School of Brown
    University
Providence, Rhode Island

Mitchel P. Goldman
Cosmetic Laser Dermatology
San Diego, California

Harriet Lin Hall
Blake Medical Center
Bradenton, Florida

Ranella Hirsch
Skin Care Doctors
Cambridge, Massachusetts

Ajay Kailas
Howard University
Washington, DC

Bridget P. Kaufman
Icahn School of Medicine at
    Mount Sinai
New York, New York

Hayley Leight
Dermatology, Laser & Vein Specialists of the
    Carolinas
Charlotte, North Carolina

Rachel Maiman
Icahn School of Medicine at
    Mount Sinai
New York, New York

Rahul C. Mehta
Allergan Aesthetics
San Marcos, California

Radha Mikkilineni
Weill-Cornell Medical School
New York Presbyterian Hospital
New York, New York

Isabelle Moseley
The Warren Alpert Medical School of Brown
    University
Providence, Rhode Island

Briana Paiewonsky
University of Minnesota
Minneapolis, Minnesota

Aleksandra J. Poole
Lineage Cell Therapeutics
San Marcos, California

Sara D. Ragi
The Warren Alpert Medical School of Brown
    University
Providence, Rhode Island

Ora Raymond
University of Minnesota
Minneapolis, Minnesota

Skylar A. Souyoul
Pennington Facial Plastics
Shreveport, Louisiana

Sarah Stierman
Dermatology Associates
Perrysburg, Ohio

Susan H. Weinkle
University of South Florida
Brandenton, Florida

1

Clinical Uses of Copper in Skin Aging and Wound Healing

Sara D. Ragi, Fadwa Ahmed, Jasmine Gibson, and Isabelle Moseley

Introduction

Copper (Cu) is a trace mineral that has well-established roles in several biological processes throughout the human body. Among these roles, copper is essential to cellular respiration, extracellular matrix formation, and neutralization of reactive oxygen species (ROS). Copper has thus been regarded as a promising dermatologic tool with applications in wound healing, photoaging, inflammatory conditions, and skin cancer.

In addition to its roles in extracellular matrix synthesis, cellular respiration, and detoxification, copper has been implicated in a number of other biological and physiological processes, including angiogenesis, skin and stem cell migration, integrin expression, and stimulation of dermal fibroblast production of extracellular matrix proteins (1–5). The wide range of well-established biochemical and physiological roles of copper have established it as a candidate for several clinical applications, including wound healing, photoaging, inflammatory conditions, and skin cancers. A range of in vitro, in vivo, and more recent clinical studies highlight the promising therapeutic and cosmetic potential of topical copper-containing compounds.

Background

Copper (Cu) is the third most abundant essential trace element in the human body. It is involved in many physiological and biological processes, including melanin production, heme synthesis, iron absorption, and bone formation (6–8). High concentrations are found in the liver, kidney, brain, and heart, but the majority is located in the skeleton and muscle tissue (9–11). The average adult body contains 50–120 mg of copper and homeostatic levels are maintained by intestinal absorption and biliary excretion (12, 13).

Foods rich in copper include shellfish, seeds, nuts, organ meats, wheat-bran cereals, whole-grain products, and chocolate (9). In the United States, the median consumption of copper from food is approximately 1.0–1.6 mg/day for adult men and women (14). The bioavailability of copper is largely determined by dietary intake and absorption is higher when copper consumption increases (14). Absorption can be as low as 12% with dietary copper intakes of 7.5 mg/day, and as high as 75% with copper intakes of 400 µg/day. Once ingested, Cu is absorbed in the proximal small intestine (15). Loosely bound to albumin and other small molecules, Cu is delivered to many tissues and organs in the body with the highest amount delivered to the liver (14, 16, 17). In the liver, Cu is incorporated into ceruloplasmin, a ferroxidase enzyme, which transports Cu to extrahepatic sites (13, 18).

The liver also plays an important role in copper excretion. Approximately two-thirds of copper that is absorbed is secreted into bile, which is produced by hepatocytes (13, 19). Excretion of copper into bile requires ATP7b, a copper-transporting P-type ATPase found in trans-Golgi network of hepatocytes (19, 20). Mutations in the gene encoding ATP7b can lead to Wilson disease, a disorder characterized by copper accumulation (19, 20).

DOI: 10.1201/9781315165905-1

Copper is an essential cofactor of several major enzymes in the human body, including cytochrome c oxidase (Cox), lysyl oxidase, and superoxide dismutase (SOD). Cox is the heme/copper enzyme at the end of the mitochondrial electron transport chain (21–23). The copper cores of the transmembrane enzyme are directly involved in electron transport in the aqueous phase of aerobic respiration and the creation of the proton electrochemical gradient that is critical for ATP production. In addition to serving as a central component of the Cox enzymatic complex, copper homeostasis appears to have a role in regulating its assembly and disassembly (23).

Lysyl oxidase, another cuproenzyme, is responsible for the conversion of lysine to aldehyde precursors of collagen and elastin (1, 24). Lysyl oxidase has been detected at high levels in the dermis and lower levels within both basal and suprabasal layers of the epidermis. While primarily known for this extracellular function, lysyl oxidase has been implicated in a number of other extracellular and intracellular processes, such as suppression of tumor proliferation, cell migration, and cell differentiation (25, 26). Decreased functions of lysyl oxidase secondary to impairments in copper transporters have been implicated in connective tissue diseases, such as Occipital Horn Syndrome and Menkes Disease (27, 28).

SOD catalyzes the neutralization of superoxide, a free radical ROS that is a byproduct of cellular respiration and metabolism (29–31). Among the SOD-family enzymes found in humans, two (SOD1 and SOD3) are copper-zinc metalloproteins. SOD1 is primarily found in the cytoplasm, while SOD3 in the extracellular matrix; both are essential for protection from oxidative stress (30).

The effects of copper on many organs, including the skin, have been well documented (32). Copper's effects on the skin include the synthesis and stabilization of skin proteins, stimulation of dermal fibroblast proliferation, increased protein expression of collagen and elastin produced by fibroblasts, and serving as a cofactor for tyrosinase, which is involved in the synthesis of melanin (2, 32, 33). Given the beneficial effects of copper on skin health, it is important to describe copper's role in wound healing, skin aging, inflammatory diseases, and skin cancer.

Clinical Applications

Wound Healing

Copper has been used in the treatment of wounds as it exerts wound healing-properties by affecting cellular processes, including angiogenesis, growth factor induction, and extracellular matrix remodeling that may improve and accelerate wound healing and tissue repair (Table 1.1). Catalytic conversion of hydrogen peroxide (H_2O_2) to toxic hydroxyl radicals ($\cdot OH$) may be used in wound sterilization (34). One study reported a pH-responsive copper peroxide-loaded wound dressing made from copper hydroxide and gelatin sponge reacted with H_2O_2 (34). In vitro experiments reveal that this wound dressing exhibited bactericidal properties against *Escherichia coli*, *Staphylococcus aureus*, and *Pseudomonas aeruginosa* (34). The wound dressing also releases OH in the bacteria-infected skin wound, as opposed to in normal tissues, and in vivo skin wound-healing experiments demonstrated that synthesized copper peroxide-loaded gelatin sponge fights *E. coli* effectively; in addition, $Cu^{2}+$ released from the gelatin sponge may incite angiogenesis and collagen deposition simultaneously (34). This wound dressing with a copper component may improve antibacterial efficacy and reduce toxic side effects of bacterial infection through the release of $\cdot OH$ via bacterial self-activation (34).

In another study, copper-loaded alginate fibers were developed and used in surgical sutures for the repair of incisional wounds in mice (37). Ninety-five percent of loaded copper ions were released from these sutures in the first day following an initial burst release (37). Copper delivered to the incision site improved recovery of tissue by increasing the biomechanical strength as compared to conventional nylon and calcium-alginate sutures at early times after surgery (37). Irradiation of copper-alginate sutures with near-infrared light leads to a strong photothermal response and may observe results in efficacies similar to those seen with non-irradiated sutures (37). Additionally, histopathology and immunohistological analyses revealed a reduced epithelial gap and a higher number of CD31+ cells, which are markers of increased angiogenesis around the incision site (37). The delivery of copper ions to incision wounds is effective in the approximation and healing of incisional wounds, and copper-eluting fibers may accelerate repair in surgical and trauma wounds (37).

TABLE 1.1

Summary of the Literature on Copper in Wound Healing

Study	Product	Subjects and Wounds	Treatment Regimen	Results
Cangul et al. (2006) (35)	Tripeptide-copper complex (TCC)	2 cm × 2 cm full-thickness skin wound on dorsum of rabbit	Daily application for 21 days	Compared to rabbits treated with topical zinc oxide and untreated rabbits; those treated with topical TCC had shorter time to coverage of the wound bed with granulation tissue and more prominent neovascularization.
Gul et al. (2008) (36)	TCC	4 cm × 4 cm full-thickness skin wound of dorsum of rabbit	Daily application for 28 days	Compared to rabbits treated with 1 J cm^{-2} He-Ne laser, rabbits treated with topical TCC or 3 J cm^{-2} He-Ne laser experienced shorter time to full coverage of the wound with granulation tissue, overall faster wound healing, and increased neutrophil counts and neovascularization.
Cui et al. (2021) (34)	Copper peroxide-loaded gelatin sponge wound dressing	1 cm, *E. coli*-infected wounds on backs of mice	Application of wound dressing for ten days	Compared to wounds dressed with Tegaderm film and unimpregnated gelatin sponge, those dressed with 2 and 4 mM CuO$_2$-impregnated gelatin sponge had faster and enhanced reduction in wound area, less erythema and exudate, and increased histopathologic re-epithelization, angiogenesis, and collagen deposition.
Ghosh et al. (2020) (37)	Copper-loaded alginate fiber sutures	1-cm long, full-thickness incision wounds on dorsum of mice	Repair of incisional wounds with copper-eluting alginate fiber as surgical sutures, removed after three days	Compared to wounds sutured with conventional nylon and calcium-alginate sutures, wounds closed with copper-alginate sutures achieved higher recovery in tissue biomechanical strengths, improved re-epithelialization, and increased angiogenesis at day 3.
Melamed et al. (2021) (38)	Copper oxide microparticle-impregnated multilayer spunbond polypropylene and absorbent wound dressing	Ten case reports of patients with comorbidities (diabetes, renal failure, sickle cell, peripheral vascular disease) with chronic or acute wounds (post-operative, necrotizing fasciitis, vascular ulcers).	Application of wound dressing with daily to weekly reapplication for one week to several months	In ten cases, use of copper oxide-impregnated dressing corresponded with reduction in wound area and/or formation of vascular granulation tissue, including six wounds with suboptimal response to prior therapy. Resolution of infection was observed in two cases.
Ogen-Shtern et al. (2021) (39)	Copper ions in saline solution	Patients 35–65 years having abdominoplasty surgery were cut into 8 × 8 mm squares, and round 0.8-mm burn wounds were inflicted on the skin explants.	Directly following the burn, and every 48 hours after, saline, or saline with 0.02, or 1 μM copper ions were applied.	Burns immediately treated with 0.02, or 1 μM copper ions preserved the zone of stasis and the increase in wound size. The copper ions also inhibited the infiltration/release of pro-inflammatory cytokines (interleukin-6 [IL-6] and IL-8) and transforming growth factor β-1 in response to burns. Re-epithelialization of skin tissue and a greater amount of collagen fibers were observed following copper treatment.

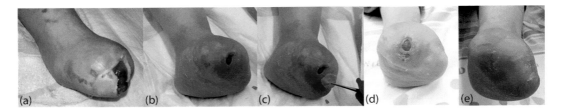

FIGURE 1.1 Closure of a six-year indolent chronic wound from insulin-dependent diabetes mellitus (IDDM) in a patient. (a) The patient underwent a trans-metatarsal amputation of the left foot in 2013; (b) the wound did not close for six years, and in June 2019, the wound was about 7-mm deep with furrow (tunneling surrounding it); (c) in June 2019, the wound was filled with copper oxide wound dressing (wound dressing was changed every three days); (d) one week later, the wound volume was reduced by approximately 90%; and (e) by August 2019, the wound was completely closed. (From 38, under Open Access Creative Common CC BY license.)

Antimicrobial dressings with copper oxide microparticles have also been tested in the treatment of acute and chronic and infected and non-infected wounds (38). The incorporation of copper oxide into wound dressings may help treat patients with wounds that are unresponsive to conventional treatments such as in those with diabetes mellitus, sickle cell disease, renal failure, and necrotizing fasciitis (Figure 1.1) (38). In infected and non-infected wounds, the application of copper oxide wound dressings resulted in significantly enhanced wound healing (38). The infected wounds cleared, fibrous and necrotic tissues were reduced, and granulation, epithelization, and wound closure were observed (38). Copper oxide wound dressings may protect wounds, accelerate regeneration/healing, and provide antimicrobial properties conferring protection (38).

After skin burning, a zone of stasis forms around the coagulation zone and may rescue the wound (39). Cells in the zone of stasis may die or survive based on the severity of the burn and treatments applied to the burn (39). Copper may improve wound healing following skin burns (39). Specifically, skin from healthy patients having abdominoplasty surgery was cut into 8×8 mm squares, and round 0.8-mm diameter burn wounds were inflicted on the skin explants (39). Burned and control skin were cultured up to 27 days post-wound (39). Directly following the burn, and after every 48 hours, saline or saline with 0.02 or 1 μM copper ions was applied to the skin explant burn wounds (39). Burns immediately treated with 0.02 or 1 μM copper ions preserved the zone of stasis and the increase in wound size (39). The copper ions also inhibited the infiltration/release of pro-inflammatory cytokines (interleukin-6 [IL-6] and IL-8) and transforming growth factor β-1 in response to burns (39). Re-epithelialization of skin tissue and a greater amount of collagen fibers were observed following copper treatment (39). Copper-ion-based therapies may protect the zone of stasis and the increase in wound size after a burn (39).

In wounds, copper may increase the expression of vascular endothelial growth factor (VEGF) that plays a central role in stimulating angiogenesis (5). Copper has been proven to directly stimulate angiogenesis, but the mechanisms have not been fully elucidated (5). The VEGF expression may be induced by copper and this may accelerate dermal wound contraction and closure (5). Topical copper sulfate at physiological levels stimulates the VEGF expression in primary and transformed human keratinocytes (5). Copper and VEGF may play roles in shared hypoxia pathways (5). Topical copper sulfate has been shown to accelerate the closure of excisional dermal wound allowed to heal by secondary intention in mice (5).

Furthermore, copper may promote wound healing and skin regeneration by stimulating endothelial cell proliferation and angiogenesis (40). A donut-like metal-organic framework (MOF) of copper-nicotinic acid (CuNA) via a solvothermal reaction was created (40). The rough surface of CuNA helps facilitate the loading/release of basic fibroblast growth factor (bFGF). CuNAs with/without bFGF may be processed into a light-responsive composite hydrogel with GelMA, which demonstrate mechanical properties, biocompatibility, antibacterial ability, and bioactivity (40). In in vivo full-thickness defect models of skin wounds, the CuNAbFGF@ GelMA hydrogels significantly accelerated wound healing by stimulating the inhibition of the inflammatory response, promoting new blood vessel formation and the deposition of collagen and elastic fibers (40). Overall, the CuNA and composite light-responsive hydrogel system promotes wound healing and tissue regeneration (40).

Skin Aging (Photoaging)

Aging of the skin is associated with loss of structural collagens and alterations in the structure and function of the extracellular matrix of the connective tissues (41). Primarily, the elastic fiber network provides physiological elasticity and durability to the skin. Collagen cross-linking and the formation of desmosines, an elastin-specific crosslink compound, are initiated by lysyl oxidase which is a copper-dependent enzyme. With aging, the elastic fiber network undergoes degradative processes that result in the loss of function of the elastic fibers. Proposed methodologies to counteract these degenerative processes include topical applications of compounds that may regenerate the elastic fiber network (41). Copper has been incorporated into cosmetics for anti-skin aging properties (41).

One clinical trial evaluated the effects of a bi-metal, 0.1% copper-zinc malonate-containing cream (41). This topical agent had previously been shown to efface wrinkles in 21 photoaged females treated with the agent for six weeks. The cream increased elastin biosynthesis and elastic tissue accumulation in skin biopsies of treated areas after six weeks as compared to baseline skin (Figure 1.2) (41). Histopathology of skin samples showed elastic fiber regeneration, including perpendicular extension toward the dermo-epidermal junction in the papillary dermis (41). Additionally, elastin biosynthesis was increased as determined by semi-quantitative immunofluorescence with an antibody recognizing newly synthesized, uncross-linked tropoelastin molecules and confirmed by assay of desmosine (41). In summary, the authors found that elastin biosynthesis was significantly enhanced following six weeks of twice daily application of the bi-metal compound suggesting that 0.1% copper-zinc malonate-containing cream has the ability to increase elastin synthesis in human skin in vivo and regenerate elastic fibers that may lead to wrinkle effacement in photoaged female facial skin (41).

The anti-aging effects of copper ions from cuprous oxide powders have also been studied (4). Specifically, dermal fibroblasts were exposed to copper and the expression of types I, III, V collagen, heat shock protein-47 (HSP-47), elastin, fibrillin-1, and fibrillin-2, TGF-β1, VEGF were determined in addition to copper ions' ability to inhibit membrane damage and lipid peroxidation (4). The direct anti-oxidant activity of copper was also determined (4). The anti-skin aging and skin regenerative properties

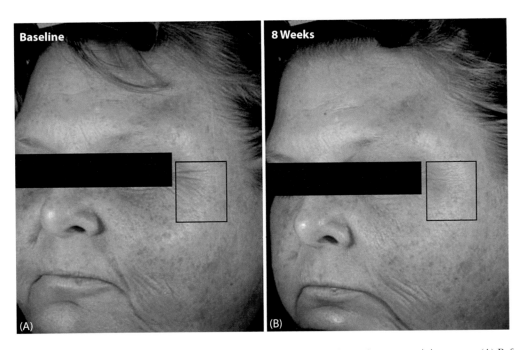

FIGURE 1.2 Clinical changes resulting from treatment with 0.1% copper-zinc malonate-containing cream. (A) Before and (B) eight weeks after treatment twice daily with a cream containing the active compound with 0.1% copper-zinc malonate. Fewer wrinkles are observed in the treated periorbital area. (Boxed, right; from 41 with permission.)

of copper were shown to be mediated by the stimulation of ECM proteins, TGF-β1, VEGF, and inhibition of oxidative stress effects at physiological concentrations and this fact supports the use of copper in cosmetics (4).

The effect of a topical galvanic zinc-copper complex (coupling elemental zinc and copper to create a biomimetic electric field) on skin photoaging was tested in a randomized, double-blind, placebo-controlled clinical trial (42). This topical agent demonstrated anti-inflammatory activity and extracellular matrix improvement in vitro including increased collagen and elastin production (42). One hundred twenty-four women (40–65 years) with mild-to-moderate photoaging were randomized to receive either a placebo topical treatment or one of three galvanic zinc-copper complex compositions (gel and activating moisturizer) (42). Clinical grading and imaging, and subject self-assessments were collected at baseline and then 15–30 minutes after topical product applications at one, two, four, and eight weeks (42). The galvanic zinc-copper complex was found to produce clinically significant improvement in photodamage, fine lines under-eye wrinkles, and to produce a lifted appearance of the eyes after application and through the eighth week of treatment (42). In summary, galvanic zinc-copper complexes, applied topically, may produce rapid and lasting anti-aging effects (42).

Exposure to copper oxide-embedded textiles (such as pillowcases) over time has been shown to reduce the depth of facial wrinkles, improve skin sagging, and enhance skin elasticity (43). Human skin explants were cultured ex vivo and exposed to saline topically or saline containing 0.02 or 1 μmol/L copper ions (43). The viability and histology of samples were determined and levels of elastin, pro-collagen 1, and TGF-β1 secretion into the culture medium were determined at different time intervals (43). Exposure to saline containing 0.02 or 1 μmol/L copper ions did not affect the viability or histology of the explants as compared to control explants treated with saline only (43). Exposure of the skin grafts to 0.02 or to 1 μmol/L of copper ions resulted in 100% and 20% increases in elastin and pro-collagen 1 concentrations, respectively, in the culture supernatants already after one day of incubation, which remained statistically significantly elevated also after six days on incubation, as compared to the control explants (43). Additionally, two- and four-fold increases in TGF-ß1 levels were observed in the culture supernatants of explants that were treated with the copper ions and were detected after four and six days of culture, as compared to the explants exposed to saline alone (43).

The effects of sodium copper chlorophyllin complexes on the expression of photoaging dermal extracellular matrix biomarkers reflecting skin repair have been studied (44). Skin biopsy samples were taken from the forearms of four healthy females with photoaged skin (44). Immunohistochemistry for biomarkers of aging skin was performed following treatment with a gel containing a liposomal dispersion of sodium copper chlorophyllin complex 0.05%, a positive control of tretinoin cream 0.025%, and an untreated negative control (44). A statistically significantly greater amount of fibrillin/amyloid P and epidermal mucins, indicating skin repair, were found in skin treated with the test material containing 0.05% sodium copper chlorophyllin complex and the reference control tretinoin 0.025% cream compared to the negative control (untreated site) (44). Expression of procollagen 1 and dermal mucin was also greater in the samples treated with the test gel although results were not statistically significant when compared to the untreated site (44). Treatment with retinoids in addition to sodium copper chlorophyllin complex may have beneficial effects on photoaged skin and increased levels of biomarkers involved in skin repair (44). Age-related decreases in skin hyaluronic acid (HA) and inhibition of the breakdown of HA may be improved by the sodium copper chlorophyllin complex by inhibition of hyaluronidase and stimulation of HA synthases by retinol (44).

Inhibitors of hyaluronidase (which break down HA) may possess anti-aging properties (45). Sodium copper chlorophyllin complex is included in many cosmetic products that purport to have reversed the effects of skin aging (45). Commercially available lots of sodium copper chlorophyllin complexes were evaluated for primary small molecule active ingredients and hyaluronidase inhibitory activity (45). Ascorbate analogs were also tested with copper chlorophyllin complexes to investigate potential synergy (45). Assays testing for hyaluronidase activity were performed and found that the hyaluronidase inhibitory activity of sodium copper chlorophyllin complex was strong and increased HA level of the dermal extracellular matrix and improved the appearance of aging facial skin (45).

Role of Copper in Inflammatory Skin Diseases and Skin Cancer

Inflammatory Skin Diseases

The role of copper as an pro-inflammatory has been well documented in the literature (46–48). In response to inflammation, serum copper levels may increase and elevated serum copper levels have been reported in inflammatory conditions, such as arthritis (49–51). However, copper has been reported to have anti-inflammatory effects when associated with non-steroidal anti-inflammatory drugs (NSAIDs) (52–56).

Elevated copper levels have been reported in many inflammatory diseases, including arthritis and psoriasis (49, 57–59). In rheumatoid arthritis (RA) patients, studies have reported higher serum copper levels and greater disease severity in patients compared to controls, and higher copper levels have been observed in RA patients in active disease compared to those in remission (49, 57–59). Elevated serum levels of copper during the inflammatory process may be attributed to increases in ceruloplasmin, an enzyme responsible for transporting copper to extrahepatic sites (51, 60). During the inflammatory process, there is an increased production of cytokines, such as IL-1 and IL-6. IL-1 and IL-6 stimulate hepatocytes leading to increased synthesis and secretion of ceruloplasmin into the blood (51, 61, 62).

Copper-lowering drugs may be useful in the treatment of inflammatory diseases (46, 63, 64). Tetrathiomolybdate, a copper chelator created to treat the neurologic presentation of Wilson's disease, has been shown to reduce inflammation by inhibiting inflammatory cytokines that utilize copper, such as tumor necrosis factor alpha (TNF-α), IL-1β, IL-6, IL-2, and nuclear factor kappa B (NF-κB) (65, 66). Penicillamine, another copper-lowering drug has been shown to positively impact disease activities in individuals with RA (67, 68). In a study by Suarez-Almazor et al. evaluating six randomized controlled trials and controlled clinical trials of D-penicillamine in patients with RA, compared to placebo, D-penicillamine was shown to have a beneficial effect on many disease outcome measures, including tender joint pain and erythrocyte sedimentation rates (ESR) (68). The disease-modifying mechanism of penicillamine is not well understood but has been attributed to decreased T-cell activity (67).

In addition to promoting inflammation, copper has been reported to enhance the anti-inflammatory effects of drugs, including NSAIDs and anticancer drugs, such as Gleevac (48, 55, 69–71). The anti-inflammatory activity of copper-NSAID complexes has been documented in numerous studies (48, 55, 69–71). Many mechanisms have been proposed to explain the anti-inflammatory activity of copper-NSAID complexes, including downregulation of SOD activity, polymorphonuclear leukocytes, and phospholipase A$_2$ (48, 72). Moreover, in a study by Hassan et al. investigating hepatocellular carcinoma-induced rats, copper was shown to enhance the anti-inflammatory activity of Gleevec, an anticancer drug for many types of cancers, including chronic myeloid leukemia and gastrointestinal tumors (69). These studies illustrate that copper may play a role in improving the anti-inflammatory activity of certain drugs.

Skin Cancer

Dysregulation of copper levels has been associated with many cancer-promoting factors, including increased proliferation, growth, angiogenesis, and metastasis (47, 73). In many cancer types, elevated copper levels have been reported (73–76). Thus, targeting copper levels has been proposed as a treatment for many cancers, including BRAF[V600]-mutated melanomas and squamous cell carcinomas (74, 76).

Increased copper levels have been reported in melanoma patients; therefore, copper suppression may aid in treatment (75). Approximately half of melanomas include BRAF mutations, a serine/threonine kinase that stimulates the MPA kinase/ERK-signaling pathway (77). Copper is involved in the MAPK pathway and reducing its availability has been proposed as a cancer therapy for BRAF[V600]-mutated melanomas (76, 78). Copper may also play a role in the prognosis and treatment of squamous cell carcinomas (79). In a study of patients with advanced esophageal squamous cell carcinomas, those expressing ATP7A, a gene responsible for the transmembrane copper-transporting P-type ATPase, had worse overall survival compared to patients not expressing ATP7A (79). To improve prognosis, reducing copper levels may be a therapy for squamous cell carcinoma. In a study by Cox et al., mice treated with tetra-thiomolybdate, a copper chelator, had a less squamous cell carcinoma tumor growth compared to the control group (74).

Though copper has many tumor-promoting factors, it may be beneficial in the treatment of skin cancers. In a case series by Klyucharvea et al., treating periorbital basal cell carcinomas in patients at the T_{1-2}, N_0, and M_0 stages with dual wavelengths, copper vapor laser was associated with an elimination of malignant cells and dysplastic vessels (80). In addition, few studies have evaluated the role of copper-nano protein complexes in skin cancer treatment (81, 82). In a study by Shi et al., copper-cysteine nanoparticles were used as a photosensitizer of X-ray-activated photodynamic therapy (X-PDT) (81). The therapy was associated with inhibited growth of XL50 cells (squamous cell carcinoma) but not B16F10 cells (melanoma) (81). In a separate study by Zhang et al. investigating the use of copper-cysteamine (Cu-Cy) nanoparticles, when activated by X-rays, the nanoparticles generated high amounts of ROS, inducing melanoma elimination (82). These studies demonstrate that copper can play a role in treating skin cancers.

Conclusion

Copper (Cu) is an essential trace mineral/element that plays a critical role in physiological and cellular processes of the human body. Although the role of copper in biological pathways and processes has been well described, the applications of copper in dermatology have not been fully described. Further, the dermocosmetic and medical benefits of topical copper treatments have yet to be fully explored. The use of copper in dermatological therapies holds a great deal of potential in treating inflammatory skin diseases, skin cancer, wound healing, and combating skin aging. Copper treatments may increase elastin, collagen fibers, and the elasticity of skin tissue. Lastly, copper may be used topically to reduce inflammation, limit damage, and improve healing in wounds. Future experiments and randomized controlled trials/studies are needed to tap into the full potential uses of copper in dermatology.

REFERENCES

1. Rucker RB, Kosonen T, Clegg MS, et al. Copper, Lysyl Oxidase, and Extracellular Matrix Protein Cross-Linking. American Journal of Clinical Nutrition. 1998;67(5):996S–1002S.
2. Chung KW, Song SH, Kim M. Synergistic Effect of Copper and Amino Acid Mixtures on the Production of Extracellular Matrix Proteins in Skin Fibroblasts. Molecular Biology Reports. 2021;48(4):3277–3284.
3. Harris ED, Rayton JK, Balthrop JE, et al. Copper and the Synthesis of Elastin and Collagen. CIBA Foundation Symposium. 1980;79:163–182.
4. Philips N, Samuel P, Parakandi H, et al. Beneficial Regulation of Fibrillar Collagens, Heat Shock Protein-47, Elastin Fiber Components, Transforming Growth Factor-β1, Vascular Endothelial Growth Factor and Oxidative Stress Effects by Copper in Dermal Fibroblasts. Connective Tissue Research. 2012;53(5):373–378.
5. Sen CK, Khanna S, Venojarvi M, et al. Copper-Induced Vascular Endothelial Growth Factor Expression and Wound Healing. American Journal of Physiology-Heart and Circulatory Physiology. 2002;282(5):H1821–H1827.
6. Barceloux, DG, Barceloux, D. Copper. Journal of Toxicology: Clinical Toxicology. 1999;37(2):217–230.
7. Bhattacharya, PT, Misra, SR, Hussain, M. Nutritional Aspects of Essential Trace Elements in Oral Health and Disease: An Extensive Review. Scientifica. 2016;2016:5464373.
8. Qu, X, He, Z, Qiao, H, et al. Serum Copper Levels Are Associated with Bone Mineral Density and Total Fracture. Journal of Orthopaedic Translation. 2018;14:34–44.
9. Burkhead, JL, Collins, JF. Nutrition Information Brief—Copper. Advances in Nutrition. 2022; 13(2):681–683.
10. Collins, JF, Klevay, LM. Copper. Advances in Nutrition. 2011;2(6):520–522.
11. Linder, MC, Wooten, L, Cerveza, P, et al. Copper Transport. American Journal of Clinical Nutrition. 1998;67(5 Suppl):965S–971S.

12. Gaetke, LM, Chow-Johnson, HS, Chow, CK. Copper: Toxicological Relevance and Mechanisms. Archives of Toxicology. 2014;88(11):1929–1938.

13. Water, N. R. C. (US) C. on C. in D. Physiological role of copper. In: Copper in Drinking Water. National Academies Press (US); 2000. Available from: https://www.ncbi.nlm.nih.gov/books/NBK225407/

14. Micronutrients, I. of M. (US) P. on. Copper. In: Dietary Reference Intakes for Vitamin A, Vitamin K, Arsenic, Boron, Chromium, Copper, Iodine, Iron, Manganese, Molybdenum, Nickel, Silicon, Vanadium, and Zinc. National Academies Press (US); 2001. Available from: https://www.ncbi.nlm.nih.gov/books/NBK222312/

15. Eom, S-Y, Yim, D-H, Huang, M, et al. Copper–Zinc Imbalance Induces Kidney Tubule Damage and Oxidative Stress in a Population Exposed to Chronic Environmental Cadmium. International Archives of Occupational and Environmental Health. 2020;93(3):337–344.

16. Adelstein, SJ, Vallee, BL. Copper Metabolism in Man. New England Journal of Medicine. 1961;265(18), 892–897.

17. Royer, A, Sharman, T. Copper toxicity. In: StatPearls. StatPearls Publishing; 2022. Available from: http://www.ncbi.nlm.nih.gov/books/NBK557456/

18. Lopez, MJ, Royer, A, Shah, NJ. Biochemistry, ceruloplasmin. In: StatPearls. StatPearls Publishing; 2022. Available from: http://www.ncbi.nlm.nih.gov/books/NBK554422/

19. Gioilli, BD, Kidane, TZ, Fieten, H, et al. Secretion and Uptake of Copper via a Small Copper Carrier in Blood Fluid. Metallomics. 2022;14(3):mfac006.

20. Hamza, I, Gitlin, JD. Hepatic copper transport. In: Madame Curie Bioscience Database [Internet]. Landes Bioscience; 2013. Available from: https://www.ncbi.nlm.nih.gov/books/NBK6381/

21. Horn D, Barrientos A. Mitochondrial Copper Metabolism and Delivery to Cytochrome C Oxidase. IUBMB Life. 2008;60(7):421–429.

22. Greiner P, Hannappel A, Werner C, et al. Biogenesis of Cytochrome C Oxidase—*In Vitro* Approaches to Study Cofactor Insertion into a Bacterial Subunit I. Biochimica et Biophysica Acta—Bioenergetics. 2008;1777(7):904–911.

23. Ruiz LM, Libedinsky A, Elorza AA. Role of Copper on Mitochondrial Function and Metabolism. Frontiers in Molecular Biosciences [Internet]. 2021;8:711227 [cited 2022 Sep 1]; p. 8. Available from: https://www.frontiersin.org/articles/10.3389/fmolb.2021.711227

24. Csiszar K. Lysyl oxidases: A novel multifunctional amine oxidase family. In: Progress in Nucleic Acid Research and Molecular Biology [Internet]. Academic Press; 2001 [cited 2022 Sep 1]. pp. 1–32. Available from: https://www.sciencedirect.com/science/article/pii/S0079660301700128

25. Ye M, Song Y, Pan S, et al. Evolving Roles of Lysyl Oxidase Family in Tumorigenesis and Cancer Therapy. Pharmacology & Therapeutics. 2020;215:107633.

26. Rodriguez-Pascual F, Rosell-Garcia T. Lysyl Oxidases: Functions and Disorders. Journal of Glaucoma. 2018;27:S15.

27. Beyens A, Van Meensel K, Pottie L, et al. Defining the Clinical, Molecular and Ultrastructural Characteristics in Occipital Horn Syndrome: Two New Cases and Review of the Literature. Genes. 2019;10(7):528.

28. Kodama H, Sato E, Yanagawa Y, et al. Biochemical Indicator for Evaluation of Connective Tissue Abnormalities in Menkes' Disease. Journal of Pediatrics. 2003;142(6):726–728.

29. Wen X, Wu J, Wang F, et al. Deconvoluting the Role of Reactive Oxygen Species and Autophagy in Human Diseases. Free Radical Biology and Medicine. 2013;65:402–410.

30. Lewandowski Ł, Kepinska M, Milnerowicz H. The Copper-Zinc Superoxide Dismutase Activity in Selected Diseases. European Journal of Clinical Investigation. 2019;49(1):e13036.

31. Elchuri S, Oberley TD, Qi W, et al. CuZnSOD Deficiency Leads to Persistent and Widespread Oxidative Damage and Hepatocarcinogenesis Later in Life. Oncogene. 2005;24(3):367–380.

32. Borkow, G. Using Copper to Improve the Well-Being of the Skin. Current Chemical Biology. 2014;8(2):89–102.

33. Solano, F. On the Metal Cofactor in the Tyrosinase Family. International Journal of Molecular Sciences. 2018;19(2):633.

34. Cui H, Liu M, Yu W, et al. Copper Peroxide-Loaded Gelatin Sponges for Wound Dressings with Antimicrobial and Accelerating Healing Properties. ACS Applied Materials and Interfaces. 2021;13(23):26800–26807.

35. Cangul, T, Gul, NY, Topal, A, Yilmaz, R. Evaluation of the Effects of Topical Tripeptide-Copper Complex and Zinc Oxide on Open-Wound Healing in Rabbits. Veterinary Dermatology. 2006;17(6):417–23. https://pubmed.ncbi.nlm.nih.gov/17083573/

36. Gul, NY, Topal, A, Cangul, TI, Yanik, K. The Effects of Topical Tripeptide Copper Complex and Helium-Neon Laser on Wound Healing in Rabbits. Veterinary Dermatology. 2008;19(1):7–14. https://pubmed.ncbi.nlm.nih.gov/18177285/

37. Ghosh D, Godeshala S, Nitiyanandan R, et al. Copper-Eluting Fibers for Enhanced Tissue Sealing and Repair. ACS Applied Materials and Interfaces. 2020;12(25):27951–27960.

38. Melamed E, Kiambi P, Okoth D, et al. Healing of Chronic Wounds by Copper Oxide-Impregnated Wound Dressings—Case Series. Medicina (Kaunas). 2021;57(3):296.

39. Ogen-Shtern N, Chumin K, Silberstein E, et al. Copper Ions Ameliorated Thermal Burn-Induced Damage in Ex Vivo Human Skin Organ Culture. Skin Pharmacology and Physiology. 2021;34(6):317–327.

40. Wang TL, Zhou ZF, Liu JF, et al. Donut-like MOFs of Copper/Nicotinic Acid and Composite Hydrogels with Superior Bioactivity for rh-bFGF Delivering and Skin Wound Healing. Journal of Nanobiotechnology. 2021;19(1):275.

41. Mahoney MG, Brennan D, Starcher B, et al. Extracellular Matrix in Cutaneous Ageing: The Effects of 0.1% Copper–Zinc Malonate-Containing Cream on Elastin Biosynthesis. Experimental Dermatology. 2009;18(3):205–211.

42. Chantalat J, Bruning E, Sun Y, et al. Application of a Topical Biomimetic Electrical Signaling Technology to Photo-Aging: A Randomized, Double-Blind, Placebo-Controlled Trial of a Galvanic Zinc-Copper Complex. Journal of Drugs in Dermatology. 2012;11(1):30–37.

43. Ogen-Shtern N, Chumin K, Cohen G, et al. Increased Pro-Collagen 1, Elastin, and TGF-β1 Expression by Copper Ions in an Ex-Vivo Human Skin Model. Journal of Cosmetic Dermatology. 2020;19(6):1522–1527.

44. McCook JP, Stephens TJ, Jiang LI, et al. Ability of Sodium Copper Chlorophyllin Complex to Repair Photoaged Skin by Stimulation of Biomarkers in Human Extracellular Matrix. Clinical Cosmetic and Investigational Dermatology. 2016;9:167–174.

45. McCook JP, Dorogi PL, Vasily DB, et al. *In Vitro* Inhibition of Hyaluronidase by Sodium Copper Chlorophyllin Complex and Chlorophyllin Analogs. Clinical Cosmetic and Investigational Dermatology. 2015;8:443–448.

46. Balsano, C, Porcu, C, Sideri, S. Is Copper a New Target to Counteract the Progression of Chronic Diseases? Metallomics. 2018;10(12):1712–1722.

47. Denoyer, D, Masaldan, S, La Fontaine, S, et al. Targeting Copper in Cancer Therapy: "Copper That Cancer." Metallomics: Integrated Biometal Science. 2015;7(11):1459–1476.

48. Weder, JE, Dillon, CT, Hambley, TW, et al. Copper Complexes of Non-Steroidal Anti-Inflammatory Drugs: An Opportunity yet to be Realized. Coordination Chemistry Reviews. 2002;232(1):95–126.

49. Berthon, G. Is Copper Pro- or Anti-Inflammatory? A Reconciling View and a Novel Approach for the Use of Copper in the Control of Inflammation. Agents and Actions. 1993;39(3):210–217.

50. Pereira, TCB, Campos, MM, Bogo, MR. Copper Toxicology, Oxidative Stress and Inflammation Using Zebrafish as Experimental Model. Journal of Applied Toxicology. 2016;36(7):876–885.

51. Strecker, D, Mierzecki, A, Radomska, K. Copper Levels in Patients with Rheumatoid Arthritis. Annals of Agricultural and Environmental Medicine: AAEM. 2013;20(2):312–316.

52. Dimiza, F, Perdih, F, Tangoulis, V, et al. Interaction of Copper(II) with the Non-Steroidal Anti-Inflammatory Drugs Naproxen and Diclofenac: Synthesis, Structure, DNA- and Albumin-Binding. Journal of Inorganic Biochemistry. 2011;105(3):476–489.

53. Hurtado, M, Sankpal, UT, Chhabra, J, et al. Copper-Tolfenamic Acid: Evaluation of Stability and Anti-Cancer Activity. Investigational New Drugs. 2019;37(1):27–34.

54. Joseph, J, Nagashri, K. Novel Copper-Based Therapeutic Agent for Anti-Inflammatory: Synthesis, Characterization, and Biochemical Activities of Copper(II) Complexes of Hydroxyflavone Schiff Bases. Applied Biochemistry and Biotechnology. 2012;167(5):1446–1458.

55. Puranik, R, Bao, S, Bonin, AM, et al. A Novel Class of Copper(II)- and Zinc(II)-Bound Non-Steroidal Anti-Inflammatory Drugs that Inhibits Acute Inflammation in Vivo. Cell & Bioscience. 2016;6(1):9.

56. Santos, ACF, Monteiro, LPG, Gomes, ACC, et al. NSAID-Based Coordination Compounds for Biomedical Applications: Recent Advances and Developments. International Journal of Molecular Sciences. 2022;23(5):2855.

57. Aldabbagh, KAO, Al-Bustany, DA. Relationship of Serum Copper and HLADR4 Tissue Typing to Disease Activity and Severity in Patients with Rheumatoid Arthritis: A Cross Sectional Study. Annals of Medicine and Surgery. 2021;73:103193.

58. Chakraborty, M, Chutia, H, Changkakati, R. Serum Copper as a Marker of Disease Activity in Rheumatoid Arthritis. Journal of Clinical and Diagnostic Research: JCDR. 2015;9(12):BC09–BC11.

59. Zoli, A, Altomonte, L, Caricchio, R, et al. Serum Zinc and Copper in Active Rheumatoid Arthritis: Correlation with Interleukin 1 Beta and Tumour Necrosis Factor Alpha. Clinical Rheumatology. 1998;17(5):378–382.

60. Gitlin, JD. Transcriptional Regulation of Ceruloplasmin Gene Expression during Inflammation. Journal of Biological Chemistry. 1988;263(13):6281–6287.

61. Di Bella, LM, Alampi, R, Biundo, F, et al. Copper Chelation and Interleukin-6 Proinflammatory Cytokine Effects on Expression of Different Proteins Involved in Iron Metabolism in HepG2 Cell Line. BMC Biochemistry. 2017;18:1.

62. Persichini, T, Maio, N, di Patti, MCB, et al. Interleukin-1β Induces Ceruloplasmin and Ferroportin-1 Gene Expression via MAP Kinases and C/EBPβ, AP-1, and NF-κB Activation. Neuroscience Letters. 2010;484(2):133–138.

63. Brewer, GJ. The Promise of Copper Lowering Therapy with Tetrathiomolybdate in the Cure of Cancer and in the Treatment of Inflammatory Disease. Journal of Trace Elements in Medicine and Biology: Organ of the Society for Minerals and Trace Elements (GMS). 2014;28(4):372–378.

64. Omoto, A, Kawahito, Y, Prudovsky, I, et al. Copper Chelation with Tetrathiomolybdate Suppresses Adjuvant-Induced Arthritis and Inflammation-Associated Cachexia in Rats. Arthritis Research & Therapy. 2005;7(6):R1174.

65. Brewer, GJ. Tetrathiomolybdate Anticopper Therapy for Wilson's Disease Inhibits Angiogenesis, Fibrosis and Inflammation. Journal of Cellular and Molecular Medicine. 2003;7(1):11–20.

66. Wang, Z, Zhang, Y-H, Guo, C, et al. Tetrathiomolybdate Treatment Leads to the Suppression of Inflammatory Responses through the TRAF6/NFκB Pathway in LPS-Stimulated BV-2 Microglia. Frontiers in Aging Neuroscience. 2018;10:9.

67. Mejias, SG, Ramphul, K. Penicillamine. In: StatPearls. StatPearls Publishing; 2022. Available from: http://www.ncbi.nlm.nih.gov/books/NBK513316/

68. Suarez-Almazor, ME, Belseck, E, Spooner, C. Penicillamine for Treating Rheumatoid Arthritis. Cochrane Database of Systematic Reviews. 2000;4:CD001460.

69. Hassan, I, Ebaid, H, Alhazza, IM, et al. Copper Mediates Anti-Inflammatory and Antifibrotic Activity of Gleevec in Hepatocellular Carcinoma-Induced Male Rats. Canadian Journal of Gastroenterology & Hepatology. 2019;2019:9897315.

70. Miche, H, Brumas, V, Berthon, G. Copper(II) Interactions with Nonsteroidal Antiinflammatory Agents. II. Anthranilic Acid as a Potential. OH-Inactivating Ligand. Journal of Inorganic Biochemistry. 1997;68(1):27–38.

71. Yassin, NZ, El-Shenawy, SM, Abdel-Rahman, RF, et al. Effect of a Topical Copper Indomethacin Gel on Inflammatory Parameters in a Rat Model of Osteoarthritis. Drug Design, Development and Therapy. 2015;9:1491–1498.

72. Sorenson, JRJ. 6 Copper complexes offer a physiological approach to treatment of chronic diseases. In: G. P. Ellis & G. B. West (Eds.). Progress in Medicinal Chemistry. Elsevier; 1989. (Vol. 26, pp. 437–568).

73. Oliveri, V. Selective Targeting of Cancer Cells by Copper Ionophores: An Overview. Frontiers in Molecular Biosciences. 2022;9:841814.

74. Cox, C, Merajver, SD, Yoo, S, et al. Inhibition of the Growth of Squamous Cell Carcinoma by Tetrathiomolybdate-Induced Copper Suppression in a Murine Model. Archives of Otolaryngology–Head & Neck Surgery. 2003;129(7):781–785.

75. Fisher, GL, Spitler, LE, McNeill, KL, et al. Serum Copper and Zinc Levels in Melanoma Patients. Cancer. 1981;47(7):1838–1844.

76. Sammons, S, Brady, D, Vahdat, L, et al. Copper Suppression as Cancer Therapy: The Rationale for Copper Chelating Agents in BRAF V600 Mutated Melanoma. Melanoma Management. 2016;3(3):207–216.

77. Ascierto, PA, Kirkwood, JM, Grob, J-J, et al. The role of BRAF V600 Mutation in Melanoma. Journal of Translational Medicine. 2012;10:85.

78. Kim, Y-J, Bond, GJ, Tsang, T, et al. Copper Chaperone ATOX1 Is Required for MAPK Signaling and Growth in BRAF Mutation-Positive Melanoma. Metallomics: Integrated Biometal Science. 2019;11(8):1430–1440.

79. Li, Z-H, Lu, X, Li, S-W, et al. Expression of ATP7A in Esophageal Squamous Cell Carcinoma (ESCC) and Its Clinical Significance. International Journal of Clinical and Experimental Pathology. 2019;12(9):3521–3525.

80. Klyuchareva, SV, Ponomarev, IV, Topchiy, SB, et al. Treatment of Basal Cell Cancer with a Pulsed Copper Vapor Laser: A Case Series. Journal of Lasers in Medical Sciences. 2019;10(4): 350–354.

81. Shi, L, Liu, P, Wu, J, et al. The Effectiveness and Safety of X-PDT for Cutaneous Squamous Cell Carcinoma and Melanoma. Nanomedicine. 2019;14(15):2027–2043.

82. Zhang, Q, Guo, X, Cheng, Y, et al. Use of Copper-Cysteamine Nanoparticles to Simultaneously Enable Radiotherapy, Oxidative Therapy and Immunotherapy for Melanoma Treatment. Signal Transduction and Targeted Therapy. 2020;5(1):58.

2

Ultrapotent Antioxidants and Anti-Inflammatories

Laurel Naversen Geraghty, Diane S. Berson, and Ranella Hirsch

Introduction

Antioxidants possess the unique ability to neutralize free radicals, which are highly reactive molecules that result from oxidative processes and may contribute to DNA damage, carcinogenesis, inflammation, and photoaging of the skin. Although the body is equipped with endogenous antioxidants, its supply may be overwhelmed by increased oxidative stress due to natural metabolic processes or exposure to ultraviolet light, pollution, or cigarette smoke. Free radicals damage dermal cells by promoting thymine dimer formation, causing the release of pro-inflammatory molecules, increasing apoptosis, and upregulating collagenase. By scavenging free radicals, antioxidants demonstrate anti-carcinogenic and anti-inflammatory activities and guard against photodamage and collagen breakdown.

By reinforcing the skin's endogenous supply of antioxidants, orally or topically administered antioxidants may help prevent an overload of oxidative stress. Antioxidants have become ubiquitous in the skin care market because they have shown promise for preventing photoaging and protecting against cellular DNA damage. Although limited research exists to support the efficacy of many commercially available antioxidants, their effects are increasingly reproducible in scientific research. This chapter will address the evidence behind some of the best-studied antioxidants and anti-inflammatory ingredients used on the skin, including vitamins A and C, coenzyme Q-10, green tea, and soy, as well as newer ingredients that show promise, including CoffeeBerry™, idebenone, feverfew, and *Polypodium leucotomos.*

Polyphenol Antioxidants

Polyphenols, or catechins, are plant-derived antioxidants with anti-inflammatory, photoprotective, and anti-carcinogenic properties (1). This family of compounds includes flavonoids, such as soy isoflavones, green tea extracts derived from the *Camellia sinensis* plant, grape seed extract, CoffeeBerry, and resveratrol.

Soy

Soy reinforces the skin's epidermal barrier, promotes collagen production and elastin repair, decreases hyperpigmentation, and inhibits hair growth (2–6). Among the active ingredients in soy are genistein and daidzein, isoflavones derived from fermented soy products, such as tofu and soy beans. These isoflavones are believed to possess chemopreventive qualities (7). Other active ingredients include essential fatty acids and amino acids; phytosterols, which strengthen and repair the skin's barrier function; and small protein serine protease inhibitors, such as Bowman-Birk inhibitor (BBI) and soybean trypsin inhibitor (STI). BBI and STI inhibit protease-activated receptor 2 to disrupt melanosome transfer to keratinocytes, thereby reducing melanin levels within the skin (2, 8–10). BBI also inhibits the hair-growth enzyme ornithine decarboxylase (11).

Clinically, soy is touted for its gentle anti-inflammatory actions. In addition to moisturization, it is used to decrease inflammation, minimize hair growth, and effect photorejuvenation, photoprotection,

DOI: 10.1201/9781315165905-2

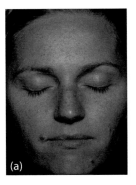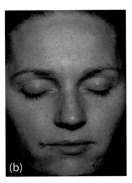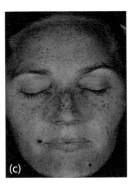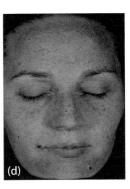

FIGURE 2.1 Baseline visible (a) and enhanced (c) images clearly demonstrate an improvement in skin tone, texture, and clarity when compared with visible (b) and enhanced (d) images after 12 weeks of use of the total soy and SPF 30 facial moisturizer. *Abbreviation*: SPF, sun protection factor. (From 10.)

skin lightening, and skin brightening (12–17). Clinical studies support the use of topical soy as a treatment for melasma and photodamage. Research suggested that, over 12 weeks, daily or twice-daily application of a topical soy formula improves overall skin tone and texture, hyperpigmentation, blotchiness, and dullness (4, 5) (Figure 2.1). In a study of six adults, genistein dose-dependently inhibited ultraviolet B (UVB)-induced erythema (18). Topical soy may also reduce the visibility and coarseness of hair, while increasing its softness and fineness (12) (Figures 2.2 and 2.3).

Tea

Although all teas are derived from the tea plant *C. sinensis*, different varieties contain different active components, due to fermentation and other processes (8).

Green tea, the most well-studied type, contains significant amounts of polyphenols, which are known to reduce DNA damage, sunburn, inflammation, and erythema. The most potent catechin contained in green tea is epigallocatechin-3-gallate (EGCG) (19). Evidence suggests that EGCG and other green tea polyphenols regulate cell growth and disrupt the carcinogenic pathway at multiple points (20). In vitro and murine research showed that EGCG may inhibit activator protein 1 (AP-1)—a transcription factor—to disrupt UV-induced tumorigenesis, suppress enzymes related to carcinogenesis, and diminish edema and hyperplasia (7, 21–24). In addition, green tea polyphenols may inhibit angiogenic factors and stimulate cytotoxic T cells in the presence of tumor cells (25).

An in vivo study suggested that topical green tea extract relieves sunburn and inhibits erythema in a dose-dependent manner (26). Topical EGCG has further been shown to reduce oxidative stress, pyrimidine dimer formation, and the infiltration of inflammatory leukocytes in humans (27). Orally consumed green tea also offers anti-tumor benefits (28). By promoting keratinocyte proliferation, green tea extracts may also increase epidermal thickness (29).

Black tea, a fermented type, has been less extensively studied for its cutaneous effects. Research suggests that oral or topical black tea inhibits tumorigenesis (30). Its mechanisms of action, as demonstrated in murine models, include the inhibition of cell proliferation, apoptosis, tumorigenic cell-signaling kinases, transcription factors, and the inflammatory protein cyclooxygenase 2 (31). Clinical study showed that the ingestion of black tea reduced the incidence of squamous cell carcinoma and decreased photodamage (8, 30, 32). Topically applied black tea extract reduced the incidence and severity of erythema and inflammation in humans following UVB exposure (33).

Rooibos tea is derived from *Aspalathus linearis*, a plant native to South Africa that may be unfermented ("green rooibos") or fermented ("red tea"). Both varieties contain high levels of polyphenols, including flavonoids and phenolic acids (34). In vitro animal studies suggested that rooibos exerts antioxidant and anti-carcinogenic effects, and topically applied rooibos extract reduces the number and size

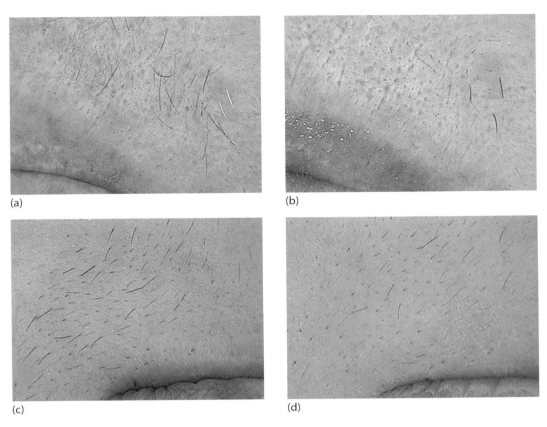

(a)   (b)

(c)   (d)

FIGURE 2.2 Video microscopic images before (a, c) and after (b, d) the use of natural soy and skin conditioner formulation. At the baseline visit, one week post-shaving, the unwanted facial hair on the upper lip area was very apparent. After eight weeks of twice-daily usage of the natural soy and skin conditioner preparation and one week post-shaving, hair appeared finer and less noticeable. Video microscopic images further verify the improvements in the appearance of unwanted facial hair as observed by the dermatologist and study participants.
(By permission of J&JCCI; J. Nebus.)

of skin tumors (35, 36). Rooibos has been used as a folk remedy for eczema, depression, nausea, and a variety of other conditions (35). However, the study of rooibos as a topical agent in humans remains limited.

Grape Seed Extract

Grape seed extract, derived from the seeds of red grapes, more effectively scavenges free radicals than vitamins C or E (37, 38). Its considerable antioxidant capacity may be attributed to its high levels of proanthocyanidins, a type of flavonoid (39). Of the nine polyphenols contained in grape seed extract, procyanidin B5-3′-gallate has the most potent antioxidant activity (7). Murine models suggested that the extract possesses chemopreventive and photoprotective abilities (7). It also promotes dermal wound healing by upregulating vascular endothelial growth factor (VEGF) expression in keratinocytes (39). Topical grape seed, which is found in many anti-aging cosmeceuticals, increases the sun protection factor of sunscreens (38) and may be of benefit in the treatment of melasma. In a study of 12 women, melasma pigmentation diminished significantly after six months of oral intake of a grape seed extract but did not improve over a longer period (40). Twice-daily application of sunscreen containing 3% GSE significantly reduced the level of melanin and erythema and improved overall skin tone (41).

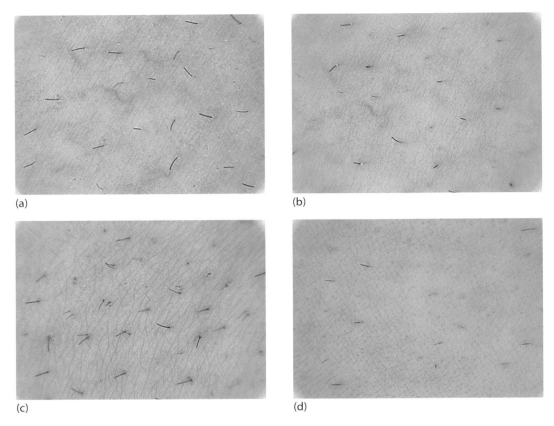

FIGURE 2.3   Video microscopic images before (a, c) and after (b, d) four weeks use of natural soy and skin conditioner formulation. At the baseline visit, subjects enrolled in the study had a moderate appearance of unwanted leg hair four days after shaving. At the four-week visit, after twice-daily application of the moisturizer containing natural soy and skin conditioners and four days after shaving the hair appeared less noticeable and finer. Video microscopic images further verified the improvements in the appearance of the unwanted leg hair.
(By permission of J&J CCI; W. Wallo.)

CoffeeBerry

Derived from the fruit of the coffee plant, *Coffea arabica*, CoffeeBerry extract (Johnson & Johnson) is rich in polyphenol antioxidants, which prevent and repair damage caused by reactive oxygen species (ROS). In an oxygen radical absorbance capacity (ORAC) test, an assessment of the free-radical scavenging ability of antioxidants, CoffeeBerry demonstrated ten times the free-radical quenching ability of green tea and even greater potency compared to pomegranate, vitamin C, vitamin E, and ferulic acid (2, 42).

Clinically, CoffeeBerry is used to combat signs of photoaging. In a proprietary trial of 30 adult women with moderate photoaging, subjects applied a 1% CoffeeBerry cream twice daily after washing with a 0.1% CoffeeBerry cleanser. Ten subjects applied CoffeeBerry formulas to one side of the face only and used a vehicle on the other half of the face, while 20 used CoffeeBerry on the entire face. After six weeks, blinded expert grading revealed a 30% mean overall skin improvement in both groups, compared to 7% improvement on the control side of the face in the split-face group; a 20–24% average reduction in fine lines and wrinkles (control: 3%) and a 15% mean improvement in pigment (control: 5%) were also observed. Immunostaining demonstrated increased collagen synthesis relative to control and decreased levels of matrix metalloproteinase-1 (MMP-1), which promotes collagen breakdown. Side effects included erythema and transient sensation of burning (43–45).

Resveratrol

Resveratrol is a polyphenol that is abundant in the skin of grapes and in red wine. This antioxidant inhibits inflammation, carcinogenesis, and platelet aggregation and upregulates sirtuin (silent information regulator) enzymes to slow the aging process in a manner similar to caloric restriction (46, 47). Preliminary research supports resveratrol's promise as a topical treatment for UV-induced photoaging. In in vitro and murine trials, resveratrol inhibited cellular proliferation and dose-dependently reduced free radicals (48, 49). In an ORAC test, a 1% resveratrol topical formula demonstrated approximately 17 times the antioxidant activity of a 1% idebenone formula (49). In a study evaluating the efficacy and safety of resveratrol combined with ablative fractional CO_2 laser system in the treatment of skin photoaging, resveratrol alone was shown to improve photoaging and both add an efficacy to the laser treatment and subside the adverse events induced by the laser (50).

Vitamin, Enzyme, and Botanical Antioxidants

Vitamin A

Vitamin A, also known as retinol, is the cosmeceutical cousin of the prescription topical drug tretinoin. Commonly used to treat acne and photoaging, and also for melasma and scars, tretinoin increases the vascularity of photoaged skin and upregulates collagen production to smooth fine lines and wrinkles (1, 51). Although less potent and efficacious than tretinoin, retinol may be used for acne and photoaging, and it is generally less irritating and better tolerated. Retinol disrupts melanogenesis to help fade lentigines and inhibits MMPs (1). Oral retinol has chemopreventive qualities (7).

As a treatment for photoaging, topical retinol reduces fine lines and wrinkles, upregulates collagen synthesis, increases dermal water content, and augments epidermal thickness (52). In a randomized, double-blind, vehicle-controlled study of 36 elderly subjects (mean age 87 years), topical 0.4% retinol was applied to one arm three times weekly. After 24 weeks, fine lines and rhytids were significantly improved in the retinol-treated arms. Histological evaluation revealed increased glycosaminoglycan expression and collagen biosynthesis compared to control (53).

Vitamin B

The vitamin B complex includes niacinamide (also known as niacin, nicotinamide, and vitamin B_3) and panthenol (provitamin B_5, dexpanthenol). B vitamins have been used to treat a variety of skin conditions, including acne, wound healing, blistering diseases, and other inflammatory conditions (1).

In an animal model, topical niacinamide prevented UVB-induced immunosuppression and skin cancer induction (54). In humans, topical niacinamide helps to reverse signs of photoaging through a variety of proposed mechanisms (55–57). First, it stimulates fibroblasts to increase collagen synthesis. Second, it inhibits melanosome transfer from melanocytes to keratinocytes, thereby decreasing hyperpigmentation. Third, it inhibits the oxidative glycation of proteins, reducing the sallow quality of photoaged skin (1). Finally, niacinamide bolsters levels of ceramides, free fatty acids, and the proteins keratin and filaggrin to enhance the skin's barrier function and reduce transepidermal water loss (1, 57). Clinically, niacinamide is non-irritating and improves skin tone and texture, decreases fine lines and wrinkles, and reduces hyperpigmentation (1, 56).

Panthenol is a humectant with anti-inflammatory and anti-pruritic effects (58–60). As a precursor to pantothenic acid—a cofactor in lipid biosynthesis—panthenol increases lipid biosynthesis, improves stratum corneum hydration, and strengthens the skin's barrier function (60). In vitro and in vivo trials showed that panthenol enhanced wound healing via fibroblast proliferation and accelerated epidermal re-epithelialization (1, 58, 60). Clinical trials found that panthenol prevented and reduced signs of irritation, including dryness, roughness, scaling, pruritus, erythema, and stratum corneum damage (60, 61). Two studies evaluating a new topical panthenol-containing emollient demonstrated sustained and deep skin moisturization in healthy adult and infant skin (62).

Vitamin C

Vitamin C, which contains the active ingredient L-ascorbic acid, is a water-soluble, photoprotective, anti-inflammatory antioxidant not produced by the human body. Because the vitamin is a required cofactor and transcriptional regulator of collagen biosynthesis, it has implications for wound healing and photoaging (1, 32). Vitamin C also reduces melanin formation via tyrosinase, inhibits elastin biosynthesis (possibly with the effect of diminishing solar elastosis in photodamaged skin), and is believed to stimulate sphingolipid production to reinforce the skin's lipid barrier (32, 63–65).

Animal studies showed that topical L-ascorbic acid decreases skin erythema, sunburn, and immunosuppression following UV exposure (66, 67). Clinically, topical vitamin C is used for photoprotection and the prevention and treatment of photoaging, hyperpigmentation, and erythema (68–70). In a small, double-blind, split-face trial, a topical solution containing 10% L-ascorbic acid and 7% tetrahexyodeyl ascorbate was compared with control. After 12 weeks, wrinkling and photodamage were significantly reduced on the cheeks, forehead, and perioral region on the treated side of the face (71). In a study of postmenopausal women, vitamin C increased pro-collagen mRNA and associated enzymes to bolster collagen synthesis (72). Because vitamin C inhibits tyrosinase and melanogenesis, it has potential clinical applications for the treatment of melasma and lentigines (1, 73). An in vivo evaluation of topical ascorbic acid application on skin aging by 50 MHz ultrasound showed significant increase in collagen synthesis after topical application (74).

Vitamin E

Vitamin E, which includes the molecular forms tocopherol and tocotrienol, is a lipid-soluble humectant and antioxidant known for its photoprotective actions. Some of these effects may be attributed to α-tocopherol's photoprotective absorption of ultraviolet light near 290 nm (75). By scavenging lipid peroxyl and oxygen radicals, vitamin E prevents the oxidation of stratum corneum proteins and inhibits lipid peroxidation, helping to preserve the integrity of cell membranes. A carrier protein selectively shuttles α-tocopherol into lipoproteins, making it the most important form of vitamin E in humans (32).

Animal models revealed that topical vitamin E protects against UV-induced erythema, lipid peroxidation, photoaging, immunosuppression, photocarcinogenesis, and the formation of pyrimidine dimers (32). In human cells, vitamin E reduced the number of sunburn cells following UV exposure and inhibits melanogenesis (1, 32, 76). Clinical reports suggested that orally administered vitamin E improves facial hyperpigmentation (76, 77).

Topically applied vitamins C, E, and ferulic acid act synergistically to compound their antioxidant and photoprotective activities. Vitamin C regenerates the active form of vitamin E, while ferulic acid stabilizes vitamins C and E (32). In a clinical trial, a combination of orally administered vitamins C and E diminished the sunburn response following UV exposure. Individually, the vitamins were not efficacious (78).

Vitamin E has historically been used to minimize the appearance of scars. However, after a 12-week, double-blind study comparing vitamin E to control, Baumann and Spencer concluded that the vitamin did not improve the cosmetic outcome of postsurgical scars and found that it caused contact dermatitis in 33% of treated subjects (79).

Ferulic Acid

Ferulic acid is a potent antioxidant ubiquitous in plant, fruit, and vegetable species, including teas, CoffeeBerry, and *P. leucotomos* (39, 80). It is touted for its ability to absorb UV energy and photoprotect the skin, stabilize vitamins C and E, and reduce thymine dimers, which may lead to DNA mutations and skin cancer (81, 82). Because ferulic acid's mechanisms of action are distinct from but complementary to the actions of sunscreens, the antioxidant may be a beneficial addition to sunscreen formulations (81).

In a small clinical study of a topical solution containing 15% L-ascorbic acid (vitamin C) and 1% α-tocopherol (vitamin E), 0.5% ferulic acid stabilized the vitamins and doubled the photoprotection of the formula, as determined by the levels of erythema and sunburn cells. Ferulic acid also reduced thymine dimers, inhibited apoptosis, and suppressed four of five pro-inflammatory and immunosuppressive cytokines tested (81).

Alpha Lipoic Acid

Mitochondria synthesize alpha lipoic acid (ALA), a lipoamide that is both water- and lipid-soluble and has the ability to cross cellular membranes. ALA quenches free radicals, prevents lipid peroxidation, and reactivates other antioxidants, including vitamins C and E, glutathione, and ubiquinol. ALA also serves as an anti-inflammatory and an exfoliant (1).

Though clinical study showed that ALA is not effective in the photoprotection of skin (83), it may have clinical applications for photoaging. In a 12-week, double-blind, split-face study of 33 women (mean age 54 years), in which a 5% topical ALA product was applied twice daily, objective and subjective evaluation revealed a significant decrease in fine lines, lentigines, and skin roughness (84). ALA has also been used in the treatment of vitiligo. In a randomized, double-blind, placebo-controlled trial of 35 patients, oral supplementation with ALA, vitamins C and E, and polyunsaturated fatty acids was administered for two months before and the six months during narrow-band ultraviolet B (NB-UVB) therapy. The oral supplement significantly improved the effectiveness of NB-UVB and diminished oxidative stress associated with vitiligo (85).

Kinetin

Kinetin (N[6]-furfuryladenine) is a botanical growth factor and antioxidant that is believed to be photoprotective. In vitro study showed that kinetin stimulates human fibroblasts and upregulates catalase, the enzyme that degrades hydrogen peroxide (86, 87).

Clinically, kinetin may restore the skin's barrier function. It has been used in the treatment of rosacea, photodamage, and dry skin. One study found that a topical 0.1% kinetin product improved fine lines, color, texture, and blotchiness over 24 weeks (88). In another trial, 59% of subjects who applied a 1% kinetin lotion twice daily for 12 weeks demonstrated moderate to marked improvements in rosacea. Subjects showed significant improvement in skin roughness and mottling, and facial erythema decreased by an average of 32% (89).

Coenzyme Q-10

Coenzyme Q-10 (CoQ-10 or ubiquinone) is an endogenous, fat-soluble antioxidant that inhibits lipid peroxidation to prevent damage to cellular and mitochondrial membranes (90). It is believed to play a role in the prevention and treatment of photoaging. Vitamin E and CoQ-10 are the only lipophilic antioxidants found within skin surface lipids and act synergistically to reduce UV-mediated depletion of cholesterol, squalene, and unsaturated fatty acids, which help to maintain the skin's barrier function (91). In vitro study indicated that CoQ-10—particularly when combined with carotenoid antioxidants—protects fibroblasts from UV-induced inflammation and photoaging, and reduces MMP levels (92). Given that CoQ-10 levels diminish with age, topical formulations may replenish the antioxidant to generate improvements in photoaging (91). Application of a CoQ-10 solution decreased wrinkle depth and inhibited UVA-induced collagenase expression and oxidative stress in human keratinocytes (93).

Idebenone

Idebenone is a synthetic cousin of coenzyme Q-10 that is believed to penetrate the skin more effectively (94, 95). Idebenone exerts photoprotective and anti-inflammatory effects; reduces sunburn cells, thymine dimers, and immunosuppression following UV irradiation; and is thought to repair mitochondrial damage (1, 96). Research demonstrated its potency relative to other common antioxidants: in a five-test comparison with tocopherol, kinetin, ubiquinone, ascorbic acid, and alpha lipoic acid, idebenone displayed the greatest overall protection against oxidative stress (96).

Idebenone may improve skin texture, hydration, and fine lines (1). In a clinical trial, 50 women with moderate photodamage were randomized to apply a 0.5% or 1.0% idebenone topical lotion twice daily. After six weeks, blinded experts noted improvements of approximately one-third in skin roughness, hydration, and fine lines and wrinkles in the 1.0% idebenone group, with more modest results seen in the 0.5% group. Histological assessment showed increased collagen levels and decreased interleukins and MMP-1 for both groups (94). No adverse events were reported in the study. However, idebenone can cause contact dermatitis (97, 98).

Polypodium leucotomos

Extract of the fern plant *P. leucotomos* is a phenolic antioxidant with photoprotective, chemoprotective, anti-inflammatory, and immune-modulating effects (99–103).

In murine models, orally administered *P. leucotomos* inhibited UVB-induced skin cancers, significantly diminished immunosuppression following UVB exposure, and reduced signs of photoaging, including dermal elastosis and skinfold thickness (104–106). In vitro study showed that, following UV exposure, *P. leucotomos* significantly improved membrane integrity, increased elastin, and inhibited lipid peroxidation and MMP-1 expression in human fibroblasts and keratinocytes. The researchers posited that *P. leucotomos* concentrations below 0.1% may protect against photoaging by reinforcing membrane integrity and inhibiting MMP-1, and concentrations greater than 0.1% may reverse elastin loss (106).

P. leucotomos has been used in the treatment of vitiligo, psoriasis, atopic dermatitis, and other inflammatory and immune-related skin conditions. It may also prove useful in the prevention and treatment of sunburn (39, 107). In a study of 21 healthy human subjects, *P. leucotomos* administered orally or topically offered photoprotection to skin and Langerhans cells and increased the UV dose required for immediate pigment darkening, the minimal erythema dose, and the minimal phototoxic dose (99). Although oral *P. leucotomos* supplements are commercially available, the authors were unaware of any topical formulations at press time.

Catalase

Catalase facilitates the degradation of hydrogen peroxide and constitutes the body's primary defense against hydrogen peroxide damage (108). Increased oxidative stress, catalase deficiency, and hydrogen peroxide accumulation appear to contribute to photoaging and inflammatory skin conditions, such as psoriasis and vitiligo (109–114). Catalase may hold promise as a therapy for these conditions.

In vitro study of human skin cells demonstrated that catalase inhibits free radicals and cytokines induced by tumor necrosis factor α (TNF-α), which contributes to inflammatory skin disease (115). Catalase significantly reduces hydrogen peroxide transfer from keratinocytes to melanocytes, promoting melanogenesis and the progression of vitiliginous lesions (116). In a randomized, double-blind trial of 25 vitiligo patients, researchers found no significant differences in repigmentation after four and ten months of consistent use of topical 0.05% betamethasone (a glucocorticoid) or a catalase/dismutase superoxide formula (111).

Additional evidence suggests that catalase may be beneficial in the prevention and treatment of dermal aging. In vitro study found significantly decreased catalase activity and increased hydrogen peroxide accumulation in fibroblasts obtained from photoaged skin. Catalase added to photoaged fibroblasts reduced hydrogen peroxide levels, suppressed MMP-1, and reversed age-related alterations in the MAP kinase signaling pathway (117).

Açai

Açai fruit (*Euterpe oleracea*) is a palm species abundant in the Brazilian Amazon. Açai and açai oil are rich in antioxidants, catechins, procyanidins, sterols, and phenolic acids (118). Preliminary in vitro study suggests that açai protects against oxidative damage, inhibits lipid peroxidation, and reduces ROS and pro-inflammatory cytokines (119). Because of açai's high stability, rich phenol content, and antioxidant activity, it is considered a promising addition to future topical skin agents (118).

Cassia alata

The leaf extract of *C. alata* (ringworm bush) has been used as a treatment for tinea infections and bites and has demonstrated anti-inflammatory and antimicrobial effects in laboratory studies (120–122).

However, limited evidence exists to support its use as a topical agent in human skin. In a controlled study of ten adults, an antioxidant formula containing *C. alata* extract and Oxynex-ST, a photostabilizer, offered significantly greater photoprotection following UV exposure compared to placebo and an even greater level of protection when combined with sunscreen, as assessed by digital photography and immunohistochemistry. (*Source*: C Oresajo et al., Evaluation of the complementary effects of antioxidants and sunscreens in reducing UV induced skin damage as demonstrated by skin biomarker expression: clinical poster, 68th Annual Meeting of the AAD, 2010.)

Anti-Inflammatory Botanicals

While all antioxidants are anti-inflammatory, only a few anti-inflammatories (including feverfew, Pycnogenol, and mushroom extract) possess antioxidant activity and therefore have the ability to improve photodamage. However, all anti-inflammatories function to reduce cutaneous erythema and irritation.

Feverfew

Feverfew, an extract of the herb *Tanacetum parthenium*, has antioxidant, anti-inflammatory, anti-irritant, and photoprotective actions (123–125). In an ORAC assessment, feverfew exerted 16 times the free-radical scavenging effects of CoffeeBerry and 288 times the effects of vitamin C (126). Research demonstrated that feverfew may reduce DNA damage, apoptosis, and epidermal hyperplasia following UV exposure and may restore cellular thiol levels after exposure to cigarette smoke (125, 127).

Feverfew contains parthenolide, a lactone that inhibits inflammation, inflammatory cytokines, and platelet aggregation (123, 125, 128, 129). Because parthenolide causes skin irritation and sensitization when ingested or applied topically, parthenolide-free feverfew extract (Feverfew PFE™) was developed as an alternative for use in skin care products (39, 125, 130, 131). In vitro and in vivo studies suggested that PFE combats erythema after UV exposure and reduces irritation (117, 127).

PFE is considered gentle enough for use on sensitive skin. Clinically, it is used as an anti-inflammatory and for photoprotection, rosacea, shaving irritation, and erythema reduction (130). In a randomized, double-blind trial, 31 women with sensitive skin applied moisturizer with PFE twice daily. After three weeks, significant improvements in erythema, roughness, and skin irritation were noted (132).

Pycnogenol®

Pycnogenol is derived from the bark of the French maritime pine tree, *Pinus pinaster*. It contains high levels of proanthocyanidins, which have a range of antimicrobial, antioxidant, anti-inflammatory, photoprotective, and anti-carcinogenic effects (133–137). This extract accelerates wound healing, reduces scar formation, stabilizes elastin and collagen, and minimizes UV-induced pigmentation and erythema (138–141). Pycnogenol's anti-inflammatory mechanisms may include the inhibition of interferon-gamma (IFN-γ), an inflammatory cytokine, and the subsequent downregulation of ICAM-1 in keratinocytes. ICAM-1 is implicated in inflammatory skin conditions, including psoriasis and atopic dermatitis (142). Pycnogenol is also believed to convert the vitamin C radical to its active form, thereby regenerating vitamin E, and to raise levels of glutathione and other free-radical quenching enzymes (1, 143).

In a mouse study, topical application of 0.05–0.2% Pycnogenol solution following UV exposure dose-dependently reduced edema, inflammation, immunosuppression, and tumor carcinogenesis (134). In another murine model, a 1–5% Pycnogenol gel significantly reduced wound-healing time compared to control (2, 138). Clinical research remains limited, but a study of 21 adults showed that oral Pycnogenol supplements taken for eight weeks reduced UV-induced cutaneous erythema (141).

Licorice Extract

Licochalcone A is the primary active ingredient in the extract of the licorice plant, *Glycyrrhiza inflata*. Glycyrrhizin and liquiritin are active components of licorice root, *Glycyrrhiza glabra*. Extracts from both plant species are touted for their anti-inflammatory and anti-tumor activities (39, 144). Evidence suggested that licochalcone A is an anti-inflammatory that reduces pro-inflammatory cytokines and prostaglandins following UV irradiation (145). *G. glabra* and glycyrrhizin inhibited skin tumors when administered orally or topically in murine models (146).

Licorice extract is used clinically for rosacea and may be found in commercial products advertising "redness relief" (1, 39). In an eight-week study of 62 adults, a topical licochalcone A formulation significantly improved subjects' rosacea and quality of life ratings (147). A liquiritin cream applied twice daily for four weeks significantly diminished melasma in a split-face controlled study of 20 women (148).

Mushroom Extract

Extracts from *Lentinus edodes* (shitake), *Grifola frontdosa* (maitake), *Ganoderma lucidum* (reishi, mannentake, and lingzhi), and other mushrooms contain a variety of compounds with antioxidant and anti-inflammatory properties (39, 149). Among their many effects, mushroom extracts scavenge free radicals, stimulate epidermal cell growth, and inhibit inflammatory cytokines, the elastin-degrading enzyme elastase, and collagen-degrading MMPs and AP-1 (2, 149, 150). Mushroom extracts may be efficacious in the treatment of dermal aging. When topical mushroom extract formulations were used to treat 31 women with moderate facial photodamage, clinicians reported significant improvements in overall photoaging, fine lines, pigmentation, and skin texture (150) (Figure 2.4). In a study of 45 human subjects who applied a mushroom extract product daily, cell turnover increased significantly compared to control (4).

Lycopene

Lycopene is a carotenoid responsible for the red color of many fruits, including tomatoes and watermelons (7). It exhibits considerable reductive potential and antioxidant activity (151). When administered orally or topically, lycopene exerts anti-carcinogenic effects, and when applied topically prior to UV exposure, it prevents apoptosis, reduces inflammation, and diminishes enzymes linked to tumor formation (7, 152). In addition, lycopene has the ability to regenerate α-tocopherol (vitamin E) (151).

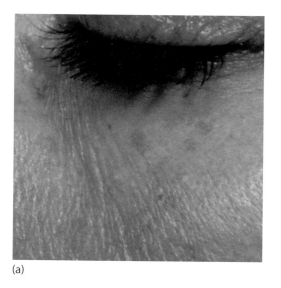
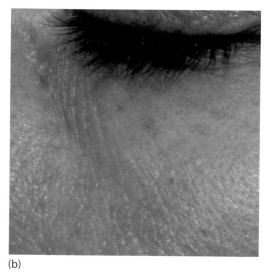

(a)   (b)

FIGURE 2.4   Digital photography before (a) and after (b) shows improvements in skin texture and fine wrinkling after 12 weeks of use of the mushroom complex serum.
(By permission of J&J CCI; D. Miller.)

Clinical study of lycopene's dermal effects remains limited. In a trial of ten volunteers, 6% topical lycopene reduced UV-induced erythema to a greater extent than a topical mixture containing vitamins C and E and offered significantly more photoprotection than control (151). The formulation of lycopene may be important to its efficacy. In a study of human fibroblasts, lycopene was not shown to offer photoprotection or reduce UVA-induced levels of MMP-1 unless combined with vitamin E (153). In some experiments, lycopene enhanced rather than reduced UVA-induced oxidative stress in human and mouse fibroblasts (153, 154).

Silymarin

Silymarin is a polyphenolic flavonoid from the milk thistle plant, *Silybum marianum*. It inhibits lipoprotein oxidation, scavenges free radicals (30), and exerts chemopreventive and anti-carcinogenic activity (7, 32, 155). It also reduces sunburn, apoptosis, and edema following UVB exposure (156, 157). Silymarin inhibits inflammatory cytokines and pyrimidine dimers and reduces edema, hyperplasia, and proliferation (155, 158).

Clinically, silymarin is used to alleviate symptoms of rosacea. In a double-blind, placebo-controlled trial, 46 subjects with rosacea were treated with a topical formulation of silymarin and methylsulfonylmethane. After one month, researchers noted statistically significant improvements in erythema, papules, itching, and hydration (159).

Chamomile

Chamomile (*Matricaria recutita*, *Chamomilla recutita*) is a member of the daisy family. This medicinal herb has been used as a soothing and moisturizing treatment for erythema, pruritus, sunburn, eczema, and allergic irritation, and it may improve skin texture and elasticity (160). Chamomile's anti-inflammatory effects may be due to its inhibition of cyclooxygenase, lipoxygenase, and histamine release (1, 161). The literature contains one study that suggests that chamomile may also serve as an antioxidant (162).

Chamomile may be found in topical formulations that claim to combat inflammation, irritation, and dryness, particularly in sensitive skin. In a clinical study, topical chamomile cream proved more effective than 0.5% hydrocortisone for decreasing wound size and healing time following dermatitis and sunburn (163).

Aloe Vera

Aloe vera is a soothing, anti-inflammatory botanical with a variety of biological effects. Study suggests that it improves wound healing, diminishes pruritus, and possesses antifungal, antibacterial, viricidal, and antioxidant properties (161, 164, 165). The plant's active ingredients include salicylic acid and gel polysaccharides, which have anti-inflammatory activity, and magnesium lactate, an anti-pruritic (161). Like chamomile, aloe vera inhibits cyclooxygenase and lipoxygenase (1).

Aloe vera has been used in the treatment of burns, wounds, leg ulcers, frostbite, pruritus, and scarring related to radiation dermatitis (30). It may be an effective agent against psoriasis. In a double-blind clinical trial, patients with mild-to-moderate psoriasis who applied 0.5% aloe vera cream three times daily demonstrated a significant reduction in psoriatic plaques (83% vs. 8% for placebo) and increased rates of clinical cure (166).

Curcumin

Curcumin (diferuloylmethane) is the primary active agent within the herb turmeric (*Curcuma domestica*, *Curcuma longa,* or Zingiberaceae). This antioxidant possesses robust anti-inflammatory capabilities, resulting from its inhibition of lipoxygenase, cyclooxygenase, prostaglandins, and pro-inflammatory cytokines (1, 160, 167).

Animal models demonstrated curcumin's chemopreventive activities, which are attributed to increased apoptosis and the inhibition of tumorigenesis (7, 160). According to other research, curcumin improves wound healing by bolstering collagen deposition, stimulating fibroblasts, and increasing angiogenesis and vascular density (167–169).

Preliminary study has explored the use of curcumin in the treatment and prevention of skin diseases, such as psoriasis, scleroderma, and skin cancer (167, 170). Although curcumin inhibits collagenase, elastase, and hyaluronidase, suggesting that it may counteract photoaging, it has not yet been proven effective for this purpose (1, 165).

Quercetin

Quercetin is an antioxidant and flavonoid found in many fruits and vegetables. Its anti-inflammatory actions may result from the inhibition of lipoxygenase, COX-2, and histamine release. By enhancing apoptosis in tumor cells, quercetin also exhibits anti-carcinogenic activity (1).

In a mouse model, quercetin reduced oxidative stress following UVA exposure (171). In vitro study found that quercetin inhibits melanoma cell growth (172). It also inhibits keloid fibroblast proliferation in a dose-dependent fashion, suggesting that it has promise for preventing and treating keloids and hypertrophic scars (173).

Allantoin

Derived from the comfrey root, allantoin is an anti-inflammatory antioxidant that accelerates the repair of cutaneous photodamage and reduces inflammation following UV radiation (1, 165). Allantoin has been used in the treatment of psoriasis (174).

Sirtuins

Though not classified as antioxidants or anti-inflammatories, silent information regulators, or sirtuins, are a family of enzymes recently acknowledged as novel potential targets for anti-aging products. Sirtuins deacetylate histones to stabilize DNA and increase the longevity of organisms, including mammals, effectively mimicking the effects of caloric restriction (46, 175). In an in vitro test of human skin keratinocytes, researchers found that UV exposure and ROS downregulate the sirtuin SIRT1 (silent mating type information regulation 2 homolog 1) (176) and theorized that reduced SIRT1 activity is linked to cellular damage caused by these insults. By acting as SIRT1 activators, resveratrol, yeast biopeptides, and other compounds may protect against this damage (176, 177). In a clinical study of 33 women (mean age 51.6), daily application of a topical formula containing 1% *Kluyveromyces* yeast biopeptides, which are SIRT1 activators, resulted in improved fine lines and wrinkles, hydration, pigmentation, firmness, and texture after four weeks (177).

Conclusion

Antioxidants and anti-inflammatories comprise a rapidly expanding and ever-evolving area of study. New antioxidants are continually being explored (178), while longer-known compounds are undergoing continued research and adjustments to maximize their cutaneous effects (177, 179). However, the U.S. Food and Drug Administration does not regulate the use of antioxidants and anti-inflammatories in cosmeceutical products or require skin-care companies to demonstrate the effectiveness of their ingredients or formulas. In vitro trials support the purported mechanisms of action outlined in this chapter, but few double-blind, vehicle-controlled studies exist to prove the benefits of antioxidants in the skin. A question that remains is the degree to which antioxidant efficacy hinges on emollient properties versus active therapeutic effects.

In summary, further study of the properties of antioxidants and anti-inflammatories is needed to elucidate their dermal effects, quantify the improvements that they may offer, and objectively review and compare the efficacy of antioxidant-containing oral and topical products.

Disclosure

Dr. Berson has consulted for the following companies: Galderma, La Roche Posay, Neutrogena, and Stiefel.

REFERENCES

1. Choi MC, Berson DS. Cosmeceuticals. Semin Cutan Med Surg 2006; 25: 163–8.
2. Berson DS. Natural antioxidants. J Drugs Dermatol 2008; 7(Suppl): s7–12.
3. Liu JC, et al. Pre-clinical and clinical evaluation of total soy preparations in improving skin physical tone parameters. In: Poster presented at the 60th Annual Meeting of the American Academy of Dermatology, February 22–27, 2002, New Orleans, LA.
4. Nebus J, et al. Clinical improvements in skin tone and texture using a facial moisturizer with a combination of total soy and SPF 30 UVA/UVB protection. In: Poster presented at the 64th Annual Meeting of the American Academy of Dermatology, March 3–7, 2006, San Francisco, CA.
5. Pierard G, et al. Effects of soy on hyperpigmentation in Caucasian and Hispanic populations. In: Poster presented at the 59th Annual Meeting of the American Academy of Dermatology, March 2–7, 2001, Washington, DC.
6. Nebus J, Wallo W, Sher D, Kurtz ES. Clinical improvement in skin tone, texture and radiance with facial moisturizers containing total soy complex. In: Poster presented at the 64th Annual Meeting of the American Academy of Dermatology, March 21–26, 2003, San Francisco, CA.
7. Wright TI, Spencer JM, Flowers FP. Chemoprevention of nonmelanoma skin cancer. J Am Acad Dermatol 2006; 54: 933–46.
8. Thornfeldt CR. Cosmeceuticals: separating fact from voodoo science. Skinmed 2005; 4: 214–20.
9. Seiberg M, et al. The protease-activated receptor 2 regulates pigmentation via keratinocytesmelanocyte interactions. Exp Cell Res 2000; 254: 25–32.
10. Wallo W, Nebus J, Leyden JJ. Efficacy of a soy moisturizer in photoaging: a double blind, vehicle controlled, 12-week study. J Drugs Dermatol 2007; 6: 917–22.
11. Seiberg M, et al. Soymilk reduces hair growth and hair follicle dimensions. Exp Dermatol 2001; 10: 405–13.
12. Nebus J, et al. Reducing the appearance of unwanted leg hair with a natural soy formulation. In: Poster presented at the 61st Annual Meeting of the American Academy of Dermatology, March 21–26, 2003, San Francisco, CA.
13. Liu JC, et al. Soy: potential applications in skin care. In: Poster presented at the 59th Annual Meeting of the American Academy of Dermatology, March 2–7, 2001, Washington, DC.
14. Zhao Y, et al. Accelerated skin wound healing by soy protein isolate-modified hydroxypropyl chitosan composite films. Int J Biol Macromol 2018; 118: 1293–302.
15. Ahn S, et al. Soy protein/cellulose nanofiber scaffolds mimicking skin extracellular matrix for enhanced wound healing. Adv Healthc Mater 2018; 7: e1701175.
16. Zhou BR, et al. Protective effects of soy oligopeptides in ultraviolet B-induced acute photodamage of human skin. Oxid Med Cell Longev 2016; 2016: 5846865.
17. Lee SM, et al. Soy milk suppresses cholesterol-induced inflammatory gene expression and improves the fatty acid profile in the skin of SD rats. Biochem Biophys Res Commun 2013; 430: 202–7.
18. Wei H, et al. Isoflavone genistein: photo-protection and clinical implications in dermatology. J Nutr 2003; 133(Suppl 1): 3811S–9S.
19. Valcic S, et al. Inhibitory effect of six green tea catechins and caffeine on the growth of four selected human tumor cell lines. Anticancer Drugs 1996; 7: 461–8.
20. Beltz LA, et al. Mechanisms of cancer prevention by green and black tea polyphenols. Anticancer Agents Med Chem 2006; 6: 389–406.
21. Barthelman M, et al. (-)-Epigallocatechin-3-gallte (EGCG) inhibition of ultraviolet B-induced AP-1 activity. Carcinogenesis 1998; 19: 2201–4.
22. Ud-Din S, et al. A double-blind, randomized trial shows the role of zonal priming and direct topical application of epigallocatechin-3-gallate in the modulation of cutaneous scarring in human skin. J Invest Dermatol 2019; 139: 1680–90 e16.

23. Li M, et al. Epigallocatechin-3-gallate augments therapeutic effects of mesenchymal stem cells in skin wound healing. Clin Exp Pharmacol Physiol 2016; 43: 1115–24.
24. Zhu W, et al. Epigallocatechin-3-gallate (EGCG) protects skin cells from ionizing radiation via heme oxygenase-1 (HO-1) overexpression. J Radiat Res 2014; 55: 1056–65.
25. Katiyar S, Elmets CA, Katiyar SK. Green tea and skin cancer: photoimmunology, angiogenesis and DNA repair. J Nutr Biochem 2007; 18: 287–96.
26. Elmets CA, et al. Cutaneous photoprotection from ultraviolet injury by green tea polyphenols. J Am Acad Dermatol 2001; 44: 425.
27. Katiyar SK. Skin photoprotection by green tea: antioxidant and immunomodulatory. Curr Drug Targets Immune Endocr Metabol Disord 2003; 3: 234–42.
28. Baumann L. Alternative medicine. In: Cosmetic Dermatology: Principles & Practice. New York: McGraw-Hill Companies, Inc., 2002: 125–235.
29. Chung JH, et al. Dual mechanisms of green tea extract-induced cell survival in human epidermal keratinocytes. FASEB J 2003; 17: 1913–5.
30. Bedi MK, Shenefelt PD. Herbal therapy in dermatology. Arch Dermatol 2002; 138: 232–42.
31. Patel R, et al. Polymeric black tea polyphenols inhibit mouse skin chemical carcinogenesis by decreasing cell proliferation. Cell Prolif 2008; 41: 532–53.
32. Pinnell SR. Cutaneous photodamage, oxidative stress, and topical antioxidant protection. J Am Acad Dermatol 2003; 48: 1–19.
33. Zhao J, et al. Photoprotective effect of black tea extracts against UVB-induced phototoxicity in skin. Photochem Photobiol 1999; 70: 637–44.
34. Krafczyk N, Glomb MA. Characterization of phenolic compounds in rooibos tea. J Agric Food Chem 2008; 56: 3368–76.
35. McKay DL, Blumberg JB. A review of the bioactivity of South African herbal teas: roobios (*Aspalathus linearis*) and honeybush (*Cyclopia intermedia*). Phythother Res 2007; 21: 1–16.
36. Marnewick J, et al. Inhibition of tumour promotion in mouse skin by extracts of rooibos (*Aspalathus linearis*) and honeybush (*Cyclopia intermedia*), unique South African herbal teas. Cancer Lett 2005; 224: 193–202.
37. Bagchi D, et al. Oxygen free radical scavenging abilities of vitamins C and E, and a grape see proanthocyanidin extract in vitro. Res Commun Mol Pathol Pharmacol 1997; 95: 179–89.
38. Bagchi D, et al. Free radicals and grape seed proanthocyanidin extract: importance in human health and disease prevention. Toxicology 2000; 148: 187–97.
39. Baumann LS. Less-known botanical cosmeceuticals. Dermatol Ther 2007; 20: 330–42.
40. Yamakoshi J, et al. Oral intake of proanthocyanidin-rich extract from grape seeds improves chloasma. Phytother Res 2004; 18: 895–9.
41. Yarovaya L, et al. Clinical study of Asian skin changes after application of a sunscreen formulation containing grape seed extract. J Cosmet Dermatol 2022; https://doi.org/10.1111/jocd.14982.
42. Downie JB, Kircik LH. Inside the science of cosmeceuticals. Pract Dermatol 2008; 5(1): 60–5.
43. Draelos ZD. CoffeeBerry: a new, natural antioxidant in professional antiaging skin care. Cosmetic Dermatol 2007; 20(10 S4).
44. Stiefel Laboratories, Inc. Clinical evaluation of antioxidant effects of REVALÉSKIN™. 2008.
45. Jancin B. Novel antioxidant shows promise as photoaging topical. Skin & Allergy News 2007; 38(1): 34.
46. Orallo F. Trans-resveratrol: a magical elixir of eternal youth? Curr Med Chem 2008; 15: 1887–98.
47. Hecker A, et al. The impact of resveratrol on skin wound healing, scarring, and aging. Int Wound J 2022; 19: 9–28.
48. Chen ML, et al. Protective effect of resveratrol against oxidative damage of UV irradiated HaCaT cells. Jhong Nan Da Xue Bao Yi Ban 2006; 31: 635–9.
49. Baxter RA. Anti-aging properties of resveratrol: review and report of a potent new antioxidant skin care formulation. J Cosmet Dermatol 2008; 7: 2–7.
50. Du YM, et al. Efficacy and safety of resveratrol combined with ablative fractional CO2 laser system in the treatment of skin photoaging. J Cosmet Dermatol 2021; 20: 3880–8.
51. Chung JH, Eun HC. Angiogenesis in skin aging and photoaging. J Dermatol 2007; 34: 593–600.
52. Draelos ZD. Retinoids in cosmetics. Cosmet Dermatol 2005; 18(Suppl): 3–5.
53. Kafi R, et al. Improvement of naturally aged skin with vitamin A (retinol). Arch Dermatol 2007; 143: 606–12.

54. Gensler HL. Prevention of photoimmunosuppression and photocarcinogenesis by topical nicotinamide. Nutr Cancer 1997; 29: 157–62.
55. Hakozaki T, et al. The effect of niacinamide on reducing cutaneous pigmentation and suppression of melanosome transfer. Br J Dermatol 2002; 147: 20–31.
56. Bissett DL, Oblong JE, Berge CA. Niacinamide: a B vitamin that improves aging facial skin appearance. Dermatol Surg 2005; 31: 860–5.
57. Bissett DL, et al. Topical niacinamide provides skin aging appearance benefits while enhancing barrier function. J Clin Dermatol 2003; 32: S9–18.
58. Bissett DL, Oblong JE. Cosmeceutical vitamins: vitamin B. In: Draelos ZD, ed. Cosmeceuticals. Philadelphia: Elsevier Saunders, 2005: 57–62.
59. Eichenfield LF, et al. Natural advances in eczema care. Cutis 2007; 80(Suppl): 2–16.
60. Ebner F, et al. Topical use of dexpanthenol in skin disorders. Am J Clin Dermatol 2002; 3: 427–33.
61. Biro K, et al. Efficacy of dexpanthenol in skin protection against irritation: a double-blind, placebo-controlled study. Contact Dermatitis 2003; 49: 80–4.
62. Stettler H, et al. A new topical panthenol-containing emollient: skin-moisturizing effect following single and prolonged usage in healthy adults, and tolerability in healthy infants. J Dermatolog Treat 2017; 28: 251–7.
63. Davidson JM, et al. Ascorbate differentially regulates elastin and collagen biosynthesis in vascular smooth muscle cells and skin fibroblasts by pretranslational mechanisms. J Biol Chem 1997; 272: 345–52.
64. Maeda K, Fukuda M. Arbutin: mechanism of its depigmenting action in human melanocytes culture. J Pharmacol Exp Ther 1996; 276: 765–9.
65. Uchida Y, et al. Vitamin C stimulates sphingolipid production and markers of barrier formation in sub-merged human keratinocytes cultures. J Invest Dermatol 2001; 117: 1307–13.
66. Darr D, et al. Topical vitamin C protects porcine skin from ultraviolet radiation-induced damage. Br J Dermatol 1992; 127: 247–53.
67. Nakamura T, et al. Vitamin C abrogates the deleterious effects of UVB radiation on cutaneous immunity by a mechanism that does not depend on TNF-alpha. J Invest Dermatol 1997; 109: 20–4.
68. Burgess C. Topical vitamins. J Drugs Dermatol 2008; 7(Suppl): s2–6.
69. Humbert PG, et al. Topical ascorbic acid on photoaged skin. Clinical, topographical and ultra-structural evaluation; double-blind study vs. placebo. Exp Dermatol 2003; 12: 237–44.
70. Traikovich SS. Use of topical ascorbic acid and its effects on photodamaged skin topography. Arch Otolaryngol Head Neck Surg 1999; 125: 1091–8.
71. Fitzpatrick RE, Rostan EF. Double-blind, half-face study comparing topical vitamin C and vehicle for rejuvenation of photodamage. Dermatol Surg 2002; 28: 231–6.
72. Nusgens BV, et al. Topically applied vitamin C enhances the mRNA level of collagens I and III, their processing enzymes and tissue inhibitor of matrix metalloproteinase 1 in the human dermis. J Invest Dermatol 2001; 116: 853–9.
73. Farris PK. Topical vitamin C: a useful agent for treating photoaging and other dermatologic conditions. Dermatol Surg 2005; 31: 814–7.
74. Vergilio MM, et al. In vivo evaluation of topical ascorbic acid application on skin aging by 50 MHz ultrasound. J Cosmet Dermatol 2022; https://doi.org/10.1111/jocd.14892.
75. Sorg O, Tran C, Saurat JH. Cutaneous vitamins A and E in the context of ultraviolet- or chemically-induced oxidative stress. Skin Pharmcol Appl Skin Physiol 2001; 14: 363–72.
76. Ichihashi M, et al. The inhibitory effect of DL-alpha tocopheryl ferulate in lecithin on melanogenesis. Anticancer Res 1999; 19: 3769–74.
77. Funasaka Y, et al. The depigmenting effect of alpha-tocopheryl ferulate on human melanoma cells. Br J Dermatol 1999; 141: 20–9.
78. Fuchs J, Kern H. Modulation of UV-light-induced skin inflammation by D-α-tocopherol and L-ascorbic acid: a clinical study using solar stimulated radiation. Free Radic Biol Med 1998; 25: 1006–12.
79. Baumann LS, Spencer J. The effects of topical vitamin E on the cosmetic appearance of scars. Dermatol Surg 1999 April; 25: 311–5.
80. Graf E. Antioxidant potential of ferulic acid. Free Radic Biol Med 1992; 13: 435–48.
81. Murray JC, et al. A topical antioxidant solution containing vitamin C and E stabilized by ferulic acid provides protection for human skin against damage caused by ultraviolet irradiation. J Am Acad Dermatol 2008; 59: 418–25.

82. Saija A, et al. In vitro and in vivo evaluation of caffeic and ferulic acids as topical photoprotective agents. Int J Pharm 2000; 199: 39–47.
83. Lin JY, et al. Alpha-lipoic acid is ineffective as a topical antioxidant for photoprotection of skin. J Invest Dermatol 2004; 123: 996–8.
84. Beitner H. Randomized, placebo-controlled, double blind study on the clinical efficacy of a cream containing 5% alpha-lipoic acid related to photoaging of facial skin. Br J Dermatol 2003; 149: 841–9.
85. Dell-Anna ML, et al. Antioxidants and narrow band-UVB in the treatment of vitiligo: a double-blind placebo controlled trial. Clin Exp Dermatol 2007 November; 32: 631–6.
86. Draelos ZD. Cosmetics and cosmeceuticals. In: Bolognia JL, Jorizzo JL, Rapini RP, eds. Dermatology. London, England: Mosby, 2003: 2361.
87. Hsiao G, et al. Inhibitory activity of kinetin on free radical formation of activated platelets in vitro and on thrombus formation in vivo. Eur J Pharmacol 2003; 465: 281–7.
88. McCullough JL, Weinstein GD. Clinical study of safety and efficacy of using topical kinetin 0.10% (kinerase) to treat photodamaged skin. Cosmetic Dermatol 2002; 15: 29–32.
89. Wu JJ, et al. Topical kinetin 0.1% lotion for improving the signs and symptoms of rosacea. Clin Exp Dermatol 2007; 32: 693–5.
90. Maroz A, et al. Reactivity of ubiquinone and ubiquinol with superoxide and the hydroperoxyl radical: implications for in vivo antioxidant activity. Free Radic Biol Med 2009; 46: 105–9.
91. Passi S, et al. Lipophilic antioxidants in human sebum and aging. Free Radic Res 2002; 36: 471–7.
92. Fuller B, et al. Anti-inflammatory effects of CoQ10 and colorless carotenoids. J Cosmet Dermatol 2006; 5: 30–8.
93. Hoppe U, Bergemann J, Diembeck W. Coenzyme Q10, a cutaneous antioxidant and energizer. Biofactors 1999; 9: 371–8.
94. McDaniel D, et al. Clinical efficacy assessment in photodamaged skin of 0.5% and 1.0% idebenone. J Cosmet Dermatol 2005; 4: 167–73.
95. Farris P. Idebenone, green tea, and CoffeeBerry extract: new and innovative antioxidants. Dermatol Ther 2007; 20: 322–9.
96. McDaniel DH, et al. Idebenone: a new antioxidant—part I. Relative assessment of oxidative stress protection capacity compared to commonly known antioxidants. J Cosmet Dermatol 2005; 4: 10–7.
97. Sasseville D, Moreau L, Al-Sowaidi M. Allergic contact dermatitis to idebenone used as an antioxidant in an anti-wrinkle cream. Contact Dermatitis 2007; 56: 117–8.
98. Natkunarajah J, Ostlere L. Allergic contact dermatitis to idebenone in an over-the-counter anti-ageing cream. Contact Dermatitis 2008; 58: 239.
99. Gonzalez S, et al. Topical or oral administration with an extract of *Polypodium leucotomos* prevents acute sunburn and psoralen-induced phototoxic reactions as well as depletion of Langerhans cells in human skin. Photodermatol Photoimmunol Photomed 1997; 13: 50–60.
100. Portillo M, et al. The aqueous extract of *Polypodium leucotomos* (fernblock (R)) regulates opsin 3 and prevents photooxidation of melanin precursors on skin cells exposed to blue light emitted from digital devices. Antioxidants (Basel) 2021; 10(3): 400.
101. Goh CL, et al. Double-blind, placebo-controlled trial to evaluate the effectiveness of *Polypodium leucotomos* extract in the treatment of melasma in Asian skin: a pilot study. J Clin Aesthet Dermatol 2018; 11: 14–9.
102. Emanuele E, Bertona M, Biagi M. Comparative effects of a fixed *Polypodium leucotomos*/pomegranate combination versus *Polypodium leucotomos* alone on skin biophysical parameters. Neuro Endocrinol Lett 2017; 38: 38–42.
103. Parrado C, et al. Fernblock (*Polypodium leucotomos* extract): molecular mechanisms and pleiotropic effects in light-related skin conditions, photoaging and skin cancers, a review. Int J Mol Sci 2016; 17(7): 1026.
104. Alcaraz MV, et al. An extract of *Polypodium leucotomos* appears to minimize certain photoaging changes in a hairless albino mouse animal model. A pilot study. Photodermatol Photoimmunol Photomed 1999; 15: 120–6.
105. Siscovick JR, et al. *Polypodium leucotomos* inhibits ultraviolet B radiation-induced immunosuppression. Photodermatol Photoimmunol Photomed 2008; 24: 134–41.
106. Philips N, et al. Predominant effects of *Polypodium leucotomos* on membrane integrity, lipid per-oxidation, and expression of elastin and matrix metalloproteinase-1 in ultraviolet radiation exposed fibroblasts, and keratinocytes. J Dermatol Sci 2003; 32: 1–9.

107. Capote R, et al. *Polypodium leucotomos* extract inhibits trans-urocanic acid photoisomerization and photodecomposition. J Photochem Photobiol 2006; 82: 173–9.

108. Maresca V, et al. UVA-induced modification of catalase charge properties in the epidermis is correlated with the skin phototype. J Invest Dermatol 2006; 126: 182–90.

109. Schallreuter KU, et al. Hydrogen peroxide-mediated oxidative stress disrupts calcium binding on calmodulin: more evidence for oxidative stress in vitiligo. Biochem Biophys Res Commun 2007; 360: 70–5.

110. Wood JM, Schallreuter KU. UV irradiated phemelanin alters the structure of catalase and decreases its activity in human skin. J Invest Dermatol 2006; 126: 13–4.

111. Sanclemente G, et al. A double-blind, randomized trial of 0.05% betamethasone vs. topical catalase/dismutase superoxide in vitiligo. J Eur Acad Dermatol Venereol 2008; 22: 1359–64.

112. Schallreuter KU, et al. Methionine sulfoxide reductases A and B are deactivated by hydrogen peroxide (H_2O_2) in the epidermis of patients with vitiligo. J Invest Dermatol 2008; 128: 808–15.

113. Sezer E, et al. Lipid peroxidation and antioxidant status in lichen planus. Clin Exp Dermatol 2007; 32: 430–4.

114. Spencer JD, et al. Oxidative stress via hydrogen peroxide affects proopiomelanocortin peptides directly in the epidermis of patients with vitiligo. J Invest Dermatol 2007; 127: 411–20.

115. Young CN, et al. Reactive oxygen species in tumor necrosis factor-alpha-activated primary human keratinocytes: implications for psoriasis and inflammatory skin disease. J Invest Dermatol 2008; 128: 2606–14.

116. Pelle E, et al. Keratinocytes act as a source of reactive oxygen species by transferring hydrogen peroxide to melanocytes. J Invest Dermatol 2005; 124: 793–7.

117. Shin MH, Rhie GE, Kim YK. H_2O_2 accumulation by catalase reduction changes MAP kinase signaling in aged human skin in vivo. J Invest Dermatol 2005; 125: 221–9.

118. Pacheco-Palencia LA, Mertens-Talcott S, Talcott ST. Chemical composition, antioxidant properties, and thermal stability of a phytochemical enriched oil from acai (*Euterpe olearacea Mart*). J Agric Food Chem 2008; 56: 4631–6.

119. Jensen GS, et al. In vitro and in vivo antioxidant and anti-inflammatory capacities of an antioxidant-rich fruit and berry juice blend. Results of a pilot and randomized, double-blinded, placebo-controlled, crossover study. J Agric Food Chem 2008; 56: 8326–33.

120. Hazni H, Ahmad N, Hitotsuyanagi Y, Takeya K, Choo CY. Phytochemical constituents from *Cassia alata* with inhibition against methicillin-resistant *Staphylococcus aureus* (MRSA). Planta Med 2008; 74: 1802–5. [Epub 2008 November 7].

121. Villaseñor IM, Sanchez AC. Cassiaindoline, a new analgesic and anti-inflammatory alkaloid from *Cassia alata*. Z Naturforsch C 2009; 64: 335–8.

122. Moriyama H, Iizuka T, Nagai M, Miyataka H, Satoh T. Antiinflammatory activity of heat-treated *Cassia alata* leaf extract and its flavonoid glycoside. Yakugaku Zasshi 2003; 123: 607–11. Erratum in: Yakugaku Zasshi 2003; 123: 716.

123. Southall M, Sallou C, Oddos T. Parthenolide-depleted tanacetum: a safe, non-irritating extract with potent anti-inflammatory activity. In: Presented at the 13th Congress of the European Academy of Dermatology and Venereology, November 17–21, 2004, Florence, Italy.

124. Gisoldi E, Walczak V, Tierney N. Parthonelide-depleted tanacetum extract: a review of safety, testing for topical use. In: Poster presented at the 13 Congress of the European Academy of Dermatology and Venereology, November 17–21, 2004, Florence, Italy.

125. Wu J. Feverfew for treatment of sensitive skin and inflammatory skin conditions. Skin and Allergy News Cosmeceutical Critique Compendium, 2008.

126. Linton GM, Anthonavage M, Southall M. Broad antioxidant activity of feverfew provides all day skin protection from oxidative stress. In: Presented at the 66th Annual Meeting of the American Academy of Dermatology, February 1–5, 2008, San Antonio, TX.

127. Martin K, et al. Parthenolide-depleted feverfew (*Tanacetum parthenium*) protects skin from UV radiation and external aggression. Arch Dermatol Res 2008; 300: 69–80.

128. Baumann L, Rodriguez D, Taylor SC, Wu J. Natural considerations for skin of color. Cutis 2006; 78(Suppl): 2–19.

129. Groenwegen WA, Heptinstall S. A comparison of the effects of an extract of feverfew and parthenolide, a component of feverfew, on human platelet activity in vitro. J Pharm Pharmacol 1990; 42: 553–7.

130. Liebel F, et al. Topical formulation containing parthenolide-free extract feverfew is highly effective in clinically reducing erythema induced by irritation or barrier disruption of the skin. J Am Acad Dermatol 2005; 52(Suppl 3): P1047.
131. Martin K, et al. Parthenolide-free extract of feverfew: An extract with effective anti-irritant activity in vitro. In: Poster presented at the 63rd Annual Meeting of the American Academy of Dermatology, February 18–22, 2005, New Orleans, LA.
132. Baumann LS, Eichenfeld LF, Taylor SC. Advancing the science of naturals. Cosmet Dermatol 2004; 18(Suppl): 2–8.
133. Torras MA, et al. Antimicrobial activity of pycnogenol. Phytother Res 1995; 19: 647–8.
134. Sime S, Reeve VE. Protection from inflammation, immunosuppression and carcinogenesis induced by UV radiation in mice by topical pycnogenol. Photochem Photobiol 2004; 79: 193–8.
135. Neves JR, et al. Efficacy of a topical serum containing L-ascorbic acid, neohesperidin, pycnogenol, tocopherol, and hyaluronic acid in relation to skin aging signs. J Cosmet Dermatol 2022; https://doi.org/10.1111/jocd.14837.
136. Zhao H, et al. Oral Pycnogenol® intake benefits the skin in urban Chinese outdoor workers: a randomized, placebo-controlled, double-blind, and crossover intervention study. Skin Pharmacol Physiol 2021; 34: 135–45.
137. Grether-Beck S, et al. French maritime pine bark extract (pycnogenol(R)) effects on human skin: clinical and molecular evidence. Skin Pharmacol Physiol 2016; 29: 13–7.
138. Blazso G, et al. Pycnogenol accelerates wound healing and reduces scar formation. Phytother Res 2004; 18: 579–81.
139. Tixier JM, et al. Evidence by in vivo and in vitro studies that binding of pycnogenols to elastin affects its rate of degradation by elastases. Biochem Pharmacol 1984; 33: 3933–9.
140. Ni A, Mu Y, Gulati O. Treatment of melasma with pycnogenol. Phytother Res 2007; 16: 567–71.
141. Saliou C, et al. Solar ultraviolet-induced erythema in human skin and nuclear factor kappa-B dependent gene expression in keratinocytes are modulated by a French maritime pine bark extract. Free Radic Biol Med 2001; 30: 154–60.
142. Bito T, Roy S, Sen CK. Pine bark extract pycnogenol downregulates INF-g-induced adhesion of T cells to human keratinocytes by inhibiting inducible ICAM-1 expression. Free Radic Biol Med 2000; 28: 219–27.
143. Draelos ZD. Botanical antioxidants. Cosmet Dermatol 2003; 16: 46–9.
144. Shibata S, et al. Inhibitory effects of licochalcone A isolated from *Glycyrrhiza inflata* root on inflammatory ear edema and tumour production in mice. Planta Med 1991; 57: 221–4.
145. Dieck K, et al. Anti-inflammatory properties of licochalcone A from *Glycyrrhiza inflata* on various human skin cells. In: Poster presented at the 63rd Annual Meeting of the American Academy of Dermatology, February 18–22, 2005, New Orleans, LA.
146. Wang ZY, Nixon DW. Licorice and cancer. Nutr Cancer 2001; 39: 1–11.
147. Weber TM, et al. Tolerance and efficacy of a skin care regimen containing licochalcone A for adults with erythematic rosacea and facial redness. In: Poster presented at the American Academy of Dermatology, February 18–22, 2005, New Orleans, LA.
148. Amer M, Metwalli M. Topical liquiritin improves melasma. Int J Dermatol 2000; 39: 299–301.
149. Silva D. Cellular and physiological effects of *Ganoderma lucidum* (reishi). Mini Rev Med Chem 2004; 4: 873–9.
150. Nebus J, et al. Clinical improvements in photoaging with topical treatments containing mushroom extracts. In: Poster presented at the 65th Annual Meeting of the American Academy of Dermatology, February 2–6, 2007, Washington, DC.
151. Andreassi M, et al. Antioxidant activity of topically applied lycopene. J Eur Acad Dermatol Venereol 2004; 18: 52–5.
152. Fazekas Z, et al. Protective effects of lycopene against ultraviolet B-induced photodamage. Nutr Cancer 2003; 47: 181–7.
153. Offord EA, et al. Photoprotective potential of lycopene, beta-carotene, vitamin E, vitamin C and carnosic acid in UVA-irradiated human skin fibroblasts. Free Radic Biol Med 2002; 32: 1293–303.
154. Yeh SL, Huang CS, Hu ML. Lycopene enhances UVA-induced DNA damage and expression of heme oxygenase-1 in cultured mouse embryo fibroblasts. Eur J Nutr 2005; 44: 365–70.
155. Singh RP, Agarwal R. Flavonoid antioxidant silymarin and skin cancer. Antioxid Redox Signal 2002; 4(4): 655–63.

156. Katiyar SK, et al. Protective effects of silymarin against photocarcinogenesis in a mouse skin model. J Natl Cancer Inst 1997; 89: 556–66.
157. Katiyar SK. Silymarin and skin cancer prevention: anti-inflammatory, antioxidant, and immunomodulatory effects (review). Int J Oncol 2005; 26: 169–76.
158. Draelos ZD. Cosmeceutical botanicals: part 1. In: Draelos ZD, ed. Cosmeceuticals. Philadelphia: Elsevier Saunders, 2005: 71–8.
159. Berardesca E, et al. Combined effects of silymarin and methylsulfonylmethane in the management of rosacea: clinical and instrumental evaluation. J Cosmet Dermatol 2008; 7: 8–14.
160. Baumann L. Botanical ingredients in cosmeceuticals. J Drugs Dermatol 2007; 6: 1084–8.
161. Wu J. Anti-inflammatory ingredients [clinical report]. J Drugs Dermatol 2008; 7(Suppl): s13–6.
162. Lee KG, Shibamoto T. Determination of antioxidant potential of volatile extracts isolated from various herbs and spices. J Agric Food Chem 2002; 50: 4947–52.
163. Yarnell E, Abacol K, Hooper CG. Clinical Botanical Medicine. Larchmont, NY: Mary Ann Liebert Inc., 2002.
164. Hamman JH. Composition and applications of aloe vera leaf gel. Molecules 2008; 13: 1599–616.
165. Thornfeldt C. Cosmeceuticals containing herbs: fact, fiction and future. Dermatol Surg 2005; 31: 873–80.
166. Syed T, et al. Management of psoriasis with aloe vera extract in a hydrophilic cream: a placebo-controlled, double-blind study. Trop Med Int Health 1996; 1: 505–9.
167. Thangapazham RL, Sharma A, Maheshwari RK. Beneficial role of curcumin in skin diseases. Adv Exp Med Biol 2007; 595: 343–57.
168. Jagetia GC, Rajanikant GK. Effect of curcumin and radiation-impaired healing of excisional wounds in mice. J Wound Care 2004; 13: 107–9.
169. Singer AJ, et al. Curcumin reduces burn progression in rats. Acad Emerg Med 2007; 14: 1125–9.
170. Hsu CH, Cheng AL. Clinical studies with curcumin. Adv Exp Med Biol 2007; 595: 471–80.
171. Erden IM, Kahraman A, Koken T. Beneficial effects of quercetin on oxidative stress induced by ultraviolet A. Clin Exp Dermatol 2001; 26: 536–9.
172. Piantelli M, et al. Tamoxifex and quercetin interact with type II estrogen binding sites and inhibit the growth of human melanoma cells. J Invest Dermatol 1995; 105: 248–53.
173. Phan TT, et al. Suppression of insulin-like growth factor signaling pathway and collagen expression in keloid-derived fibroblasts by quercetin: its therapeutic potential use in the treatment and/or prevention of keloids. Br J Dermatol 2003; 148: 544–52.
174. Young E. Allantoin in treatment of psoriasis. Dermatologica 1973; 147: 338–41.
175. Su S, et al. Mitochondrial sirtuins in skin and skin cancers. Photochem Photobiol 2020; 96: 973–80.
176. Cao C, et al. SIRT1 confers protection against UVB- and H_2O_2-induced cell death via modulation of p53 and JNK in cultured skin keratinocytes. J Cell Mol Med 2008; [Epub ahead of print]. Postprint; https://doi.org/10.1111/j.1582-4934.2008.00453.x.
177. Moreau M, et al. Enhancing cell longevity for cosmetic application: a complementary approach. J Drugs Dermatol 2007; 6(Suppl): s14–9.
178. Gelo-Pujic M, et al. Synthesis of new antioxidant conjugates and their in vitro hydrolysis with stratum corneum enzymes. Int J Cosmet Sci 2008; 30: 195–204.
179. Perugini P, et al. Efficacy of oleuropein against UVB irradiation: preliminary evaluation. Int J Cosmet Sci 2008; 30: 113–20.

3

Cosmeceutical Peptides

Susan H. Weinkle and Harriet Lin Hall

Introduction

Cosmeceuticals are topical creams and lotions designed to improve the appearance of aging skin. These products are not tested and approved as drugs, but rather appear in the consumer arena based on theoretical benefits from in vitro studies of active ingredients. Peptides, which are short chain sequences of amino acids, are perhaps the most popular topical anti-aging product in the market. There are three main categories of cosmeceutical peptides: signal peptides, carrier peptides, and neurotransmitter-affecting peptides. The active ingredient must be delivered to the target in a stable form and be able to have the desired biologic effect in vivo.

Background

Cosmeceuticals are topical product formulas designed to improve the appearance of the skin. The 1938 Food, Drug and Cosmetic Act differentiated clearly between drugs and cosmetics and charged the US Food and Drug Administration with regulating these products. This document allows the use of raw materials and ingredients in cosmetics for "cleansing, beautifying, promoting attractiveness, or altering the appearance" without approval from a government agency; however, no therapeutic claims for these products may be made (1, p. 1). In 1984, Albert Kligman, MD, PhD, coined the term "cosmeceutical" to describe products that combine the concepts of "cosmetic" and a "drug" (a product designed to mitigate or prevent disease). Dr. Kligman believes that a "cosmeceutical" should represent a product that "does something more than coloring the skin and something less than a therapeutic drug" (2, p. 890). Thus, cosmeceuticals have a unique niche in dermatology and some 90% of cosmetics now fall into this growing category.

The differences between cosmeceuticals and drugs may involve a simple difference in terminology. For example, although a drug and a cosmeceutical may contain the same active ingredient, the drug may be marketed as an anti-aging substance, while the cosmeceutical must be marketed as an agent that may "improve the appearance of wrinkles," given that therapeutic claims may be made only for drugs (1, p. 2). More than cosmetics that adorns or camouflage, but not categorized as drugs that alter cellular functions, cosmeceuticals have grown in popularity in the past two decades. Both the peptides and their degradation products are key players in the field of cosmetics and dermatology. One of the most popular categories is the peptide group (3, p. 343).

Small-sequence amino acid chains are being incorporated in cosmetic formulas to improve the signs of aging skin. According to Lupo (4), chronologically aged skin demonstrates lower procollagen type I messenger RNA and protein resulting in decreased production of new collagen (5, p. 1218). In addition, aging skin, and particularly aging skin that is exposed to ultraviolet (UV) light, overexpresses a proteolytic activity of matrix meralloproteinase-1, also known as interstitial collagenase (6, p. 43). Additionally, aging fibroblasts have a lower rate of proliferation than do fetal fibroblasts (7, p. 99). Much of the research demonstrating the role of amino acids and peptides in reversing the cutaneous signs of aging has been a secondary benefit of research on wound healing. These peptides are small-sequence amino acid chains

DOI: 10.1201/9781315165905-3

TABLE 3.1

Cosmeceutical Peptides

Type	In Vitro	Expected In Vivo Clinical Benefit
Signal peptides	Triggers wound-healing mechanisms that activate fibroblasts in response to fragmented chains of elastin and collagen	Increased collagen production to improve skin appearance
Carrier peptides	To deliver copper into skin, resulting in activation of enzymatic wound-healing pathways	Enhanced copper production, resulting in smoother skin
Neurotransmitter-inhibiting peptides	Interferes with stabilization step in neurotransmitter release	Decreases muscle movement

Source: Adapted from 4.

that may stimulate angiogenesis, production of granulation tissue, and new collagen synthesis. These classes of peptides have been designed with these goals in mind (Table 3.1).

Signal Peptides

Peptides with the ability to increase fibroblast production of collagen or decrease collagenase breakdown of existing collagen should potentially improve the clinical appearance of fine and course wrinkles visible in both chronologically and photoaged skin. Advanced research into the cellular and biochemical processes of aging and wounded skin results in new strategies to manipulate these processes for a therapeutic clinical effect. As wound healing and genomic research continue, certain bioactive amino acid chains have been discovered, which stimulate human skin dermal fibroblast growth in vitro. The use of signal peptides in commercial products has significantly risen in recent years (8). Peptides in the skin have been shown in vitro to (i) stimulate the production of extracellular matrix components, including collagen, elastin, and fibronectin and (ii) decrease the production of glycosaminoglycans (GAGs) as illustrated in Figure 3.1.

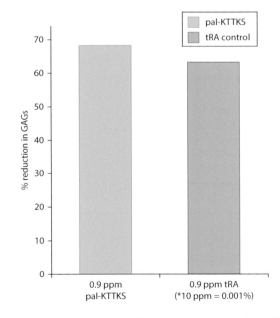

FIGURE 3.1 In in vitro cell culture experiments, pal-KTTS reduces glycosaminoglycan (GAG) comparably at 1/10th the dose of tRA (10 ppm = 0.001%).
(From 9 and P&G Beauty.)

Additionally, in the variations in amino acid sequence, number of amino acids, and use of derivatives of these acids, there are limitless combinations of possible peptides. By testing the effect of multiple peptides on the synthesis of collagen in culture, scientists at the University of Tennessee narrowed the field of possible amino acid combinations to a pentapeptide fragment of procollagen, KTTS (lysine, threonine, threonine, lysine, serine). This peptide retained 80% of the collagen-stimulating activity of the original, much larger than the 34–44 amino acid procollagen peptides from which it was delivered (9).

According to Kamoun (10) and Tajima (11), the linking of valine-glycine-valine-alanine-proline-glycine (VGVAPG) peptide was discovered in one study of elastin-derived peptides, which significantly stimulated human dermal skin fibroblast production and simultaneously downregulated elastin expression. Trans-dermal delivery of ionic peptides is likely to pose a significant issue for delivery of bioactive peptide into the skin. The signal peptide is combined with palmitic acid to aid in peptide penetration of the epidermis and is marketed currently in many cosmeceutical products under the name of palmitoyl oligopeptide (12).

In another study, Njieha et al. (13, p. 758) examined a different linking of peptides. Turosine-trosine-argine-alanineaspartame-aspartame-alanine sequence inhibited procollagen-C proteinase, which cleaves C-propeptide from type I procollagen, thus leading to decreased collagen breakdown.

The most prevalent and widely published signal peptide is the sequence lysine-threonine-threonine-lysine-serine (KTTKS) found on type I procollagen. This pentapeptide has been demonstrated to stimulate feedback regulation of new collagen synthesis and results in an increased production of extracellular matrix proteins such as types I and II collagen and fibronectin (3, p. 344). Like VGVAPG, KTTS is linked to palmitic acid in order to enhance delivery through the epidermis for engagement in the dermis. In a 12-week, double-blind, placebo-controlled, split-face, randomized clinical study of 93 Caucasian women between 35 and 55 years of age, Robinson and others found that pal-KTTS was well tolerated and significantly reduced fine lines by both qualitative technical and expert grader image analyses (Figure 3.2) (3, p. 344). Of importance to mention, Robinson et al. (14) also found pal-KTTS to be both efficacious and gentle on the skin barrier, as assessed by trans-epidermal water loss (TEWL) measurements. Maxtrixyl, the most common signal peptide currently in the market, is an ingredient in Olay Regenerist® and Stivectin-SD®.

The tripeptide glycyl-l-histadyl-l-lysine (GHK) is primarily known as carrier peptides but has also been shown to have some signal peptide effects. GHK without copper has been shown to enhance collagen production by stimulating fibroblasts (3, p. 344). GHK has also been linked with palmitic acid and marketed as Biopeptide-CL. In vitro and in vivo studies have been performed by the company (12).

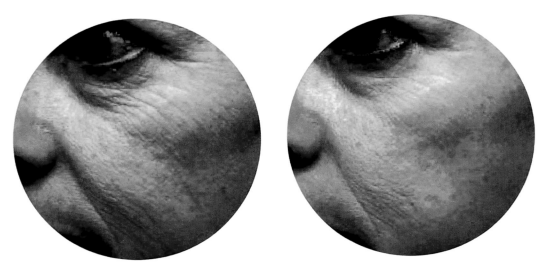

FIGURE 3.2 A significant improvement in the appearance of fine lines and wrinkles is observed following 12 weeks of treatment with moisturizer containing pal-KTTS.
(From 14 and P&G Beauty.)

Carrier Peptides

Carrier peptides function to stabilize and deliver important trace elements necessary for wound healing and enzymatic processes. In cosmeceuticals, the most common carrier peptide used is the delivery of copper into the cells (15, 16). Copper is an elemental metal that enhances wound healing, enzymatic processes, and angiogenesis. There are several mechanisms whereby copper may have beneficial effects on the skin. Lysyl oxide is an important enzyme in collagen and elastin production. It is dependent upon the action of copper. Tyrosinase and cytochrome-c oxidase require copper as well. Superoxide dismutase acts as an important antioxidant and requires copper and a cofactor. Copper is an essential cofactor for collagen and elastin formation, downregulates MMPs, and reduces the activity of collagenase. The tripeptide complex, glycyl-l-histidyl-l-lysine (GAK), spontaneously complexes with copper and facilitates the uptake of copper by cells (17, p. 715). This peptide sequence is found in proteins of the extracellular matrix such as the alpha chain of collagen, and it is believed to be released during wounding and inflammation. Prepared as a cosmeceutical, copper peptide is thought to improve skin firmness and texture, fine lines, and hyperpigmentation. GHK–copper complex increases levels of MMP/TIMPs and aids in dermal tissue remodeling (18, p. 2257). It also causes stimulation of collagen I, GAGs, cytochrome-c oxidase, and tyrosinase (19, p. 962; 20, p. 345). As mentioned earlier in this section, a feedback stimulation of collagen repair has also been proposed for this peptide (3), but the main benefit to photoaged skin is believed to be its ability to enhance delivery of copper. Both the tripeptide alone and copper tripeptide complex have been found to have beneficial effects on collagen stimulation. This carrier peptide–copper combination has also been found to increase levels on MMP-2 and MMP-2 mRNA, as well as TIMP-1 and -2. As such, it could function in collagen remodeling (18, p. 2257). Experiments using GHK–Cu have demonstrated stimulation of both type I collagen and the GAG's dermatan sulfate and chondroitin sulfate in rat wounds as well as cultured rat fibroblasts (19, p. 962). Human fibroblast cultures showed increased synthesis of dermatan sulfate and heparin sulfate after addition of the tripeptide–copper complex (21, p. 1049). Limited clinical trials with patients using a facial cosmeceutical product containing the complex as the active ingredient did demonstrate improvement in the appearance of fine lines as well as increase skin density and thickness (22).

Neurotransmitter-Affecting Peptides

Multi-chain peptides have generated interest for potential wrinkle-fighting properties. Pentapeptides may be more popular with patients and physicians; matrixyl acetate or Pal-KTTKS pentapeptide coupled with palmitic acid is a widely available drugstore product (Regenerist, Proctor & Gamble). However, the neurotransmitter-affecting peptides currently incorporated into cosmeceutical products were developed as topical mimics of the botulinum neurotoxins. Currently, only botulinum neurotoxin type A (BTX-A) has been approved for subcutaneous, intradermal, and intramuscular injection for facial wrinkles (23, p. 543). All botulinum neurotoxin serotypes (A–G) are single-chain polypeptides which inhibit acetylcholine release at the neuromuscular junction (NMJ) in a three-step process. The single-chain polypeptides are activated by proteases and cleaved into a double chain consisting of heavy- and light-chain moieties. Upon cleavage, the heavy chain binds to a high-affinity receptor on the presynaptic nerve terminal, which enables internalization of the bound toxin into the cell. The light-chain moiety is a zinc-dependent endopeptidase that cleaves membrane proteins that are responsible for docking acetylcholine vesicles on the inner sides of the nerve terminal membrane. The cleavage of these proteins inhibits the fusion to the vesicles with nerve membrane, thereby preventing release of acetylcholine into the NMJ. The intracellular target of BTX-A is synaptosome-associated protein of molecular weight 25 kDa (SNAP-25), which is a protein essential for successful docking and release of acetylcholine vesicles with the presynaptic vesicle. In contrast, botulinum neurotoxin type B (BTX-B) cleaves vesicle-associated membrane protein (VAMP), which is known as synaptobrevin. Like SNAP-25, VAMP is essential for the docking and fusion of the synaptic vesicle to the presynaptic membrane for the release of acetylcholine. The use of these polypeptides inhibits the repetitive contraction of the intrinsic muscles of facial expression and thereby reduces hyperkinetic facial lines (24, p. 34). The topical neurotransmitter-affecting peptides that are currently marketed in cosmeceuticals reportedly function to decrease facial muscle contraction and thus reduce lines and wrinkles by raising the threshold for a minimal muscle activity, requiring more signals to achieve movement and reducing subconscious muscle movement over time. Most of these peptides act on the soluble *N*-ethylmaleimide-sensitive factor attachment protein receptors (SNARE) complex, whereas others target different parts of the NMJ or certain neurotransmitters. Although it sounds like botulinum neurotoxin in a jar, it has yet to be proven whether these topical neurotransmitter-affecting proteins can penetrate to the level of the NMJ. The most popular cosmeceutical peptide in this category is acetyl hexapeptide-3 marketed as Argireline (McEit International Trade Co, Ltd; Tianjin, China).

Leuphasyl® (Lipotec S.A.), a pentapeptide of unpublished amino acid sequence, is proposed to modulate calcium channels by mimicking enkephalins. Enkephalins are endogenous opioids that inhibit neuronal activities. Their receptors are on the outside of neurons, couples to inhibitory G-proteins (Gi). The docking of enkephalins on these receptors results in the release of G-protein subunits (alpha, beta, or gamma) in the cell. These subunits close calcium ion channels and open potassium ion channels. Preventing the entry of calcium ions into the neuron avoids vesicle fusion and consequently inhibits acetylcholine release across the synapse to the muscle (25, 26). This enkephalin-like peptide couples to the enkephalin receptor on the outside of nerve cells and a conformational change initiates a cascade inside the neuron that results in a decrease of excitability and modulates the release of acetylcholine, thus diminishing muscle contraction. In vivo and in vitro placebo-controlled cosmeceutical studies performed by the company (Lipotec) reportedly confirm efficacy at reducing neurotransmitter release and decreasing wrinkle depth as assessed by a skin topography analysis of silicon imprints. The studies also showed a synergistic effect when both Leuphasyl and Argireline® were applied together (Centerchem). Tripeptide-3(β-Ala-Pro-Dab-NH-Benzyl*2AcOH), marketed as Syn®-Ake (Lipotec S.A.) (27), is proposed to act similarly to Walglerin-1. Walglerin-1 is a neurotoxin found in the venom of the temple viper, which causes reversible antagonism of muscular nicotinic acetylcholine receptors (mnAChR) at the postsynaptic membrane. It is proposed to bind to the epsilon subunit of the mnAChR which prevents binding of acetylcholine to the receptor, preventing it from opening. In the closed state, there is no uptake of sodium ions so that no depolarization takes place and the muscles remain relaxed (23). The company (Pentapharm) has performed their own in vitro and in vivo tests confirming its efficacy in decreasing muscle contraction and reducing wrinkle depth (Centerchem). A combination of peptides that include Tripeptide-3 has been patented in a cream named HydroPeptide Nimni Cream. In a single-center, double-blind, placebo-controlled study to evaluate the safety and efficacy of Nimni Cream by Hydropeptide® on skin quality and wrinkles, it was found to be safe and effective for improving skin quality in the face and can be considered a satisfactory therapeutic option adjuvant to aesthetic procedures (28).

Clinical Testing of Peptide Products

In 2006, a randomized, investigator-blinded, parallel study of 77 female subjects compared four products that purported to improve wrinkles—BTX type A (BTX-A), StriVectin-SD, DDF Wrinkle Relax, and Hydroderm™—with a placebo injection (29, p. 191). This study, supported by Allergan, Inc., evaluated the products based on the safety and efficacy of treating moderate-to-severe glabellar rhytids. The products were assessed according to blinded investigators' assessments of glabellar line severity on the facial wrinkle scale (FWS) and subjects' global assessments of overall change in appearance, ratings of glabellar-related self-perception before and after treatment, and satisfaction with the results. Figure 3.3 illustrates results based upon the FWS (29, p. 191). Statistically significant reductions in wrinkle severity on the FWS were found with the use of BTX-A which resulted in statistically significant improvements in subject-reported outcomes and satisfaction.

New Innovations in Technology and Clinical Testing

The past decade has witnessed remarkable advances in the field of biology. Disciplines such as genomics and proteomics have emerged to exploit our growing knowledge of the human genome and have

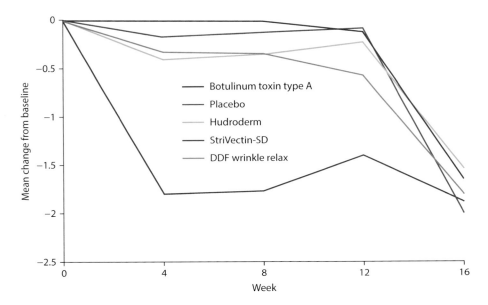

FIGURE 3.3   Changes in facial wrinkle scale.
(From 29.)

drastically accelerated our ability to understand how the human body responds to its environment. Genomics is a branch of biotechnology which applies genetic and molecular biology techniques to the genetic mapping and DNA sequencing of sets of genes or the complete genomes of selected organisms, whereas proteomics applies the techniques of molecular biology, biochemistry, and genetics to analyze the structure, function, and interactions of the proteins produced by the genes of a particular cell, tissue, or organism. The development of genomics and bioinformatics capabilities today enables a comprehensive assessment of skin aging and photoaging at the fundamental level of gene expression. Bioinformatics tools also enable an integrated analysis of gene expression themes and pathways, which provide new insights into the mechanisms of skin aging and possible interventions (30). Robinson et al. conducted a combined study of chronologic skin aging and photoaging to address several questions: (*i*) How does gene expression compare between young and old skin? (*ii*) How does gene expression compare between UV-exposed skin and UV-protected skin? (*iii*) Can genomics help dermatologists understand the skin aging process? (*iv*) Can genomics help dermatologists identify important biomarkers of skin aging and perhaps new targets to intervene in the skin aging process (p. s8)? At the conclusion of the study, a strong knowledge base was derived that provided new insight into the mechanism of skin aging.

One of the most important technologies in the genomics toolbox is the gene chip or microarray. The gene chip allows dermatologists to determine which genes are turned on/up or turned off/down in response to different biological conditions. Previously, if researchers were interested in measuring these gene changes, it would have to be done one gene at a time. However, with the gene chip, tens of thousands of genes can be monitored in a single experiment, allowing the entire genome to be examined in less than a week's time. If one gene at a time was monitored, each trial would take nearly 150 years.

Genomics tools such as gene chips have become well established in the medical field over the past 15 years and most universities have instituted some form of genomics curriculum in their biomedical programs. Additionally, this platform has proven to be very useful for learning how the skin responds to microbial infection, including malassezia (31). Furthermore, pharmaceutical companies have seen the potential of this capability and exploit it to develop new drugs and therapeutics. While the close connection between genomics technologies and medicine has been well established over the years, there are other realms of biology that are showing the benefits of incorporating genomics technologies into their research programs. The advent of next-generation DNA- and RNA-sequencing technologies is poised to significantly impact the study of skin. The Next-Gen RNA platforms like RNA-Seq (also known as Digital Gene Expression Profiling) promise to replace microarrays in the future by providing even more information about the transcription process (31). Once the information is received, dermatologists can provide greater individualized patient skin care.

Peptides: What Is to Come?

To further explore the power of peptides for anti-aging applications, Procter and Gamble Beauty Science continues diligent research on the matter. Osborne et al. (32) indicated how human skin equivalents provide useful in vitro models to identify and evaluate cosmetic technologies based on knowledge gained via gene expression profiling of aged skin. A series of acyl-modified di-, tri-, and tetra-peptides were synthesized and screened in vitro for their capacity to stimulate production of collagen I as well as other skin structural proteins, including procollagen-C, collagens III, IV, and VI, elastin, fibronectin, CD44, vimentin and laninins I and IV in both dermal fibroblasts and human skin equivalent cultures.

Of the peptides evaluated, palmitoyl-lysine-threonine (pal-KT) stimulated skin biomarkers to the greatest extent. RT-PCR analysis of mRNA from the human skin equivalent cultures revealed significantly increased expressions of the skin structural proteins. The results illustrated in Figure 3.4 suggest that pal-KT is a promising candidate for cosmetic ingredients, either alone or in combination with other peptides.

According to a recent P&G genomic study (34), a regimen approach provides the greatest treatment flexibility as well as enhanced opportunity to use optimum levels of potentially incompatible anti-aging ingredients. After eight weeks of daily application, more than 70% of subjects showed some improvement. Computer image analysis showed that the periorbital region was significantly reduced (Figure 3.5). Unlike the daily application of a tretinoin, considering the benchmark prescription, neither dryness nor TEWL increased significantly during the study (33).

Cosmeceutical peptides are a major player in the anti-aging market. Dermatologists are trained adequately to guide patients in maintaining a youthful appearance and lessen any confusion over the bombardment of anti-aging claims. Clearly, peptides play various roles in combating the signs of aging. The potential for new treatment option, as represented by cosmeceutical peptides, is a developing field with most ongoing research occurring within the industry. In some of the marketing arenas, some peptide-containing cosmeceuticals cost much more than the average peptide bought at the drug store instigating many questions from patients on which product is better. It is important that the final marketed product is stable in formula, deliverable to its target dermal site and biologically active at this target site. As dermatologists well know, these results do not always translate into in vivo actions. It is not an easy task to penetrate the barrier of the skin. Double-blind, placebo-controlled drug study is lacking, as it is with all cosmeceuticals as a result of regulatory concerns by the industry (3, p. 348). Consumer demand for products that improve appearance and counteract the signs of aging likely will lead to more research and development into cosmeceutical peptides for primary and adjunctive treatments of the signs of aging.

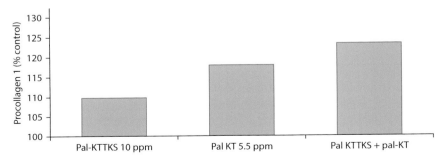

FIGURE 3.4 In in vitro cell studies, pal-KT increases collagen synthesis to a greater extent than pal-KTTS. Further, the combination of both peptides has an even more profound effect on collagen synthesis than either peptide alone. (From 32 and P&G Beauty.)

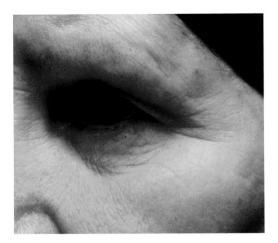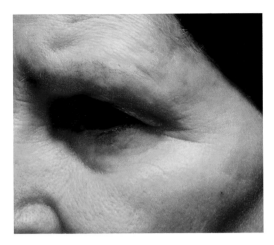

FIGURE 3.5   Used Olay Professional ProX 3-product wrinkle regimen for eight weeks: SPF 30 lotion during day; night cream at bedtime; wrinkle treatment twice daily.
(From 33 and P&G Beauty.)

REFERENCES

1. Vleugels R. Cosmeceuticals: From topical antioxidants to peptides. Dermatol Rep 2008; 2: 1–10.
2. Draelos Z. The future of cosmeceuticals: An interview with Albert Kligman, MD, PhD. Dermatol Surg 2005; 31: 890–91.
3. Lupo M, Cole A. Cosmeceutical peptides. Dermatol Therapy 2007; 20: 343–49.
4. Lupo M. Cosmeceutical peptides. Dermatol Surg 2005; 31: 832–36.
5. Chung JH, Seo JY, Choi HR, et al. Modulation of skin collagen metabolism in aged and photoaged human skin in vivo. J Invest Dermatol 2001; 117: 1218–24.
6. Brennan M, Bhotti H, Nerusu KC, et al. Matrix metalloproteinase I is the major collagenolytic enzyme responsible for collagen damage in UV-radiated human skin. Photochem Photobiol 2003; 78: 43–8.
7. Khorramizadeh MR, Tredget EE, Telasky C, et al. Aging differentially modulates the expression of collagen and collagenase in dermal fibroblasts. Mol Cell Biochem 1999; 194: 99–108.
8. Skibska A, Perlikowska R. Signal peptides: Promising ingredients in cosmetics. Curr Protein Pept Sci 2021; 22: 716–28.
9. Lintner, K. Promoting production in the extracellular matrix without compromising barrier. Cutis 2002; 70S: 13–6.
10. Kamoun A, Landeau JM, Godeau G, et al. Growth stimulation of human skin fibroblasts by elastin-derived peptides. Cell Adhes Commun 1995; 3: 273–81.
11. Tajima S, Wachi H, Uemura Y, Okamoto K. Modulation by elastin peptide VGVAPG of cell proliferation and elastin expression in human skin fibroblast. Arch Dermatol Res 1997; 289: 489–92.
12. Croda, Snaith, UK. Palmitoyl oligopeptide. Accessed 2022 at: https://www.crodapersonalcare.com/en-gb/product-finder/product/2954-Biopeptide_1_CL
13. Njieha FK, Morikawa T, Tuderman L, et al. Partial purification of a pro-collagen C proteinase. Inhibition by synthetic peptides and sequential cleavage of type 1 procollagen. Biochemistry 1982; 21: 757–64.
14. Robinson L, Fitzgerald N, Doughty D, et al. Topical palmitoyl pentapeptide provides improvement in photoaged human facial skin. Int J Cosmetic Sci 2005; 27: 155–60.
15. Dou Y, Lee A, Zhu L, et al. The potential of GHK as an anti-aging peptide. Aging Pathobiol Ther 2020; 2: 58–61.
16. Pickart L, Vasquez-Soltero JM, Margolina A. The human tripeptide GHK-Cu in prevention of oxidative stress and degenerative conditions of aging: Implications for cognitive health. Oxid Med Cell Longev 2012; 2012: 324832.
17. Pickart L, Freedman JH, Loher WJ, et al. Growth modulating plasma tripeptide may function by facilitating copper uptake into cells. Nature 1980; 288: 715–17.

18. Simeon A, Emonard H, Horneback W, et al. The tripeptide copper complex glycyl-ʟ-histidyl-L-lysine-Cu2+ stimulates matrix metalloproteinase-2 expression by fibroblast cultures. Life Sci 2000; 67: 2257–65.
19. Simeon A, Wegrowski Y, Bontemps J, et al. Expression of glycosaminoglycan and small proteoglycans in wounds: Modulation by the tripeptide-copper complex glycyl-L-histidyl-L-lysine-Cu2+. J Invest Dermatol 2000; 115: 962–68.
20. Buffoni F, Pino R, Dal Pozzo A. Effect of tripeptide–copper complexes on the process of skin wound healing and on cultured fibroblasts. Arch Int Pharacodyn Ther 1995; 330: 345–60.
21. Wegrowski Y, Maquart FX, Borel JP. Stimulation of sulfated glycosaminoglycan synthesis by the tripeptide–copper complex glycyl-L-histidyl-L-lysine-CU2+. Life Sci 1992; 51: 1049–56.
22. Leyden JJ. Skin care benefits of copper peptide containing facial cream. In: Paper presented at the American Academy of Dermatology 60th Annual Meeting, February, 2002, New Orleans, Louisiana.
23. McArdle JJ, Lentz TL, Witzemann V, et al. Walglerin-1 selectively blocks the epsilon form of the muscle nicotinic acetylcholine receptor. J Pharm Exp Ther 1999; 289: 543–50.
24. Yamauchi P, Lowe N. Botulinum toxin types A and B: Comparison of efficacy, duration, and dose-ranging studies for the treatment of facial rhytides and hyperhidrosis. Clin Dermatol 2004; 22: 34–9.
25. Wikipedia. Enkephalin. http://www.wikipedia.org/wiki/Enkephalins; accessed 2022.
26. Hughs J, Smith TW, Kosterlitz HW, et al. Identification of two related pentapeptides from the brain with potent opiate agonist activity. Nature 1975; 258: 577–80.
27. Centerchem, Basel, Switzerland. Syn®-Ake. Product information accessed 2022 at: https://www.centerchem.com/products/syn-ake/
28. Sadick N, Bohnert K, Serra M, et al. Single-center, double-blind, randomized, placebo-controlled, study of the efficacy and safety of a cream formulation for improving facial wrinkles and skin quality. J Drugs Dermatol 2018; 17: 664–69.
29. Beer K. Comparative evaluation of the safety and efficacy of botulinum toxin type A and topical creams for treating moderate-to-severe glabellar rhytids. Dermatol Surg 2006; 32: 184–92.
30. Robinson M, Binder R, Griffiths C. Genomic-driven insights into changes in aging skin. J Drugs Dermatol 2009; 8: s8–11.
31. Tiesman J. From bench to beauty counter: Using genomics to drive technology development for skin care. J Drugs Dermatol 2009; 8: s12–14.
32. Osborne R, Mullins L, Jarrold B. Understanding metabolic pathways for skin anti-aging. J Drugs Dermatol 2009; 8: s4–7.
33. Kaczvinsky J, Grimes P. Practical applications of genomics research for treatment of aging skin. J Drugs Dermatol 2009; 8: s15–18.
34. Fu J, Hillebrand G, Raleigh P, et al. A randomized controlled comparative study of the wrinkle reduction benefits of a cosmetic niacinamide/peptide/retinyl propionate product regimen versus a prescription 0.02% tretinoin product regimen. Br J Dermatol 2010; 162: 647–54.

4

Growth Factors, Cellular Secretome and Exosomes

Rahul C. Mehta and Mitchel P. Goldman

What Are Growth Factors, Cellular Secretome and Exosomes?

Intercellular communication is one of the critical functions of all cells to maintain homeostasis and facilitate skin repair and regeneration. Until recently, it was believed that secreted soluble growth factors and cytokines are primary mediators of intercellular communications (1). However, whole cellular secretome (all soluble and insoluble materials secreted by a cell) and extracellular vesicles also play an important part in cellular communication (2). Exosomes are the smallest of the extracellular vesicles ranging in size from 30 to 100 nm and contain proteins, mRNA, miRNA and lipids. They play an integral part in all stages of wound healing and skin repair (3).

Biochemistry of Skin Aging and Repair

Intrinsic aging is primarily caused by excess free radical production from the mitochondrial energy generation processes. Exposure to solar radiation and environmental toxins as well as lifestyle choices such as diet, sleep, stress and exercise (collectively defined as exposome) is primarily responsible for extrinsic aging. Biological pathways for both intrinsic and extrinsic aging are now being identified and understood (4, 5).

The process of wound healing provides a complete picture of epidermal repair. Wound healing occurs in four stages: hemostasis, inflammation, proliferation and remodeling, each with its own characteristic cellular and molecular fingerprint (2). Table 4.1 shows the predominant cells involved in different stages of wound healing. After a wound has been inflicted, a rapid influx of platelets initiates hemostasis. Addition of secretome from monocytes and endothelial cells transitions wound healing into an inflammation phase when neutrophils and monocytes are recruited to eliminate potential pathogens, foreign bodies and necrotic tissue from the wound. In the next phase, pro-inflammatory secretome activates fibroblast and keratinocytes to rapidly proliferate, producing an unorganized extracellular matrix to achieve wound closure. Recruitment of neutrophils, lymphocytes and platelets starts angiogenesis in the new wound bed. In the remodeling phase of wound healing, the initial unorganized extracellular matrix is replaced by a more functional matrix by the actions of fibroblasts, keratinocytes and endothelial cells. In each phase, secretome of different predominant cell types with a unique blend of growth factors, cytokines, and exosomes is responsible for intercellular communication leading to wound healing and skin repair.

Sources of Growth Factors and Secretome for Cosmeceutical Use

Dermal Fibroblasts

Dermal fibroblasts are a critical component of skin repair and regeneration process. They produce and maintain extracellular matrix and communicate with other cells to maintain skin homeostasis and therefore considered ideal for use as a source of anti-aging products. The first cosmeceutical product containing

DOI: 10.1201/9781315165905-4

TABLE 4.1

Selection of Clinical Studies Using Products Containing Cellular Secretome, Platelet-Rich Plasma and Synthetic Growth Factors

Secretome Source	Study Design	Summary of Results	Ref.	Year	Authors
Fibroblast Conditioned Medium					
Neonatal Fibroblasts	N-14, open-label, 60 days, aged skin	Reduction in fine lines, wrinkles and periorbital photodamage by IA and profilometry; increase in Grenz-zone thickness in biopsy	6	2003	Fitzpatrick and Rostan
Neonatal Fibroblasts	N-60, double-blind, vehicle-controlled, 90 days, aged skin	Reduced periorbital fine lines and wrinkles over vehicle using IA and profilometry	7	2008	Mehta et al.
Neonatal Fibroblasts	N-37, open-label, 90 days, aged skin	Reductions in fine and coarse wrinkles and improvements in skin texture, tone and radiance	10	2010	Atkin et al.
Neonatal Fibroblasts	N-35, double-blind, vehicle-controlled, 90 days, aged skin	Improvements in overall photodamage and in fine and coarse wrinkles over vehicle control	8	2017	Kadoya et al.
Hypoxic Fibroblast Conditioned Medium					
Neonatal Foreskin Fibroblasts	N-42 open-label, 90 days, post-laser resurfacing	Accelerated wound healing and more normal skin recovery	12	2012	Zimber et al.
Neonatal Foreskin Fibroblasts	N-40 open-label, 90 days, aged skin	Improvement in skin hydration and in global investigator and subject assessments	13	2017	Draelos et al.
Stem Cell Conditioned Medium					
Endothelial Precursor	N-15, split-face, inv-blind, 12 weeks, with microneedeling, aged skin	Skin roughness was different from saline microneedeling; all other parameters show no difference from saline microneedeling	33	2013	Seo at al.
Endothelial Precursor	N-25, split-face, inv-blind, 12 weeks, with microneedeling, aged skin	Improvement in wrinkles and pigmentation over saline microneedling by IA and instrumental measurements	34	2014	Lee et al.
Adipose	N-22, 30 days, with fractional laser resurfacing	Increased elasticity, hydration, and decreased TEWL, roughness, and melanin index. Increased dermal collagen density, elastin density in biopsy	19	2016	Zhou et al.
Adipose, Placenta	N-22, 15 days, double-blind, very superficial injection of Adipose CM, Placenta CM or saline	Improved erythema, hydration, gloss and melanin indices over baseline, Melanin index better for Adipose-CM over Placenta-CM	21	2016	Xu et al.
Adipose	N-35, double-blind, FB-CM-controlled, three months, aged skin	Improvement in wrinkles, texture and firmness by IA and SA from baseline. No statistical difference from FB-CM.	20	2017	Wu et al.

(Continued)

TABLE 4.1 *(Continued)*

Secretome Source	Study Design	Summary of Results	Ref.	Year	Authors
Amniotic Membrane	N-48, double-blind, vehicle-controlled, eight weeks, microneedling, aged skin	Improvement in pore, wrinkle, spot and skin tone compared to vehicle	22	2019	Prakoeswa et al.
Red Deer Placenta	N-40, split-face, double-blind, vehicle-controlled, three months, aged skin	Improvements in photoaging parameters in both groups	23	2019	Alhaddad et al.
Umbilical Cord	N-24, split-face, double-blind, vehicle-controlled, 12 weeks, aged skin, microneedling	Improvements in brightness and skin texture compared to vehicle group	35	2022	Liang et al.
Platelet-Rich Plasma					
Autologous PRP	N-20, inv-blind, vehicle-controlled, eight weeks, aged skin	Improved dryness, smoothness, softness, luminosity, and radiance for both groups. Improved rete peg architecture and collagen upregulation	27	2019	Draelos et al.
Autologous PRP vs Plasma gel	N-40, split-face, double-blind, PRP vs Plasma gel, 16 weeks, injection	Improvement of periorbital wrinkles after two treatments but results not maintained for three months	28	2022	Diab et al.
Ameotic Collagen Matrix vs PRP	N-20, split-face, double-blind, PRP vs amniotic collagen matrix, 12 weeks, microneedling	More improvement in clinical, pathological and photographic method over PRP	29	2022	Basyoni et al.
Synthetic					
TGF-β	N-31, open-label, 90 days, aged skin	Improvement in facial wrinkle scores by IA	36	2006	Ehrlick et al.
TGF-β vs FB-CM	N-60, split-face, double-blind, FB-CM-controlled, 12 weeks, aged skin	Improved smoothness, firmness, fine lines, radiance and overall appearance in both groups	37	2016	Draelos et al.
Recombinant GFs	N-11, open-labeled, three months	Improvement in skin texture, wrinkles, redness, brown spots	38	2022	Quinlan et al.

human growth factors, TNS (Tissue Nutrient Serum, SkinMedica, Irvine, CA), was launched in 2001 with clinical data showing new collagen formation, epidermal thickening and clinical appearance of smoother skin with less visible wrinkling after 60 days of topical use (6). The growth factor blend used in this product was a concentrated conditioned medium from human dermal fibroblasts culture used for production of diabetic wound-healing products. At that time, eight growth factors were initially identified in the product. Subsequent analysis of the same product identified over 110 growth factors, cytokines and active proteins (7) and a more recent analysis identified over 350 active proteins (8). It is believed that the process of collecting conditioned media without further processing or purification retained the entire secretome of activated fibroblasts as a physiologically balanced mixture of everything fibroblasts can make and secrete in the cell culture (9). Subsequent multiple larger, controlled clinical studies confirm the activity of this product in combination with antioxidants for skin rejuvenation and post-procedure recovery (7, 8, 10).

Advanced analytical techniques identify extracellular vesicles and the presence of exosomes in this conditioned medium and the product (Figure 4.1).

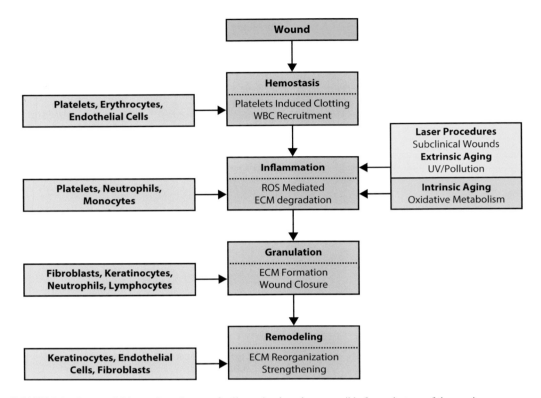

FIGURE 4.1   Stages of skin repair and types of cells predominantly responsible for each stage of the repair process.

The composition of any growth factor mixture varies with cell phenotype and environmental variables. Growing dermal fibroblasts under hypoxia leads to upregulation of genes associated with pluripotent stem cells and secretion of known stem cell markers (11). The conditioned media from such a process has different biological activities with greater anti-inflammatory and wound-healing properties and lower extracellular matrix production (12). A product containing hypoxic conditioned media applied immediately after ablative and non-ablative laser resurfacing produces accelerated wound healing and enhanced skin recovery (12). Combining it with antioxidants in a moisturizing base shows statistically significant improvement in skin hydration and in global investigator and subject assessments in 90 days (13).

Mesenchymal Stem Cells

Mesenchymal stem cells (MSC) abundant in skin and its secretome are essential in skin repair (14). Secretome from adipose-derived MSC is shown to increase collagen production, protection against oxidative damage, skin repair and downregulate tyrosinase (15, 16); adipose MSC also secrete exosomes to regulate extracellular matrix composition and fibroblast differentiation to mitigate scar formation (17, 18). Secretome from adipose MSC used after fractional carbon dioxide (CO_2) laser resurfacing results in increased elasticity, hydration and decreased trans-epidermal water loss (TEWL), roughness and dyspigmentation. Histological analysis shows increased dermal collagen density and elastin density (19). In another split-face comparison of adipose MSC secretome-based product with fibroblast secretome-based product, the latter showed slightly better, but not statistically different, improvement in wrinkles, texture and firmness (20).

The source of MSC also affects its composition and function. Adipose MSC secretome is more adept at cell adhesion, migration, wound healing and tissue remodeling, while placental MSC secretome is more adept at angiogenesis, cell proliferation, differentiation, cell survival, immunomodulation and collagen degradation (21). In a head-to-head clinical comparison using very superficial injection, both sources showed improved erythema, hydration, gloss and pigment normalization compared to control, and adipose MSC secretome was better in improving dyspigmentation (21). Amniotic membrane MSC secretome assessed in a vehicle-controlled study showed a statistically significant improvement in photoaging compared to vehicle when applied with microneedling (22).

MSC secretome from non-human sources have also been used in skin care. Red Deer umbilical cord lining stem cell conditioned medium containing product was tested in a split-face, vehicle-controlled, investigator-blinded study. Significant improvements were seen in photoaging parameters in both groups (23).

Platelet-Rich Plasma

Platelets are critical first source of growth factors and exosomes after skin damage (24). Autologous platelet-rich plasma (PRP) can be easily prepared in clinic using commercially available kits. It has been used in many skin care applications, especially after microneedle treatment (25). An autologous PRP topical serum was found to promote cell proliferation, chemotactic activity and stimulation of collagen and hyaluronic acid (26). Clinical effects of another topically delivered PRP in a cosmetic base show improved rete peg architecture and collagen upregulation after eight weeks of use (27). Additional studies show benefits of PRP-based products after injection or microneedling in clinical efficacy face and periorbital region (28, 29).

Synthetic Growth Factors

Individual growth factors and cytokines can be made via recombinant technology using bacterial or yeast cultures modified to include DNA sequence for growth factors. Many growth factors of cosmeceutical interest are produced by this technique, including TGF-β, VEGF, EGF, various FGFs, PDGF and more (30). While clinical studies have shown a marginally beneficial effect of some of the individual growth factors, more studies must be performed to understand the role for combination of growth factors in skin rejuvenation. Combinations of growth factors in cell secretome that complement effects of each other are likely to be more effective as multiple components of the secretome are involved in most biochemical processes, including wound healing (31).

Desirable Attributes of a Topical Growth Factor Product

Cell secretome containing growth factors produce anti-aging benefits by virtue of their biological role to maintain healthy skin structure and function. Together with cytokines, growth factors and exosomes provide constant communication between cells of the immune system, keratinocytes and fibroblasts throughout the process of wound healing, skin repair and regeneration. During the final remodeling phase of wound healing, a number of different growth factors, cytokines and exosome constituents interact with each other and with surrounding cells in concert to improve the quality of the extracellular matrix. The use of individual growth factors is unlikely to duplicate these complex interactions essential for remodeling of skin. Therefore, a physiologically balanced cell secretome proven to have a role in skin remodeling should provide superior benefits than individual growth factors. Ideal growth factor and secretome products should contain this unique mixture obtained from natural sources.

Cosmeceutical products containing mixtures of natural substances such as cellular growth factors, cytokines and exosomes are generally difficult to analyze for concentrations of "active" ingredients. Even products manufactured with a single growth factor are not labeled with growth factor content which makes it difficult to compare product strengths. More analytical efforts are needed to ensure that consumers know that the products they are using have reliable quality standards. In addition, most biologically active molecules and structures are inherently unstable in a non-physiologic environment, unless they are stored frozen at temperatures below −20°C. The presence of surface-active additives, alcohols and other protein-denaturing excipients further decreases product stability and compromises product efficacy during the claimed shelf life of the product. One published study shows the presence of high levels of growth factors and cytokines in a commercial product stored at room temperature throughout its two-year shelf life (7). If quantitative analysis is not possible due to complexity of the formulation, measurement of biological activity should be performed using appropriate techniques to ensure product stability throughout the labeled shelf life. Such a model is now available using reconstituted skin for in-vitro assessment of upregulation of genes critical for skin repair and rejuvenation (8). This model is also used to compare multiple products and multiple sources of secretome.

Risks Associated with Growth Factors

Growth factors are key molecules that affect cellular proliferation and differentiation which, if unregulated, can lead to carcinogenic transformation of cells. The presence of receptors for some growth factors in melanoma cells and expression of certain growth factors by cancerous cells (32) has raised concerns about the potential for topically applied growth factors to stimulate the development of cancer. Whether presence of receptors or increased expression contributes to tumor growth is uncertain. However, a recent finding suggests that chronic administration of high concentrations of PDGF directly into debrided diabetic pressure wounds may result in increased mortality from cancer. It is unlikely that growth factors applied topically to intact skin would affect tumor proliferation as the protein molecules are too large to be absorbed in large quantities (7). All commercial products manufactured from whole secretome have a composition similar to what the cells would produce in their natural environment. Therefore, it is unlikely that the levels of growth factors in skin after topical application are significantly higher than those following inflammation-causing event such as chemical peel, lasers or skin infections. Finally, no reports of epidermal or dermal cancers have been seen or reported in the world's medical literature in over 20 years of use of the original SkinMedica TNS serum.

Conclusion

Topical products containing growth factors have been used in skin care for over 20 years. We now know that some of these products actually contain cellular secretome, including exosomes, rather than only growth factors. Exosomes may play a critical role in producing the biological and clinical activities seen with these products. Functions of secretome containing growth factors and exosomes in the natural wound-healing process are complex and incompletely understood; however, it appears that wound healing is dependent on the synergistic interaction of many secreted components from multiple cell types. The use of whole secretome topical formulations provides a good first-line treatment for mild-to-moderate photodamaged skin. Table 4.1 lists a sample of clinical studies using products containing secretome from different sources. The most promising research suggests that secretome products stimulate the growth of collagen, elastin and glycol amino glycans leading to reduction in fine lines and wrinkles. Clinical studies demonstrate that dermal collagen production and clinical improvement in photodamage are significant. More research is needed to understand the role of all secretome components, including exosomes, in the reversal of skin aging.

REFERENCES

1. Werner S, Krieg T, Smola H. Keratinocyte-fibroblast interactions in wound healing. *J Invest Dermatol* 2007 May;127(5):998–1008.
2. Laberge A, Arif S, Moulin VJ. Microvesicles: Intercellular messengers in cutaneous wound healing. *J Cell Physiol* 2018 August;233(8):5550–5563.
3. Stahl AL, Johansson K, Mossberg M, Kahn R, Karpman D. Exosomes and microvesicles in normal physiology, pathophysiology, and renal diseases. *Pediatr Nephrol* 2019 January;34(1):11–30.
4. Gilchrest BA. Skin aging and photoaging: An overview. *J Am Acad Dermatol* 1989;21:610–613.
5. Mehta RC, Fitzpatrick RE. Endogenous growth factors as cosmeceuticals. *Dermatol Ther* 2007; 20:350–359.
6. Fitzpatrick RE, Rostan EF. Reversal of photodamage with topical growth factors: A pilot study. *J Cosmet Laser Ther* 2003;5:25–34.

7. Mehta RC, Smith SR, Grove GL, et al. Reduction in facial photodamage by a topical growth factor product. *J Drugs Dermatol* 2008;7:864–871.

8. Kadoya K, Makino E, Jiang LJ, et al. Upregulation of extracellular matrix genes collaborate clinical efficacy of human fibroblast-derived growth factors in skin rejuvenation. *J Drug Dermatol* 2017;16(12):611–617.

9. Sundaram H, Mehta RC, Norine JA, et al. Topically applied physiologically balanced growth factors: A new paradigm of skin rejuvenation. *J Drugs Dermatol* 2009 May;8(5 Suppl Skin Rejuvenation):4–13.

10. Atkin DH, Trookman NS, Rizer RL, et al. Combination of physiologically balanced growth factors with antioxidants for reversal of facial photodamage. *J Cosmet Laser Ther* 2010;12:14–20.

11. Pinney E, Zimber M, Schenone A, et al. Human embryonic-like ECM (hECM) stimulates proliferation and differentiation in stem cells while killing cancer cells. *Int J Stem Cells* 2011;4(1):70–75.

12. Zimber MP, Mansbridge JN, Taylor M, et al. Human cell-conditioned media produced under embryonic-like conditions result in improved healing time after laser resurfacing. *Aesthetic Plast Surg* 2012;36:431–437.

13. Draelos ZD, Karnik J, Naughton G. The anti-aging effects of low oxygen tension generated multipotent growth factor containing serum. *J Drugs Dermatol* 2017;16(1):30–34.

14. Golchin A, Farahany TZ, Khojasteh A, et al. The clinical trials of mesenchymal stem cell therapy in skin diseases: An update and concise review. *Curr Stem Cell Res Ther* 2019;14:22–33.

15. Park BS, Jang KA, Sung JH, et al. Adipose-derived stem cells and their secretory factors as a promising therapy for skin aging. *Dermatol Surg* 2008;34:323–326.

16. Kim WS, Park BS, Sung JH. Protective role adipose-derived stem cells and their soluble factors in photoaging. *Arch Dermatol Res* 2009;301:329–336.

17. Wang L, Hu L, Zhou X, et al. Exosomes secreted by human adipose mesenchymal stem cells promote scarless cutaneous repair by regulating extracellular matrix remodelling. *Sci Rep* 2017;7:13321.

18. Wu P, Zhang B, Shi H, et al. MSC-Exosome: A novel cell-free therapy for cutaneous regeneration. *Cytotherapy* 2018;20:291–301.

19. Zhou BR, Zhang T, Bin Jameel AA, et al. The efficacy of conditioned media of adipose-derived stem cells combined with ablative carbon dioxide fractional resurfacing for atrophic acne scars and skin rejuvenation. *J Cosmet Laser Ther* 2016;18(3):138–148.

20. Wu DC, Goldman MP. Topical human growth factors for the rejuvenation of aging face. *J Clin Aesthetic Dermatol* 2017;10(5):31–35.

21. Xu Y, Guo S, Wei C, et al. The comparison of adipose stem cell and placental stem cell in secretion characteristics and in facial antiaging. *Stem Cells Int* 2016:1–14. https://pubmed.ncbi.nlm.nih.gov/27057176/

22. Prakoeswa CRS, Pratiwi FD, Herwanto N, et al. The effects of amniotic membrane stem cell-conditioned medium on photoaging. *J Dermatol Treat* 2019;30(5):478–482.

23. Alhaddad M, Boen M, Wu DC, et al. Red Deer umbilical cord lining mesenchymal stem cell extract cream for rejuvenation of the face. *J Drugs Dermatol* 2019;18(4):363–366.

24. Van der Meijden PEJ, Hemmskerk JWM. Platelet biology and functions: New concepts and clinical perspectives. *Nat Rev Cardiol* 2018;16:166–179.

25. Wand 2020 PRP-Stem-Cell-Collagen-Skincare. *J Clin Aesthet Dermatol* 2020;13(1):44–49.

26. Anitua E, Troya M, Pino A. A novel protein-based autologous topical serum for skin regeneration. *J Cosmet Dermatol* 2020;19:705–713.

27. Draelos ZD, Rheins LA, Wootten S, et al. Pilot study: Autologous platelet-rich plasma used in a topical cream for facial rejuvenation. *J Cosmet Dermatol* 2019;18:1348–1352.

28. Diab HM, Elhosseiny R, Bedair NI, Khorkhed AH. Efficacy and safety of plasma gel versus platelet-rich plasma in periorbital rejuvenation: A comparative split-face clinical and Antera 3D camera study. *Arch Dermatol Res* 2022 September;314(7):661–671. doi: 10.1007/s00403-021-02270-7. Epub July 6, 2021. PMID: 34231136.

29. Basyoni RRH, Hassan AM, Mohammed DA, Radwan NK, Hassan GFR. Facial rejuvenation by microneedling with irradiated amniotic collagen matrix compared to platelet rich plasma. *Dermatol Ther* 2022 September;35(9):e15739. doi: 10.1111/dth.15739. Epub 2022 August 5. PMID: 35899486.

30. Gottscha TE, Bailey JE (Eds). *International cosmetic ingredient dictionary and handbook*. Washington DC: Toiletry and Fragrance Association, pp. 1170–1174 (2008).

31. Eming SA, Krieg T, Davidson JM. Inflammation in wound repair: Molecular and cellular mechanisms. *J Invest Dermatol* 2007;127(3):514–525.

32. Liu B, Earl HM, Baban D, et al. Melanoma cell lines express VEGF receptor KDR and respond to exogenously added VEGF. *Biochem Biophys Res Commun* 1995;217(3):721–727.
33. Seo KY, Kim DH, Lee SE, et al. Skin rejuvenation by microneedle fractional radiofrequency and a human stem cell conditioned medium in Asian skin: A randomized controlled investigator blinded split-face study. *J Cosmet Laser Ther* 2013;15:25–33.
34. Lee HJ, Lee EG, Kang S, et al. Efficacy of microneedling plus human stem cell conditioned medium for skin rejuvenation: A randomized, controlled, blinded split-face study. *Ann Dermatol* 2014;26(5):584–591.
35. Liang X, Li J, Yan Y, et al. Efficacy of microneedling combined with local application of human umbilical cord-derived mesenchymal stem cells conditioned media in skin brightness and rejuvenation: A randomized controlled split-face study. *Front Med (Lausanne)* 2022 May 24;9:837332. doi: 10.3389/fmed.2022.837332.
36. Ehrlich M, Rao J, Pabby A, Goldman MP. Improvement in the appearance of wrinkles with topical transforming growth factor beta(1) and l-ascorbic acid. *Dermatol Surg* 2006 May;32(5):618–625. doi: 10.1111/j.1524-4725.2006.32132.x. PMID: 16706755.
37. Draelos ZD. The effect of a combination of recombinant EGF cosmetic serum and a crosslinked hyaluronic acid serum as compared to a fibroblast-conditioned media serum on the appearance of aging skin. *J Drugs Dermatol* 2016;15(6):738–741.
38. Quinlan DJ, Ghanem AM, Hassan H. Topical growth factors and home-based microneedling for facial skin rejuvenation. *J Cosmet Dermatol* 2022 August;21(8):3469–3478. doi: 10.1111/jocd.14650. Epub 2021 December 23. PMID: 34951101.

5

Stem Cell-Derived Cosmetics and Their Use in Clinical Practice

Mary D. Lupo, Aleksandra J. Poole, and Skylar A. Souyoul

Introduction

Stem cells remain the Holy Grail of regenerative medicine, due to their limitless ability to divide and proliferate in order to regenerate or repair any organ. What distinguishes stem cells from any other cell type is their ability to self-renew and, under certain physiologic or experimental conditions, to give rise to any specific cell type. The use of stem cells is one of the most rapidly developing fields of regenerative medicine and already several stem cell-based therapies have been approved by the FDA for the treatment of various diseases and medical conditions. In recent years, multiple publications demonstrated exciting possibilities for stem cell-derived products to target skin renewal and regeneration. Skin regeneration and rejuvenation have become a major focus in the dermatological field as an aging population, which has been overexposed to the sun, seeks non-invasive treatment and topical products to improve wrinkles and the appearance of photoaged skin (1).

Types of Stem Cells and Their Source

Stem cells differ based on their origin and they can be found in embryos and adult organisms. Two main stem cell types in humans are embryonic stem cells (hESCs) and adult stem cells (or somatic stem cells). hESCs are isolated from preimplantation-stage embryos and have the greatest capacity of becoming any cell type under the right conditions. Because embryonic stem cells can proliferate without limit and may contribute to any cell type, hESCs offer an unprecedented supply of human cells for transplantation or in basic research seeking to test and improve the safety and efficacy of human drugs. Since these cells have the potential to form so many different cell types, they are also called pluripotent ("pluri" = many, "potent" = potential) stem cells. The potency of cells decreases during development: The highest level of potency is found in zygotes (totipotent) and embryonic stem cells (pluripotent), then hematopoietic stem cells (multipotent), myeloid stem cells (oligopotent), and highly specialized cells of specific tissues (unipotent) (Zakrzewski). However, the discovery of induced pluripotent stem cells (iPSCs) by Shinya Yamanaka changed the way we think about cell potency hierarchy. In the past several years, iPSCs have gained popularity since they are produced in the lab by reprogramming adult cells to express characteristics of young stem cells.

Adult or somatic or tissue-specific stem cells are specialized cells found in tissues of adults, children, and fetuses. These cells are committed to becoming a cell from their tissue of origin. Unlike embryonic stem cells, researchers have not been able to grow adult stem cells indefinitely in the lab.

Skin stem cells are of special interest because they are easily targeted by topical products. These cells are found near hair follicles, sweat glands, and in the basal layer of the epidermis and lie dormant until they receive appropriate signals to start the regeneration process. Skin stem cells are also found in the dermis, but these cells are less likely to be activated by topical products.

Similar to humans, organisms of the plant kingdom also have stem cells. Groups of non-differentiated plant stem cells, called a callus, form after mechanical damage to a plant's surface (2). This callus

DOI: 10.1201/9781315165905-5

maintains the potential to produce growth in culture or regenerate an adult plant, provided the appropriate nutrients or hormonal stimulation, respectively (2). In topical products, plant-derived stem cell extracts are now being used for their potential to improve fine lines.

Stem Cells in Skin Care Products

The use of stem cells has recently become popular in the skin care world, whether those stem cells are derived from plants, animals, or humans. It is necessary to clarify that most stem cell-derived topical products do not contain stem cells, but rather stem cell extracts such as growth factors, cytokines, and proteins, that can lead to renewal, regeneration, and repair of the skin. Growth factors and cytokines are proteins that can mediate signaling pathways both between the cells in the tissue and within the cells themselves. Growth factors have been used both in topically applied cosmetic products and in injected autologous platelet-rich plasma (PRP). It is of importance to understand how these growth factors work at the cellular level and how they can counteract physiological skin aging. PRP is separated from the subjects' own blood and although it does not involve actual stem cells, it contains a cytokines-rich fraction that can induce the regeneration of skin or hair follicles by inducing cell proliferation and extracellular matrix synthesis. Since PRP is from an autologous source, it is tolerated well but large controlled clinical trials are still lacking to demonstrate its clinical efficacy.

Daily exposure to environmental stressors, including ultraviolet (UV) light and pollution, increases oxidative stress and leads to a decline in the restorative properties of skin. These extrinsic factors amplify the skin's intrinsic, age-related decline in antioxidant capacity coupled with increased production of ROS from oxidative metabolism in cells of the skin (3). Together, extrinsic and intrinsic aging of the skin results in collagen and elastin breakdown, loss of elasticity, and overall skin atrophy.

The use of stem cell-derived growth factors was based on the premise that the extrinsic aging process of skin is like that of wound healing (4, 5). For instance, the role of epidermal growth factor (EGF) has been extensively investigated in normal and pathological wound healing. It is implicated in keratinocyte migration, fibroblast function, and the formation of granulation tissue. Since the discovery of EGF, growth factor therapy has progressed into clinical practice for the treatment of acute and chronic wounds (6). Besides EGF, additional topical and injectable growth factors have emerged as therapeutic candidates that can be harnessed for cosmetic and medical purposes.

In the skin, GFs are synthesized by fibroblasts, keratinocytes, platelets, lymphocytes, and mast cells and they mediate inter- and intracellular signaling pathways that control cell growth, proliferation, and differentiation. The role of growth factors in skin varies as depicted in Table 5.1. Just like endogenous GFs, topical and injectable GFs have the same potential to modulate complex cellular communications.

Once topical GFs successfully penetrate the stratum corneum, they can bind to specific receptors on keratinocytes and initiate a signaling cascade. After GF-receptor binding, GFs secreted by the keratinocytes can stimulate fibroblasts to synthesize GFs that stimulate the effects in the dermis. However, the penetration of GFs through the stratum corneum is typically difficult to achieve for proteins that have a molecular weight greater than 500 Da (7). GFs are large, hydrophilic molecules with a molecular weight over 15,000 Da. Therefore, it is unlikely that they could penetrate intact epidermis in sufficient quantities to produce clinically significant effects. One route by which topical GFs could reach epidermal keratinocyte receptors is via hair follicles and sweat glands or by using vehicle molecules that can capture the GFs and transport them into the skin. Another consideration is that the barrier function of aging skin is somewhat compromised, and this may permit better penetration. Once GFs have traversed the stratum corneum, their interaction with specific receptors on keratinocytes can initiate a cytokine signaling cascade that affects fibroblasts, resulting in induction of collagen production (8).

One proprietary product contains human stem cells that were cultivated in balanced conditions and differentiated into skin lineage precursors and shown to secrete large amounts of fetuin, a glycoprotein only secreted in large quantity by young cells, as well as multiple growth factors beneficial for human skin development and maintenance (9). These cell secretions were incorporated in two simple cosmetic formulations (serum and lotion) and investigated in an IRB-approved 12-week human trial that included

TABLE 5.1

Roles of Growth Factors and Cytokines in the Skin

Growth Factor, Cytokine, Protein	Role in Skin Biology
Bone morphogenetic protein 5 (BMP-5)	Regulates number and size of keratinocytes
Collagen, type I	Part of skin ECM
Epidermal growth factor (EGF)	Most potent mitogen of fibroblasts and keratinocytes
Fibroblast growth factor (FGF)	Induces proliferation of fibroblasts and keratinocytes. Induces collagen synthesis in dermis
Fibronectin	Part of skin ECM
Granulocyte-macrophage colony-stimulating factor (GM-CSF)	Secreted by keratinocytes shortly after injury to induce wound healing Cytokine for fibroblasts in skin
Growth differentiation factor 15 (GDF-15)	Regulation of keratinocyte differentiation
Growth hormone (GH)	Induces growth of keratinocytes and fibroblast Induces wound healing
Hepatocyte growth factor (HGF)	Involved in tissue regeneration and wound healing
Heparin-binding epidermal growth factor	Mitogen for fibroblasts and keratinocytes
Insulin-like growth factor and binding proteins 1 and 2 (IGF, IGF-BP1, IGF-BP1)	Mitogen for fibroblasts and endothelial cells
Keratinocyte growth factor (KGF)	Stimulates re-epithelization and hair growth
Placenta growth factor (PGF)	Mitogen for fibroblasts and promotes growth of endothelial cells
Platelet-derived growth factor-AA, and receptors (PDGF-AA)	Induces fibroblast migration and matrix production
Transforming growth factor-β1, -β2 (TGF-β1, TGF-β2)	Induces keratinocyte, fibroblast, macrophage migration Regulates angiogenesis Initiates collagen and fibronectin synthesis
Vascular endothelial growth factor (VEGF)	Mediates angiogenesis
IL-1α and IL-1β	Activates growth expression in macrophages, keratinocytes and fibroblasts
IL-6	Regulates wound-healing process
IL-10	Anti-inflammatory
Tumor necrosis factor-α (TNF-α)	Activates growth expression in macrophages, keratinocytes and fibroblasts
Interferon-γ	Anti-inflammatory

Source: From 9, with permission.

25 subjects in each group (Figure 5.1). Subjects were examined at 2, 4, 8, and 12 weeks by a dermatologist to evaluate safety, trans-epidermal water loss, wrinkles, firmness, radiance, texture, softness, and overall appearance. A sub-group of subjects from each group consented for biopsies for histological analyses. The clinical investigation demonstrated significant amelioration of the clinical signs of intrinsic and extrinsic skin aging, findings that were confirmed by significant changes in skin morphology, filaggrin, aquaporin 3, and collagen I content (9).

In another clinical study, a GF-containing serum was applied to the facial skin of 14 patients twice a day for 60 days. Patients were evaluated by a 9-point scale for clinical signs of photodamage, optical profilometry, and histopathologic evaluation of a punch biopsy from treated skin. Approximately 78.6% of patients with photodamaged skin showed clinical improvement at 60 days (1). Using the same GF mixture, another randomized, vehicle-controlled, double-blind study was performed in 60 patients (mean age 55 years). Improvements were seen in preauricular fine rhytids, skin tone and texture, and hyperpigmentation ($p = 0.012$ at three months) (7).

Fetal skin tissue-derived growth factors in processed skin cell proteins (PSP) were investigated for six months, in a study of 12 subjects who applied the cream twice daily. Results were assessed by standardized photography and clinical evaluation of treated skin using a 5-point visual wrinkle scale. After

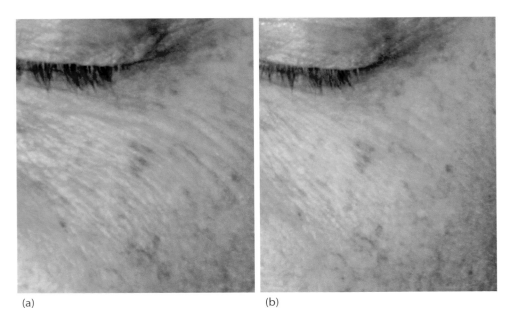

(a)   (b)

FIGURE 5.1 Twice-daily application of Aivita's proprietary human skin stem cell progenitor-derived growth factor formulation over 12 weeks demonstrated significant amelioration of the clinical signs of extrinsic skin aging. (a) Subject 44, baseline; (b) subject 44, 12-week post-treatment.
(Lead investigator, Hans S. Keirstead; by courtesy of Aivita Biomedical, Inc.)

treatment, the mean clinical improvements in the appearance of periorbital and perioral wrinkles were 33% and 25%, respectively (10).

A double-blind study on a natural ingredient extracted from the eggs of snails included 25 patients that received serum on the one side of the face and placebo cream on the other. This product's mechanism of action is the activation of innate stem cells located in the hair follicle bulge (11). Patient and physician assessments were performed at baseline and at 8, 12, and 14 weeks (Figure 5.2). At 12 weeks, there was a significant improvement in coarse periocular rhytides on the side treated with the GF active (12).

A preparation containing the extract from the Uttwiler Spätlauber apple tree's stem cells is of particular interest. Apples from this variety were cultivated in the 18th century as they produced apples with a longer shelf life than other apple varieties (13). Plant stem cells from the Uttwiler Spätlauber were tested on cell viability of umbilical cord stem cells; at a concentration of 0.1%, the extract increased cell proliferation by 80% (13). In another experiment, the Uttwiler Spätlauber stem cells improved the viability of

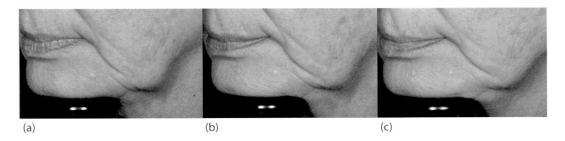

(a)   (b)   (c)

FIGURE 5.2 Twice-daily application of Tensage Stem Cell and Tensage Stem Cell Eye Cream, along with a gentle cleanser and sunscreen in a single center evaluation of the ability of Tensage® with stem cells to improve the visible signs of aging. (a) Baseline; (b) 8 weeks; (c) 12 weeks.
(Lead investigator, Zoe Diana Draelos; by courtesy of Biopelle, Inc.)

the umbilical cord stem cells after exposure to UV irradiation (13). ISDIN Laboratories has developed a product containing apple stem cells in addition to urea, creatine, and palmitoyl tripeptide-38. The product was studied in the crow's feet area of 32 women. After 28 days of using the product twice a day, the study participants had an average of 27% increase in dermal density and 68% of them had a visible improvement in wrinkles (14).

Role of Exosomes in Skin Biology

Exosomes, previously considered to be a way for cells to expel waste, are now becoming an attractive approach to skin care. These nanosized membrane vesicles are loaded with cytokines, growth factors, nucleic acid, and lipids and are involved in many biological activities of skin cells. Despite the challenges in isolating bioactive exosomes, few recent studies have shown the efficacy of exosomes in aging, atopic dermatitis, and wound healing. Once isolated, exosomes are highly stable, non-immunogenic, and able to induce multiple therapeutic effects, such as angiogenesis, collagen synthesis, and reduction of inflammation. The exosomes can be derived from multiple cell sources, and they can regulate various effector cells. So far, the exosomes from mesenchymal stem cells (MSCs), keratinocytes, endothelial cells, immune cells, and bodily fluids were found to have wound-healing abilities through different mechanisms (15).

One study showed that human keratinocytes can release exosomes that play an important role in the regulation of pigmentation in melanocytes and these exosomes can modulate the amount of pigment by changing melanocytes' gene expressions (16). In another study, exosomes derived from macrophages were able to inhibit inflammation and accelerate diabetic wound healing (17).

Zhao et al. published the role of human umbilical cord-derived MSC exosomes in treating the cutaneous wound in vivo by enhancing epidermal re-epithelialization and dermal angiogenesis (18). Exosomes can also aid in the engraftment and survival of skin flaps used in aesthetics by promoting angiogenesis and vascularization (19). Exosomes derived from human dermal fibroblasts or pluripotent cells (iPS and hES cells) have all inhibited photoaging and underlying inflammation and induce collagen biosynthesis in several studies (20–22).

Conclusion

Topical and injectable growth factors and cytokines have the potential to address skin aging through stimulation of skin stem cell regeneration, as demonstrated by several studies in which topically applied factors stimulated collagenases and epidermal thickening. The use of injectable GFs in PRP is on the rise and reports on their efficacy, while promising are limited. In addition, since this is a review of cosmeceutical growth factors, PRP is out of the scope of this cosmeceutical discussion. All data generated so far supports that the use of GFs is not only safe but efficacious as well. However, the bioavailability of GFs, their preservation in the formulation, and their delivery system may present a challenge to manufacturers. Recently, exosomes become attractive in dermatology and for cutaneous medical aesthetics, due to their paracrine mediator roles in multiple physiological and pathological processes of the skin. However, there are still some limitations of exosomes in clinical skin applications and those are mainly related to isolation techniques, purity, yield, and characterization. In human studies, immunogenicity, dose, route of administration, and long-term side effects are yet to be determined.

REFERENCES

1. Fitzpatrick RE, Rostan EF. Reversal of photodamage with topical growth factors: a pilot study. J Cosmet Laser Ther. 2003; 5: 25–34.
2. Moruś M, Baran M, Rost-Roszkowska M, Skotnicka-Graca U. Plant stem cells as innovation in cosmetics. Acta Pol Pharm. 2014; 71: 701–7.
3. Martin P. Wound healing—aiming for perfect skin regeneration. Science. 1997; 276: 75–81.

4. Sundaram H, Mehta RC, Norine JA, Kircik L, Cook-Bolden FE, Atkins DH, et al. Role of physiologi-cally balanced growth factors in skin rejuvenation. J Drugs Dermatol. 2009; 8(Suppl 5): 4–13.

5. Watson RE, Griffiths CE. Pathogenic aspects of cutaneous photoaging. J Cosmet Dermatol. 2005; 4: 230–6.

6. Hardwicke J, Schmaljohann D, Boyce DE, Thomas DW. Epidermal growth factor therapy and wound healing–past, present and future perspectives. Surgeon. 2008; 6: 172–7.

7. Mehta RC, Fitzpatrick RE. Endogenous growth factors as cosmeceuticals. Dermatol Ther. 2007; 20: 350–9.

8. Fabi S, Sundaram H. The potential of topical and injectable growth factors and cytokines for skin reju-venation. Facial Plast Surg. 2014; 30: 157–71.

9. Nistor G, Poole AJ, Draelos Z, Lupo MP, Tzikas M, et al. Human stem cell-derived skin progenitors produce alpha 2-HS glycoprotein (fetuin): a revolutionary cosmetic ingredient. J Drugs Dermatol. 2016; 15: 583–98.

10. Hussain M, Phelps R, Goldberg DJ. Clinical, histologic, and ultrastructural changes after use of human growth factor and cytokine skin cream for the treatment of skin rejuvenation. J Cos and Laser Ther. 2008; 10: 104–9.

11. Sundaram H. The mechanism and potential impact of stem cell activation in skin rejuvenation: an evidence-based analysis. J Drugs Dermatol. 2017; 16(4): 378–84.

12. Fabi SG, Cohen JL, Peterson JD, Kiripolsky MG, Goldman MP. The effects of filtrate of the secretion of the *Cryptomphalus aspersa* on photoaged skin. J Drugs Dermatol. 2013; 12: 453–7.

13. Schmid D, Schürch C, Blum P, Belser E, Zülli F. Plant stem cell extract for longevity of skin and hair. SOFW J. 2008; 134: 30–5.

14. Sans MT, Campos C, Milani M, Foyaca M, Lamy A, et al. Biorevitalizing effect of a novel serum containing apple stem cell extract, pro-collagen lipopeptide, creatine, and urea on sign aging signs. J Cosmet Dermatol. 2016 March; 15(1): 24–30.

15. Xiong M, Zhnag Q, Hu W, Zhao C, Lv W, et al. The novel mechanisms and applications of exosomes in dermatology and cutaneous medical aesthetics. Pharmacol Res. 2021 April; 166: 105490.

16. Cicero A, Delevoye C, Gilles-Marsens F, et al. Exosomes released by keratinocytes modulate pigmenta-tion. Nat Commun. 2015; 6: 7506.

17. Li M, Wang T, Tian H, Wei G, et al. Macrophage-derived exosomes accelerate wound healing through their anti-inflammatory effects in a diabetic rat model. Artif Cells Nanomed Biotechnol. 2019; 47(1): 37933803.

18. Zhao G, Liu Z, Liu K, Zuo B, Wang Y, et al. MSC-derived exosomes attenuate cell death through sup-pressing AIF nucleus translocation and enhance cutaneous wound healing. Stem Cell Res Ther. 2020; 11: 174.

19. Xie L, Wang Y, Zhnag H, Chen D, Lin J, et al. The effects of local injection of exosomes derived from BMSC's on random skin flap in rats. Am J Transl Res. 2019; 11: 7063–73.

20. Hu S, Li J, Cores K, Huang T, Su P-U, et al. Needle-free injection of exosomes derived from human dermal fibroblast spheroid ameliorates skin photoaging. ACS Nano. 2019; 13: 11273–82.

21. Oh J, Lee Y, Kim W, et al. Exosomes derived from human induced pluripotent stem cells ameliorate the aging of skin fibroblasts. Int J Mol Sci. 2018; 19: Article 1715.

22. Bae Y-U, Son C-H, Kim KS, Kim SH, et al. Embryonic stem cell derived mmu-miR-291a-3p inhibits cellular senescence in human dermal fibroblasts through the TGF-B receptor 2 pathway. J Gerontol Ser A. 2019; 74: 1359–67.

6

Matrix Metalloproteinases

Macrene Alexiades

Introduction

Matrix metalloproteinases (MMPs) are zinc-containing endopeptidases, enzymes that break peptide bonds other than terminal ones in a peptide chain. Ultraviolet (UV) radiation is known to induce MMPs in human skin. MMPs degrade extracellular matrix (ECM) proteins, including collagen, fibronectin, elastin, and proteoglycans. Such degradation is a major contributing factor in the manifestations of photoaging. MMPs are also important factors in carcinogenesis, playing a role in tumor progression, angiogenesis, and metastasis. In humans, there are 23 MMPs; they are regulated by activation of precursor zymogens and inhibition by tissue inhibitors of metalloproteinases (TIMPs).

MMP Structure

MMPs share a common structure consisting of a pro-peptide, catalytic, and hemopexin-like C-terminal domain (Figure 6.1). They are first synthesized as inactive zymogens and the pro-peptide domain is removed to activate the enzyme. A conserved cysteine residue that interacts with zinc in the active site prevents activity. The catalytic domain contains an enzymatically important zinc ion, thus a zinc-binding motif. The C-terminal domain is structurally similar to hemopexin, a serum protein. This domain determines substrate specificity and is the target site of TIMPs.

MMP Classification

A number of classification systems exist for the MMPs, the most common being a numbering system with named groupings. The common named groups include the collagenases, gelatinases, stromyelysins, matrilysins, and membrane-type MMPs, including transmembrane type and GPI-anchored and others (Table 6.1). The human collagenases, MMP-1, -8, and -13, cleave interstitial collagens I–III. MMP-1 also activates protease-activated receptor (PAR) 1, which promotes growth and invasion of breast carcinoma cells (Nagase et al. 2006). Gelatinases (MMP-2 and 9) digest gelatin, types IV, V, and XI collagens, laminin, and aggrecan core protein. Matrilysins (MMP-7 and -26) process cell surface molecules such as pro-α-defensin, Fas-ligand, pro-tumor necrosis factor α, and E-cadherin (Nagase et al. 2006). Stromelysins (MMP-3, MMP-10, and MMP-11). MMP-3 and -10 digest a number of ECM molecules and participate in pro-MMP activation. MMP-11 evinces a weak activity toward ECM molecules but cleaves serpins (Nagase et al. 2006).

Role of MMPs in Skin Aging

UV light exposure in skin upregulates MMP expression. Cumulative exposure results in continuous ECM degradation. Degradation of collagen is normally regulated by MMPs and by the activity of their

DOI: 10.1201/9781315165905-6

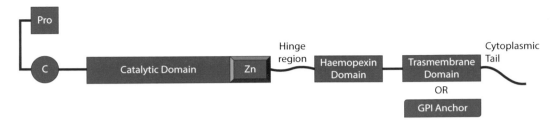

FIGURE 6.1   Common structure of MMPs. MMPs share a common structure consisting of a pro-peptide, catalytic, and hemopexin-like C-terminal domain.
(By courtesy of Macrene Alexiades, MD, PhD.)

TABLE 6.1

Matrix Metalloproteinases (MMPs)

Group	Classification Number	Name	Substrate
Interstitial Collagenases	MMP-1	Fibroblast	Collagen I, fibronectin
	MMP-8	Neutrophil	Fibrillar collagen
	MMP-13	Collagenase-3	Collagen I
Gelatinases	MMP-2	Gelatinase A	Collagen I, IV, V, gelatin, chondroitin sulfate proteoglycan, fibronectin
	MMP-9	Gelatinase B	Collagen IV, V, gelatin
Stromelysins	MMP-3	Stromelysin-1	Laminin, fibronectin, non-helical collagen, basement membrane, E-cadherin, plasminogen
	MMP-7	Matrilysin	Fibronectin, laminin, non-helical collagen
	MMP-10	Stromelysin-2	Laminin, fibronectin, non-helical collagen
	MMP-11	Stromelysin-3	Collagen IV, Gelatin, Laminin
MT-MMPs	MMP-14	MT1-MMP	Collagen I, II, III, gelatin
	MMP-15	MT2-MMP	MMP-2, gelatin
	MMP-16	MT3-MMP	MMP-2
	MMP-17	MT4-MMP	Unknown
Elastase	MMP-12	Metalloelastase	Elastin, fibronectin

natural inhibitors, TIMPs. Increased MMP activity is an important factor influencing the development of age-related changes in skin.

Cutaneous findings of photoaging have been defined and categorized by the author with a validated scale. These categories include rhytids, laxity, dyspigmentation, erythema-telangiectasia, solar elastosis, poor texture, and keratoses (Alexiades et al. 2008). In skin aging, MMPs play a prominent role in transforming the cutaneous structure. A clinical example of solar elastosis, characterized by yellow-white pebbly papules which correlate histologically with degraded elastotic material in the dermis, is shown in Figure 6.2.

Mechanism of UV Induction of MMPs

Within the cell, UV-induced reactive oxygen species (ROS) activate mitogen-activated protein kinases (MAPKs) and nuclear factor-kappa B (NF-κB), culminating in the transcriptional regulation of MMPs (Pittayapruek et al. 2016). This eventuates into the degradation of collagen and elastin, leading to photoaging. Moreover, AP-1 inhibits transforming growth factor beta (TGF-β) signaling, causing a reduction in procollagen synthesis.

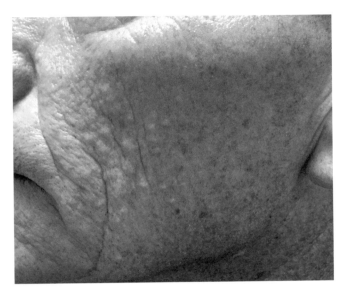

FIGURE 6.2   Solar elastosis. A clinical example of solar elastosis, characterized by yellow-white pebbly papules which correlate histologically with degraded elastotic material in the dermis, is shown. It is due to the degradative effects of UV exposure and MMP activity, particularly MMP-12.

Cutaneous Changes Mediated by MMPs

Histological and ultrastructural features of photoaging include epidermal hyperplasia, damaged and disorganized collagen fibrils, and abnormal elastic material in papillary dermis (Chiang et al. 2013; Parkinson et al. 2015). An imbalance between ECM accumulation and degradation results in a breakdown of the structural and functional support to the skin. Accumulated photo-exposure results in ongoing degradation of ECM proteins, including collagen and elastin, and a decreased rate of neocollagenesis (Chiang et al. 2013; Parkinson et al. 2015).

Collagen Degradation

Epidermal keratinocytes and dermal fibroblasts secrete MMP-1 (collagenase 1), which digests fibrillar collagen types I and III into fragments further hydrolyzed by gelatinases. The functions of the collagens are thus compromised in the dermis (Pittayapruek et al. 2016). Concurrent with induction of MMP-1 synthesis by dermal fibroblasts, UV light also induces intracellular ROS such as singlet oxygen ($^{1}O_2$), superoxide anion (O_2^{-}), hydrogen peroxide (H_2O_2), and hydroxyl radicals (OH) (Chiang et al. 2013). ROS subsequently activates the MAPK family, proline-directed Ser/Thr kinases comprising extracellular signal-regulated kinases (ERKs), p38, and c-Jun NH2-terminal kinase (JNK). ERK stimulates the c-Fos expression; p38 and JNK result in c-Jun expression. c-Jun and c-Fos form transcription factor AP-1, which transcriptionally regulates MMP-1, -3, and -9, ultimately resulting in the degradation of collagen (Pittayapruek et al. 2016). AP-1 inhibits TGF-β signaling, thereby decreasing its stimulation of procollagen type I (Chen et al. 2015).

AP-1 activation upregulates the expression of MMP-1, -3, and -9. MMP-3 (stromelysin-1) degrades types IV, V, IX, and X collagens, gelatin, fibrillin-1, fibronectin, laminin, and proteoglycans. MMP-3 activates pro-MMPs such as collagenases, gelatinase B, and matrilysins during ECM turnover. MMP-10 (stromelysin-2) cleaves several ECM proteins and also activates pro-MMPs (Pittayapruek et al. 2016). UV irradiation also induces NF-κB, which is reported to induce the MMP expression in dermal fibroblasts (Lee et al. 2012).

MMP-9 (gelatinase B or 92-kDa type IV collagenase) is produced by human keratinocytes and degrades collagen type IV, a basement membrane component critical in epidermal-dermal adhesion and regulating epidermal differentiation (Onoue et al. 2003; Sbardella et al. 2012). MMP-2 (gelatinase A or 72-kDa type IV collagenase) also digests collagen type IV. Both gelatinases can also degrade collagen types V, VII, and X, fibronectin, and elastin. Importantly, after fibrillar collagens are initially degraded by collagenases, the gelatinases degrade the fibrillar collagen fragments (Pittayapruek et al. 2016). Collagenases, including MMP-1 (interstitial collagenase), MMP-8 (neutrophil collagenase), and MMP-13 (collagenase 3), are attributed with the ability to digest collagen without first unwinding the triple helix (Sbardella et al. 2012).

Thus, MMP-1 is critical in a photoaging process, as compared to MMP-8 and -13 which play a small role in collagen degeneration in skin.

Elastin Degradation

MMPs not only degrade cutaneous collagens but also impact the quality and levels of elastin during photoaging. Elastin is a major dermal component which confers the properties of recoil and resilience to the skin. While elastin comprises only 2–4% of the total protein content of skin, its degradation contributes significantly to facets of skin aging such as laxity and solar elastosis.

MMP-12 (macrophage metalloelastase) has the most potent negative impact on elastin. Following UV exposure, macrophages and fibroblasts secrete MMP-12, which results in the accumulation of elastotic material in the upper dermis of photodamaged skin (Fortino et al. 2007).

Solar elastosis is the result of damaged elastotic material accumulating in the papillary dermis as a result of UV irradiation and MMP-12 activity (Tewari et al. 2014; Figure 6.2). MMP-12 degrades other ECM substances, including collagen type IV fragments, fibronectin, fibrillin-1, laminin, entactin, vitronectin, heparin, and chondroitin sulfates. It also activates other pro-MMPs, including pro-MMP-1, -2, -3, and -9. Another MMP that targets elastin is MMP-7 (matrilysin). UV-induced MMP-7 also degrades collagen type IV, entactin, fibronectin, laminin, and cartilage proteoglycan aggregates (Sbardella et al. 2012).

Neutral endopeptidase (NEP, neprilysin), a 94-kDa membrane-bound metalloprotease, is reported to be identical to fibroblast-derived elastase (Morisaki et al. 2010). Dermal fibroblast NEP activity is an important mediator in the UV-induced rhytids and laxity. It is responsible for the degradation of the structure of elastic fibers and the subsequent loss of skin elasticity and resilience (Imokawa et al. 2015).

UV irradiation activates keratinocytes to secrete interleukin-1 alpha (IL-1α), which in turn induces a granulocyte macrophage colony stimulatory factor (GM-CSF) expression. IL-1α and GM-CSF are secreted into the dermis, consequently stimulating fibroblast upregulation of NEP. NEP then degrades elastic fibers resulting in impairment of skin elasticity and increased skin laxity (Imokawa et al. 2015).

MMP Inhibitors

MMP inhibition is an important target for the treatment of rhytids, laxity, and photoaging, but finding effective inhibitors has been challenging (Laronha et al. 2020). Plant-derived active ingredients have been shown to decrease MMP activity. These include resveratrol, Butcher's broom rhizome (*Ruscus aculeatus*), *Galla chinensis*, *Neonauclea reticulata*, white and green tea, which have all been reported to inhibit MMPs in normal human dermal fibroblasts. *Neonauclea* significantly decreases the expression of MMP-1, -3, and -9 by suppressing ERK, p38, and JNK phosphorylation. *Ixora parviflora* and *Coffea arabica* inhibit the expression of MMP-1, -3, and -9 and MAPK activity.

Conclusion

The upregulation of MMPs due to photo-exposure plays an essential role in the degradation of collagen and elastin, leading to rhytids, laxity, and photoaging. Targeted inhibition of MMPs provides a therapeutic opportunity for the treatment of the findings of skin aging.

REFERENCES

Alexiades MR, Dover J, Arndt K. The spectrum of laser skin resurfacing: Nonablative, fractional, and ablative laser resurfacing. J Am Acad Dermatol. 2008;58(5):719–737.

Chen B, Li R, Yan N, Chen G, Qian W, Jiang HL, Ji C, Bi ZG. Astragaloside IV controls collagen reduction in photoaging skin by improving transforming growth factor-β/Smad signaling suppression and inhibiting matrix metalloproteinase-1. Mol Med Rep. 2015;11:3344–3348.

Chiang HM, Chen HC, Chiu HH, Chen CW, Wang SM, Wen KC. Neonauclea reticulata (Havil.) merr stimulates skin regeneration after UVB exposure via ROS scavenging and modulation of the MAPK/MMPs/collagen pathway. Evid Based Complement Altern Med. 2013;2013:1–9. doi: 10.1155/2013/324864.

Fortino V, Maioli E, Torricelli C, Davis P, Valacchi G. Cutaneous MMPs are differently modulated by environmental stressors in old and young mice. Toxicol Lett. 2007;173:73–79. doi: 10.1016/j.toxlet.2007.06.004.

Imokawa G, Nakajima H, Ishida K. Biological mechanisms underlying the ultraviolet light-induced formation of skin wrinkling and sagging II: Over-expression of Neprilysin/Neutral endopeptidase via epithelial-mesenchymal interaction plays an essential role in wrinkling and sagging. Int J Mol Sci. 2015;16:1–25. doi: 10.3390/ijms16047776.

Laronha H, Carpinteiro I, Portugal J, et al. Challenges in matrix metalloproteinases inhibition. Biomolecules. 2020;10(5):717. doi:10.3390/biom10050717. Published May 5, 2020

Lee YR, Noh EM, Han JH, et al. Brazilin inhibits UVB-induced MMP-1/3 expressions and secretions by suppressing the NF-κB pathway in human dermal fibroblasts. Eur J Pharmacol. 2012;674:80–86. doi: 10.1016/j.ejphar.2011.10.016.

Morisaki N, Moriwaki S, Sugiyama-Nakagiri Y, Haketa K, Takema Y, Imokawa G. Neprilysin is identical to skin fibroblast elastase. J Biol Chem. 2010;285:39819–39827. doi: 10.1074/jbc.M110.161547.

Nagase H, Visse R, Murphy G. Structure and function of matrix metalloproteinases and TIMPs. Cardiovasc Res. February 2006;69(3):562–573. doi: 10.1016/j.cardiores.2005.12.002. https://academic.oup.com/cardiovascres/article/69/3/562/272258

Onoue S, Kobayashi T, Takemoto Y, Sasaki I, Shinkai H. Induction of matrix metalloproteinase-9 secretion from human keratinocytes in culture by ultraviolet-B irradiation. J Dermatol Sci. 2003;33:105–111. doi: 10.1016/j.jdermsci.2003.08.002.

Parkinson LG, Toro A, Zhao H, Brown K, Tebbutt SJ, Granville DJ. Granzyme B mediates both direct and indirect cleavage of extracellular matrix in skin after chronic low-dose ultraviolet light irradiation. Aging Cell. 2015;14:67–77. doi: 10.1111/acel.12298.

Pittayapruek P, Meephansan J, Prapapan O, Komine M, Ohtsuki M. Role of matrix metalloproteinases in photoaging and photocarcinogenesis. Int J Mol Sci. 2016;17(6):868. doi: 10.3390/ijms17060868. Published 2016 June 2

Sbardella D, Fasciglione GF, Gioia M, et al. Human matrix metalloproteinases: An ubiquitarian class of enzymes involved in several pathological processes. Mol Asp Med. 2012;33:119–208. doi: 10.1016/j.mam.2011.10.015.

Tewari A, Grys K, Kollet J, Sarkany R, Young AR. Upregulation of MMP12 and its activity by UVA1 in human skin: Potential implications for photoaging. J Invest Dermatol. 2014;134:2598–2609. doi: 10.1038/jid.2014.173.

7

Retinoids

Briana Paiewonsky, Ora Raymond, Sarah Stierman, and Ronda Farah

Introduction

Vitamin A, in its various forms and derivatives, is a common additive in cosmeceutical products. Vitamin A exists in two major forms: retinol and carotenoids (1; see Figure 7.1). Retinol, also known as preformed vitamin A, is commonly found in nature in animal products (2), while carotenoids, referred to as provitamin A, are more frequently found in plant products. Carotenoids can be converted into the more active form, retinols, via oxidation reactions within the body (3).

Retinols can also undergo various conversion reactions resulting in natural derivatives with varying degrees of biological activities, including retinoic acid (tretinoin), retinol, retinaldehyde (retinal), retinyl esters (such as retinyl palmitate and retinyl acetate), and oxoretinoids (Figure 7.2) (3). Synthetic retinol derivatives have also been created and include tazarotene, acitretin, etretinate, adapalene, and isotretinoin (Table 7.1). The term "retinoids" is used to describe retinol and its synthetic and natural products.

Retinoids have various treatment applications in dermatology, including treatment of acne, psoriasis, rosacea, photoaging, dermatitis, ichthyosis, and more (4). In this chapter, we will discuss the use of retinoids in cosmeceutical preparations.

History of Retinoids and the Beginning of Their Use in Cosmeceuticals

The use of retinol for medicinal purposes dates back to Ancient Egypt, when liver enzymes, which contain high quantities of vitamin A, were used topically to treat night blindness (5, 8). In the early 1900s, vitamin A in egg yolks was discovered to have an integral role in chick and mice growth and development (5, 8). Shortly after this, the importance of vitamin A for proper epithelization and gland function was discovered in the mouse model (9). Further research developed during World War I found that vitamin A deficiency resulted in xerosis and hyperkeratosis (5, 10, 11). In 1947, vitamin A was synthesized by Isler and colleagues (8, 12). The "retinoid project" was initiated in the 1960s and was aimed at developing vitamin A derivatives with clinical safety and efficacy (5, 10). Not long after, researchers found evidence for the efficacy of topical retinoids in the treatment of acne vulgaris, and FDA approval for topical tretinoin followed shortly thereafter (8, 13). As topical retinoid use became more prevalent, improved general appearance of skin was observed in older populations, leading to the investigation of topical retinoids for photoaging (14). There is a large quantity of scientific evidence supporting the use of tretinoin, among other prescription retinoids, for treatment of photoaging (Table 7.2). However, cosmeceutical preparations do not contain retinoids that are considered drugs by the FDA—we will discuss these in detail separately.

Classifying Retinoids

Four generations of retinoids exist. The first generation are natural retinoids that are not aromatic. The second generation includes the monoaromatic retinoids that contain a ring rather than a cyclic end group (15).

DOI: 10.1201/9781315165905-7

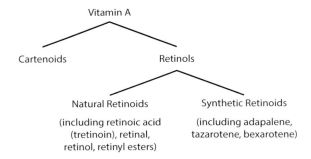

FIGURE 7.1   Forms of vitamin A.

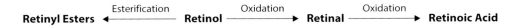

FIGURE 7.2   Conversion of retinoids (3, 5, 6).

TABLE 7.1

Classification of Select Retinoids

Natural Retinoids[a]	Synthetic Retinoids
All-trans retinol (Retinol)	Tazarotene
All-trans retinoic acid (Tretinoin)	Adapalene
13-cis-retinoic acid (Isotretinoin)	Trifarotene
9-cis-retinoic acid (Alitretinoin)	Bexarotene
Retinyl esters (Retinyl acetate and Retinyl palmitate)	
Retinaldehyde (Retinal)	

[a]   Of note, some naturally occurring retinoids now have synthetic versions available.

Source: From (7).

TABLE 7.2

Topical Retinoids Classified as Drugs

FDA Considered Drugs
Tretinoin
Alitretinoin
Tazarotene
Adapalene

The third generation are the polyaromatic retinoids that are tailored to interact with specific receptors (16). The fourth and newest generation contains a structurally unique retinoid that has recently been approved by the FDA for the treatment of acne (16–19).

Mechanism of Action

The mechanism of action of retinoids has been elucidated through studies evaluating retinoic acid, which is the most biologically active form of vitamin A (17). Topical retinoids function primarily through their role in the regulation of epithelial cells and dermal components (20). In general, active retinol metabolites function through alteration of nuclear processes, most notably of which is gene regulation.

TABLE 7.3

Classification of Synthetic Retinoids

Generation	Retinoids
First Generation	• All-trans retinol • All-trans retinoic acid • 13-cis-retinoic acid • 9-cis-retinoic acid
Second Generation	• Acitretin • Etretinate
Third Generation	• Adapalene • Tazarotene • Bexarotene
Fourth Generation	• Trifarotene

The retinoid family is composed of lipophilic molecules that are consequently able to diffuse through cellular membranes of keratinocytes into the intracellular and intranuclear compartments (7, 21). Specifically, retinoic acid enters the nucleus via cellular retinoic acid-binding proteins (CRABPs) (17). CRABP II is found to be the most predominant CRABP in the skin (22). The retinoid molecule then binds to nuclear receptors, binding and activating the family of receptors known as the retinoic acid receptors (RAR) and retinoid X receptors (RXR) (17, 23). Three isotypes exist for both RAR and RXR, including alpha, beta, and gamma (13). Though all of these isotypes are expressed in the skin, RAR-gamma and RXR-α dominate the epidermis (24). Additionally, RXR levels are significantly greater in the epidermis compared to RAR levels (24). Various retinoids selectively bind and activate different isotypes of these receptors, the details of which are further discussed below.

Once activated, the retinol metabolites and their respective receptors form homo- or heterodimers and bind to DNA response elements called retinoic acid response elements (RARE) (24). This allows for regulation of gene expression and influence on cellular differentiation, proliferation, and apoptosis (25–27), the results of which affect collagen production and degradation, epidermal hyperplasia, and keratinocyte differentiation (28–30).

It is important to note, however, that some of the topical retinoid effects may occur through a nongenomic pathway, and as such, do not require alteration of gene transcription (15, 31, 32). These pathways include ultraviolet (UV) light protection, protection from free radicals, and alterations in pigmentation (7). The mechanisms behind these nongenomic pathways have not been fully elucidated yet; however, it is thought that many signaling pathways may be involved (15). For example, it is thought that retinoids reduce signs of photoaging through blocking the activation of transcription factor AP-1, thereby inhibiting matrix metalloproteinase-mediated collagen damage (24). Of note, some of these nongenomic pathways can also influence or even amplify the gene transcription effect of retinoids, suggesting that there is interplay between these two mechanisms of action (15).

How to Use Topical Retinoids

Some formulations of retinoids, typically generic tretinoins, are not stable in light (33). Keeping this in mind, topical retinoids used for photoaging should be applied at night (33). Many dermatologists suggest the application of retinoid products 20–30 minutes after washing the face. A pea-sized amount is typically required for facial application, and patients should be counseled to avoid the delicate skin surrounding the eyes. As topical retinoids may be irritating, one clinical pearl is to recommend using these products every other night and to slowly increase use to nightly as tolerated. Irritation is most likely to occur within the first two weeks of initiating treatment but can occur off and on for months and even years (34). If irritation occurs, the patient may discontinue the retinoid or decrease frequency of use (e.g., three times weekly) until the irritation subsides (35). Other options for irritation include decreasing the strength of the retinoid or using another topical vehicle, such as an emollient cream rather than a drying

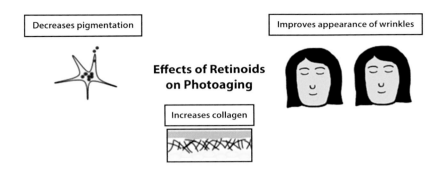

FIGURE 7.3 Effects of retinoids on photoaging.
(By courtesy of Briana Paiewonsky and Ora Raymond.)

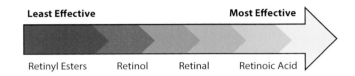

FIGURE 7.4 Efficacy of the natural retinoids.
(By courtesy of Briana Paiewonsky.)

gel. It is important to avoid significant irritation, especially in darker skin types, as this can lead to erythema, scale, hyperpigmentation, hypopigmentation, and in some rare instances, even scarring from severe irritant dermatitis (35).

To help mitigate irritation, moisturizers may be used in concert with topical retinoids, whether applied before or after. Controlled studies examining the impact of emollient use with retinoids are lacking. Regardless, it is best to use a non-comedogenic or oil-free moisturizer to avoid inducing acne. The physician should screen for other active ingredients in the patient's skin care regimen, such as benzoyl peroxide, which may oxidize or inactivate the retinoid when they are used together (33). Combining over-the-counter retinols with prescription retinoids can compound skin irritation; therefore, at-home products should be reviewed prior to writing a prescription. Additionally, retinoids have been linked with photosensitivity, further supporting the use of topical retinoids at night. Patients starting a retinoid should be counseled on the increased risk of sunburn and should be encouraged to wear sunscreen appropriately (33). See further Figures 7.3 and 7.4.

Types of Retinoids

The topical retinoids – their properties and their role in cosmetics, including use for photoaging and pigmentation – are described below.

Synthetic Retinoids

Adapalene

Adapalene is a synthetic retinoid and naphthoic derivative that is currently FDA approved for acne (36, 37). Adapalene is available by prescription and over the counter in the United States. It can be formulated into a variety of vehicles, including cream, gel, and lotion. Over the counter, it is only sold as a 0.1% gel. As a prescription, it is available up to 0.3% in any of the vehicles mentioned above (33, 34). It is a relatively stable molecule, including when it is exposed to light (17). Adapalene selectively binds to RAR-β and -γ (33). In addition to influencing cellular differentiation, this retinoid has anti-inflammatory effects (38–40).

The use of adapalene for photoaging has few studies to date. In 2003, Kang and colleagues performed a prospective, randomized, controlled, parallel-group study conducted at two centers with the investigators masked (41). The 90 participants were divided into three equal groups, including 30 in the adapalene gel 0.1% treatment group, 30 in the adapalene gel 0.3% treatment group, and 30 in the gel vehicle or control group. The face, ears, and scalp were treated for nine months. Assessment of solar lentigines before and after treatment showed a statistically significant decrease in pigmentation with both adapalene gel 0.1% and adapalene gel 0.3% when compared to the gel vehicle. Investigators conducted a global assessment of the solar lentigines, also finding significant improvement in color of the lesions treated with adapalene versus the gel vehicle. They did not find any difference between the adapalene gel 0.1% and adapalene gel 0.3% groups. General photoaging effects were assessed with global photography in 42 of the participants (41). The blinded evaluations showed significant improvement in mottled hyperpigmentation, fine rhytides, and overall facial appearance. There was no significant reduction in the appearance of coarse wrinkles. Furthermore, histological evaluation showed decreased diffuse melanin in the epidermis, increased granular epidermal layers, and decreased cellular atypia in the adapalene treatment groups. Another study from Bagatin et al. compared the efficacy of adapalene gel 0.3% and tretinoin cream 0.05% in a parallel-group comparison study with blinded investigators (42). One hundred twenty-eight participants were randomly assigned to treatment groups and treated for 24 weeks. The study found that both treatment groups showed a significant improvement in photoaging, based on the cutaneous photoaging assessment (ECPA). There was no significant difference among both treatment groups, showing that adapalene gel 0.3% and tretinoin cream 0.05% may have similar efficacy in the treatment of photoaging. Similar safety profiles between the two were also noted (42). A final open-label study evaluating adapalene gel 0.3% for photoaging included 35 Chilean females with facial photoaging (Glogau classification 2–3) (43). The study showed statistically significant improvement in rhytides in participants, determined by a scaled clinical assessment from two blinded dermatologists and by a complexion analysis system (VISIA Complexion Analysis System [Canfield Scientific Inc., Fairfield, NJ, USA]. The study also found a statistically significant improvement in skin tone with adapalene use (43). A study assessing adapalene use in 65 African patients found that it was effective in reducing the appearance of hyperpigmentation (44). Though these studies show that adapalene may have some effect on the reduction of photoaging signs and hyperpigmentation, more studies are needed.

Overall, adapalene has a low risk of irritation and has been shown to be better tolerated than tretinoin and tazarotene (45–51). Mild-to-moderate dermatitis, burning sensation, pruritus, erythema, skin dryness, skin scaling, and photosensitivity have been reported (45–47, 52). Serious allergic reactions have occurred but are extremely rare (46, 53). See also Figure 7.5.

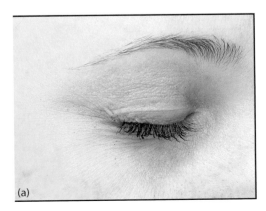 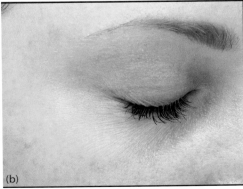

FIGURE 7.5 (a) Before and (b) after 11 months of nightly adapalene treatment. (By courtesy of Sarah Stierman, MD, FAAD.)

Tazarotene

Tazarotene is a synthetic retinoid that is currently FDA approved for acne and plaque psoriasis. It is also approved for use in the reduction of facial fine rhytides, mottled pigmentation, and benign lentigines. Similar to the previous retinoids, tazarotene can be formulated into a variety of vehicles, including cream, gel, lotion, and even a foam (54, 55). Tazarotene is not sold over the counter in the United States. It is available as a prescription in doses of 0.05% or 0.1% (33). Tazarotene is converted in the skin to tazarontenic acid. This active metabolite preferentially binds to RAR-beta and -gamma, similar to adapalene (56).

Tazarotene has been well studied for use in photoaging and hyperpigmentation. Multiple randomized, double-blind, controlled trials have shown that daily use of tazarotene cream 0.1% results in a statistically significant improvement (at least one grade via a 5- or 6-point scale) in the appearance of rhytides, mottled hyperpigmentation, irregular pigmentation, skin elasticity, skin tactual roughness, and overall clinical appearance (57–59). Results were mixed as to whether there was improvement in the appearance of pore size and lentigines, and there were no significant changes in the appearance of telangiectasias in two of the aforementioned studies (58). The studies showed improvement in some of these signs of photoaging as early as week 2 of treatment (57). Another randomized, double-blind, controlled trial evaluated tazarotene cream 0.01%, 0.025%, 0.05%, and 0.1% compared to a control vehicle and tretinoin cream 0.05% (60). This study found significant improvement in fine rhytides, mottled hyperpigmentation, and overall clinical assessment via a 6- or 7-point scale in groups treated with tazarotene cream 0.05%, and 0.1%, with 0.1% being superior. No significant differences in coarse rhytides, tactual roughness, pore size, or appearance of telangiectasia were found. Effects were seen as early as week 8 and lasted through re-evaluation 2 weeks after the 24-week treatment period ended (60). A fifth randomized, double-blind, controlled trial compared tazarotene cream 0.1% to tretinoin cream 0.05% (61). This study found that tazarotene offered superior improvements in facial fine rhytides and mottled hyperpigmentation compared to tretinoin. The tazarotene treatment group also experienced more skin irritation compared to the tretinoin group (61). Investigation into tazarotene effects on post-inflammatory pigmentation has shown that tazarotene cream 0.1% was more effective than the control vehicle in decreasing the intensity of the post-inflammatory hyperpigmentation (62).

Adverse effects of tazarotene are commonly related to skin irritation, as is common with the use of any retinoid product; however, these side effects may be more intense with tazarotene when compared with other retinoids. They include desquamation, erythema, pruritus, burning or stinging sensation, and dermatitis (57–59). Higher concentrations of tazarotene have higher risks of these local side effects (63).

Trifarotene

Trifarotene is a fourth-generation synthetic retinoid that was approved by the FDA for the treatment of acne in 2019. It was also given Orphan Drug Designation by the FDA in 2014 for the treatment of lamellar ichthyosis (64). It is only available as a prescription and in the form of a 0.05% cream as of 2021. Trifarotene is the only retinoid that selectively targets RAR-gamma, which was previously mentioned to be one of the most predominant RAR within the epidermis (64, 65). It is postulated that this receptor selectivity increases trifarotene's efficacy in dermatologic conditions; however, there are currently no studies that compare trifarotene to the other retinoids. As trifarotene is relatively new to the market, its use for photoaging and dyspigmentation is an exciting new area that should be investigated in the future.

Bexarotene

Bexarotene is a synthetic retinoid that is currently FDA approved for the treatment of cutaneous T-cell lymphoma. The topical formulation in the United States is a 0.1% gel and is only sold as a prescription. It is not considered a cosmeceutical product. Bexarotene selectively binds to the RXR isotypes (66). Investigation into the use of bexarotene for photoaging and dyspigmentation is not available.

Natural Retinoids

Retinal Esters (Retinyl Acetate, Retinyl Palmitate, Retinyl Propionate)

Retinal esters are often found in cosmeceutical products and are generally considered to be the weakest topical retinoids since they require multiple chemical reactions before conversion into biologically active molecules (5, 67–70). They are often found in combination with other active ingredients, such as hydroxy acids, since retinal esters are not very effective in treating photoaging as monotherapy (7, 71, 72). A study assessing retinyl propionate cream found no statistically significant differences in clinical or histological evaluation of photoaging after use for 48 weeks when compared to controls (73). Retinyl palmitate has been shown to increase epidermal thickness in human studies – it may have some effect on increasing fibrillin-1 and procollagen-I deposition in the skin, but studies remain inconclusive (70, 74). No clinical studies in humans have assessed the effects of these retinyl esters on pigmentation. Overall, more studies are needed to assess the efficacy and role of retinal esters in the treatment of photoaging and dyspigmentation.

Retinol

Retinol is a naturally occurring retinoid molecule that can be metabolized into retinal and then further into retinoic acid. Similar to retinal, retinol is not considered a drug in the United States and is often found in cosmeceutical products. Retinol is available in concentrations ranging from 0.075% to 1% (72). Studies have assessed its use for photoaging and shown promising results; however, it is important to note that retinol is very susceptible to degradation via light exposure.

Many mid- to late 1990s studies assessed the efficacy and tolerability of retinol. Two studies showed that topical retinol use resulted in increased epidermal thickening (75, 76). Moreover, retinol was shown to be significantly less potent than tretinoin, requiring increased concentrations to achieve comparable results (76). It is thought that the less potent nature of retinol is likely related to retinol requiring conversion into retinoic acid for biological effects (76, 77). Accordingly, topical retinol was shown to cause less irritation than topical retinoic acid (tretinoin) (76, 78). During this same time frame, a randomized, double-blind controlled clinical study was conducted assessing the effects of retinol on fine lines and rhytides (79). The trial showed that retinol 0.04% improved the appearance of these aging signs (79). Additional studies found increased collagen with retinol use (80, 81).

In 2007, *JAMA Dermatology* published a randomized, double-blind, controlled trial assessing the efficacy of retinol 0.4% lotion by applying it topically to one arm, while comparing it to a vehicle applied to the other arm (82). Though this was a small study with only 23 completing participants, it showed an improvement of fine lines and wrinkles via blinded dermatologist evaluation with retinol use after 24 weeks (82). Another double-blind, controlled study was conducted in Japan with 54 participants (83). The study involved applying retinol cream to half of the face and a control vehicle to the other half. It showed that retinol cream 0.075% use resulted in significant improvement in signs of photoaging, including improvements in appearance of fine and deep rhytides and decreased dyspigmentation. The study went on to investigate retinol cream 0.04% use in 36 participants, finding that it improved the appearance of fine rhytides in 13 weeks (83). An additional half-face study that evaluated a moisturizer containing 0.1% stabilized retinol highlighted improvement of photoaging, including rhytides and dyspigmentation with retinol use (84), achieving similar results with retinol 1% and 0.5% (85). A third half-face study of 27 participants evaluated 0.025% retinol cream and found similar results to those previously mentioned, including improvement in appearance of photodamage via photographic assessment (86). The longest study involved 62 participants and found that the use of stabilized retinol 0.1% resulted in decreased appearance of crow's feet rhytides and mottled pigmentation compared to the control (87).

A more recent double-blind, controlled study was conducted to assess the efficacy of retinol serum in comparison to tretinoin cream (80). The 12-week study found that the use of retinol serum and tretinoin cream had similar effects on clinical appearance via photographic assessment. Retinol, however, also showed improvement in skin texture and dryness that was not experienced by participants in the tretinoin group. This study suggests that retinol may be a more tolerable and effective treatment for photoaging compared to tretinoin (80).

Overall, there is evidence via small clinical trials supporting the use of retinoids for treatment of photoaging and dyspigmentation. Retinol, though very unstable, may be a very tolerable over-the-counter treatment option.

Retinaldehyde (Retinal)

Retinal is a naturally occurring retinoid molecule that is metabolized into retinoic acid when applied topically to the skin (88). Retinal is not considered to be a drug by the FDA and is commonly found in over-the-counter cosmeceutical products. It is not available as a prescription in the United States. Topical retinal concentrations range from 0.015% to 0.1% (72). Retinal has been shown to be efficacious in reducing signs of photoaging, as we will discuss below.

In 1999, Creidi and Humbert performed an open trial assessing the effect of six months of retinal cream 0.05% among 32 participants (89). The study found that treatment with retinal resulted in a decrease in rhytide intensity, facial redness, and facial telangiectasias. Additionally, there was an improvement in facial skin appearance, specifically noted as shinier skin with decreased roughness, improved pigmentation, and increased skin hydration (89). The same authors also conducted two more studies on retinal. The next was a randomized, double-blind, vehicle-controlled study using the same retinal cream 0.05% with 85 participants (89). This study found a decrease in rhytid severity with retinal use. The results were most significant at week 18, although the study went on until week 44 (89). The final study assessed not only the retinal cream 0.05%, but also retinoic acid (tretinoin) in 125 patients for 44 weeks (90). The study found that both the retinaldehyde and retinoic acid reduced the appearance of rhytides compared to the control; however, by the end of the study, retinal was shown to have a smaller effect compared to retinoic acid, though it was still significant (90). Topical retinal 0.05% was further shown to significantly increase the thickness of the epidermal skin layer and improve skin elasticity after one year of use in a study with 40 photoaged participants utilizing ultrasound measurements (91). However, there were no significant improvements in dermal thickness or skin stiffness with retinal use in this study (91).

Another study assessing the effectiveness of retinal cream compared two different concentrations, 0.1% and 0.05%, via twice daily use over three months on 40 Korean participants (92). The results showed that both groups had significant improvement in the overall clinical signs of photoaging, fine rhytides, skin texture, and skin hydration. There was no significant difference among the two groups in these factors (92). A randomized, blinded, split-face study similarly assessed retinal 0.1% and 0.05% multilamellar vesicle containing retinal cream, but compared the two to 0.1% and 0.05% retinol cream (93). The study found that after eight weeks of use among 22 participants, retinal had significantly better improvement in rhytid depth, skin elasticity, and skin hydration (93).

As for tolerability, retinal has been shown to be generally tolerated by participants (89, 90). One double-blind clinical trial with six participants compared the tolerability of retinal, retinol, and retinoic acid, finding that retinol and retinal resulted in less erythema compared to retinoic acid (78). Additionally, they found that retinal and retinoic acid caused similar amounts of scaling, while retinol treatment participants had less scaling comparatively. The study also highlighted the fact that retinal did not cause any burning or pruritus among participants, while retinol and retinoic acid did. A second clinical arm of this study with 355 participants, showed that retinal was considerably more tolerable than retinoic acid (78).

Overall, retinal has been shown to be effective in reducing signs of photoaging in small clinical trials. Though it may not be as effective as tretinoin, retinal is less irritating and better tolerated. Retinal therapy provides a good over-the-counter option for the treatment of photoaging, but larger studies would be beneficial. Additionally, more studies are needed to assess its efficacy on reduction of pigmentary changes associated with photoaging.

All-Trans Retinoic Acid (Tretinoin)

Retinoic acid is a natural retinoid found in the skin and is the most studied of the retinoids. A topical synthetic version of all-trans retinoic acid called tretinoin has been synthesized and is FDA approved for acne in 1971 and palliation of rhytides, mottled hyperpigmentation, and skin coarseness in 1995 (13, 94). Though tretinoin is only FDA approved for photoaging and acne, it is often used off-label for melasma, scarring, actinic keratoses, striae, and numerous other skin diseases (13). All-trans retinoic acid (tretinoin) is only available by prescription in the United States. It can be formulated into a variety of vehicles, including cream, gel, gel microsphere, among numerous others. Dosing from 0.025% to 0.1% is available (33).

Several prospective studies analyzed the use of tretinoin for reducing the appearance of photoaging and dyspigmentation. Selected and relevant studies are described in Table 7.4. Overall, tretinoin has been proven to be effective in treating signs of photoaging, including improving the appearance of rhytides, skin texture, and pigmentation changes (Table 7.4).

13-cis-Retinoic Acid (Isotretinoin)

Isotretinoin is a naturally occurring retinoid molecule and isomer of tretinoin. Once sold as a prescription topical useful for the treatment of signs of photoaging, isotretinoin is now only sold in the United States in an oral, systemic form. Given its systemic nature, a discussion of isotretinoin is beyond the scope of this chapter.

Alitretinoin

Alitretinoin is a naturally occurring retinoid molecule. A synthetic version is currently FDA approved for use in topical treatment of Kaposi's sarcoma (110). The topical formulation in the United States is a 0.1% gel and is only sold as a prescription. It is theoretically thought to be effective in reducing signs of photoaging as it binds to all RAR and RXR isotypes (72, 111). One open-label pilot study assessed the efficacy of topical alitretinoin gel 0.1% for photoaging in 20 participants, finding an improvement in appearance of photodamage and skin lesions such as actinic and seborrheic keratoses (112). The treatment was well tolerated (112). Although alitretinoin seems promising for the treatment of photoaging, larger clinical trials are needed. One study suggests that alitretinoin and other RXR agonists influence melanogenesis and thus may be useful in treating pigmentation disorders (113). However, additional investigation into the use of alitretinoin for dyspigmentation is needed as no human clinical trials currently exist.

Systemic Agents

Systemic agents beyond the scope of this chapter, primarily utilized for medical dermatologic diseases such as acne and psoriasis, include oral isotretinoin, acitretin, bexarotene, and alitretinoin.

Side Effects of Retinoids

As mentioned above, common side effects from topical retinoids include skin dryness, pruritus, erythema, and peeling or scaling, often referred to as a retinoid reaction or retinoid dermatitis. Dermatologists may encourage slow use of topical retinoids with slow up titration through increased frequency of use in order to build a bit of a tolerance to the retinoid and hopefully avoid over-treatment and resultant retinoid dermatitis. Other less common side effects include discoloration of the skin and acne flares with first use (114, 115).

The prescription as well as the over-the-counter retinoids that have a higher biological activity tend to have decreased tolerability and thus increased irritation with use (6). For example, tretinoin, which is more biologically active than retinol, may cause more irritation than its weaker counterpart (Figure 7.6).

Topical retinoids are not commonly used in pregnant women. The initial concern regarding the use of topical retinoids in pregnancy stems from three reports of patients who used topical retinoids delivered neonates with holoprosencephaly in the 1980s (34). A recent review of the teratogenic effects of topical

TABLE 7.4

Clinical Studies Supporting Tretinoin

Authors	Study Design	Number of Subjects	Study Duration	Intervention	Results	Adverse Side Effects
Babcock et al. (2015) (95)	Randomized, double-blind, split-face study	65	12 weeks	Tretinoin (0.025%, 0.05%, and 0.1%) versus retinol (0.025%, 0.05%, and 0.1%) applied to the face	• Clinical assessment showed significant improvement in appearance of overall photoaging, rhytides, mottled pigmentation, and skin texture and tone in both treatment groups • No significant difference was found between treatment groups	Twenty-two cases of peeling, dryness, erythema, and burning sensation were reported. Three subjects withdrew from the study due to adverse events.
Ellis et al. (1990) (96)	Randomized, blinded, controlled study	30	4 months	0.1% tretinoin versus vehicle cream applied to either face and/or forearms	• Clinical assessment showed significant improvement in skin texture and coarse and fine rhytides in the original and open-label studies • Histologic assessment also showed significant thickening of the epidermis	Peeling, dryness, and erythema were reported.
	Open-label study	21	10 months	0.1% versus 0.05% tretinoin cream applied to either face and/or forearms		
	Open-label study	16	22 months	0.1% versus 0.05% tretinoin cream applied to either face and/or forearms		
Griffiths et al. (1994) (97)	Randomized, double-blind trial	45	40 weeks	0.01% tretinoin cream versus vehicle	• Clinical assessment showed significant improvement in hyperpigmentation with tretinoin use • Colorimetric and histologic assessment also showed significant improvement in hyperpigmentation with tretinoin use compared to vehicle	No study withdrawals due to adverse events. Erythema, burning sensation, and scaling were noted.
Griffiths et al. (1995) (98)	Double-blind, controlled trial	99	48 weeks	0.01% tretinoin cream versus 0.025% tretinoin cream versus control vehicle applied to the face	• Clinical assessment showed significant improvement in appearance of overall photoaging in both tretinoin groups compared to the control • No significant difference was found between the tretinoin groups	One study withdrawal due to scaling and severe erythema

(Continued)

TABLE 7.4 (*Continued*)

Clinical Studies Supporting Tretinoin

Authors	Study Design	Number of Subjects	Study Duration	Intervention	Results	Adverse Side Effects
Ho et al. (2012) (99)	Randomized, double-blind, controlled trial	34	3 months	0.025% tretinoin cream versus 1.1% tri-retinol gradual release cream	• Clinical assessment showed significant improvement in appearance of overall photoaging, periocular rhytides, skin firmness, tone, and texture, and pigmentation in both treatment groups • No significant difference was found between treatment groups	One study withdrawal due to scaling and severe erythema, not in the tretinoin group. Other reported adverse effects included burning sensation, pruritus, and skin tightness.
Kligman et al. (1986) (100)	Controlled study	16	3 months	0.05% tretinoin cream versus vehicle	• Histologic and electron micrograph assessment showed epidermal hyperplasia, decreased dysplasia and atypia, increased collagen, eradication of actinic keratosis, and angiogenesis	In about 25% of subjects, mild irritation was noted in the first month
Kligman et al. (1993) (101)	Controlled study	6	9 months	0.025% tretinoin cream to the thigh versus vehicle	• Tretinoin increased epidermal thickness	No participants withdrew due to adverse events
Kligman and Draelos (2004) (102)	Prospective study	32	1 month	0.25% tretinoin solution	• Clinical assessment showed significant improvement in overall appearance of photoaging, rhytides, pigmentation, and texture with tretinoin use	Desquamation and erythema, which subsided
Leyden et al. (1989) (103)	Randomized, double-blind, controlled trial	40	6 months	0.05% tretinoin cream versus vehicle	• Clinical assessment showed significant decrease in hyperpigmentation, sallowness, and fine and coarse rhytides was noted via photographic assessment with tretinoin use	One patient withdrew due to skin irritation
Olsen et al. (1992) (104)	Randomized, multicenter, double-blind trial	296	24 weeks	0.05% tretinoin emollient cream versus 0.01% tretinoin emollient cream versus 0.001% tretinoin emollient cream	• Clinical assessment showed improvement in overall appearance of photoaging, rhytides, pigmentation, and skin texture with 0.05% tretinoin use • No significant difference was found between vehicle and tretinoin emollient cream 0.01% or 0.001%.	Erythema, burning, peeling were most commonly reported

(*Continued*)

TABLE 7.4 *(Continued)*

Clinical Studies Supporting Tretinoin

Authors	Study Design	Number of Subjects	Study Duration	Intervention	Results	Adverse Side Effects
Olsen et al. (1997) (105)	Double-blind extension study	259	48 weeks	0.05% tretinoin emollient cream versus 0.01% tretinoin emollient cream versus 0.001% tretinoin emollient cream	• Clinical assessment shows maintenance of photoaging results from prior study or continued improvement	Seventeen percent of participants withdrew due to adverse events
Rafal et al. (1992) (106)	Randomized, double-blind, controlled trial	58	10 months	0.1% tretinoin versus control vehicle applied to face, forearms, or both	• Clinical assessment showed significant improvement in appearance of hyperpigmentation after one month of treatment with tretinoin use • Biopsy showed significantly decreased epidermal pigmentation, increased epidermal thickness, increased granular layer thickness, and further compaction of the stratum corneum with tretinoin use • Additional 6 months of use in 6/7 subjects, showed continued improvement in photoaging signs with tretinoin use	Erythema and scaling were reported. One participant withdrew due to contact dermatitis.
Weiss et al. (1988) (107)	Randomized, double-blind, controlled trial	30	16 weeks	0.1% tretinoin versus control vehicle applied to face and forearms	• Clinical assessment showed statistically significant improvement photoaging • Biopsy showed increased epidermal thickness and specifically increased granular layer thickness with tretinoin use	Ninety-two percent of participants experienced dermatitis, 3 withdrew due to dermatitis
Weinstein et al. (1991) (108)	Multicenter, randomized, controlled study	251	24 weeks	0.05% tretinoin emollient cream versus 0.01% tretinoin emollient cream versus vehicle	• Clinical assessment showed statistically significant improvement photoaging in both tretinoin groups • Histologic assessment showed a significant increase in epidermal and granular layer thickness in both tretinoin groups • Histological assessment also showed an decrease in melanin with 0.05% tretinoin use	Twelve participants withdrew due to adverse skin reactions. Skin reactions included burning sensation, peeling, and erythema, which were more common in the 0.05% tretinoin group.
Woodley et al. (1990) (109)	Double-blind, controlled trial	6 underwent biopsy	4 months	0.1% tretinoin cream versus control?	• Biopsy showed statistically significant increase in anchoring fibrils with tretinoin use	N/A

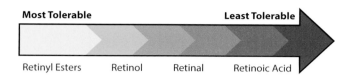

Most Tolerable   **Least Tolerable**

Retinyl Esters   Retinol   Retinal   Retinoic Acid

FIGURE 7.6 Tolerability of natural retinoids.
(From 3, 6. By courtesy of Briana Paiewonsky.)

retinoids highlights the safety of topical retinoid use in the pregnant animal mode and the nominal effect on retinoid blood levels (116). Although the system absorption of topical retinoids is minimal, there is a lack of human epidemiologic studies on this topic and thus some topical retinoids are not recommended for use during pregnancy. Of note, tazarotene and bexarotene were previously considered pregnancy category X (33, 117). In fact, the American College of Obstetricians and Gynecologists currently recommends avoiding topical retinoid use during pregnancy (118). As with all medications, patients should be counseled regarding the risks of treatment with topical retinoids and should utilize shared decision making with their healthcare team when considering use.

REFERENCES

1. Zussman, J., Ahdout, J., & Kim, J. (2010). Vitamins and photoaging: do scientific data support their use? *Journal of the American Academy of Dermatology, 63*(3), 507–525. https://doi.org/10.1016/j.jaad.2009.07.037
2. *Office of Dietary Supplements—Vitamin A.* (n.d.). Retrieved October 7, 2021, from https://ods.od.nih.gov/factsheets/VitaminA-HealthProfessional/
3. Sorg, O., Antille, C., Kaya, G., & Saurat, J. H. (2006). Retinoids in cosmeceuticals. *Dermatologic therapy, 19*(5), 289–296. https://doi.org/10.1111/j.1529-8019.2006.00086.x
4. Scheinfeld, N. (2006). Schools of pharmacology: retinoid update. *Journal of drugs in dermatology: JDD, 5*(9), 921–922.
5. Mukherjee, S., Date, A., Patravale, V., Korting, H. C., Roeder, A., & Weindl, G. (2006). Retinoids in the treatment of skin aging: an overview of clinical efficacy and safety. *Clinical interventions in aging, 1*(4), 327–348. https://doi.org/10.2147/ciia.2006.1.4.327
6. Draelos, Z. D. (2007). Cosmeceuticals. In D. J. Goldberg (Ed.), *Facial Rejuvenation: A Total Approach* (pp. 167–183). Springer: Berlin Heidelberg. https://doi.org/10.1007/978-3-540-69518-9_8
7. Babamiri, K., & Nassab, R. (2010). Cosmeceuticals: the evidence behind the retinoids. *Aesthetic surgery journal, 30*(1), 74–77. https://doi.org/10.1177/1090820X09360704
8. Khalil, S., Bardawil, T., Stephan, C., Darwiche, N., Abbas, O., Kibbi, A. G., Nemer, G., & Kurban, M. (2017). Retinoids: a journey from the molecular structures and mechanisms of action to clinical uses in dermatology and adverse effects. *Journal of dermatological treatment, 28*(8), 684–696. https://doi.org/10.1080/09546634.2017.1309349
9. Wolbach, S. B., & Howe, P. R. (1925). Tissue changes following deprivation of fat-soluble A vitamin. *Journal of experimental medicine, 42*(6), 753–777. https://doi.org/10.1084/jem.42.6.753
10. Ramos-e-Silva, M., Hexsel, D. M., Rutowitsch, M. S., & Zechmeister, M. (2001). Hydroxy acids and retinoids in cosmetics. *Clinics in dermatology, 19*(4), 460–466. https://doi.org/10.1016/s0738-081x(01)00189-4
11. Ellis, C. N., & Voorhees, J. J. (1987). Continuing medical education (therapy): etretinate therapy. *Journal of the American Academy of Dermatology, 16*(2, Part 1), 267–291. https://doi.org/10.1016/S0190-9622(87)70037-1
12. Roels, O. A. (1970). Vitamin A physiology. *JAMA, 214*(6), 1097–1102. https://doi.org/10.1001/jama.1970.03180060075015
13. Baldwin, H. E., Nighland, M., Kendall, C., Mays, D. A., Grossman, R., & Newburger, J. (2013). 40 years of topical tretinoin use in review. *Journal of drugs in dermatology: JDD, 12*(6), 638–642.
14. Thorne, E. G. (1990). Topical tretinoin research: an historical perspective. *Journal of international medical research, 18*(Suppl 3), 18C–25C.

15. Szymański, Ł., Skopek, R., Palusińska, M., Schenk, T., Stengel, S., Lewicki, S., Kraj, L., Kamiński, P., & Zelent, A. (2020). Retinoic acid and its derivatives in skin. *Cells, 9*(12), 2660. https://doi.org/10.3390/cells9122660

16. Vahlquist, A., & Duvic, M. (Eds.). (2007). Retinoids and Carotenoids in Dermatology (1st ed.). Boca Raton, FL: CRC Press. https://doi.org/10.3109/9781420021189

17. Karadag, A. S., Aksoy, B., & Parish, L. C. (Eds.). (2019). Retinoids in Dermatology (1st ed.). https://www.taylorfrancis.com/books/edit/10.1201/9780429456732/retinoids-dermatology-ayse-serap-karadag-berna-aksoy-lawrence-charles-parish

18. Vahlquist, A., & Rollman, O. (1987). Clinical pharmacology of 3 generations of retinoids. *Dermatology, 175*(1), 20–27. https://doi.org/10.1159/000248850

19. Scott, L. J. (2019). Trifarotene: first approval. *Drugs, 79*(17), 1905–1909. https://doi.org/10.1007/s40265-019-01218-6

20. Orfanos, C. E., Ehlert, R., & Gollnick, H. (1987). The retinoids. A review of their clinical pharmacology and therapeutic use. *Drugs, 34*(4), 459–503. https://doi.org/10.2165/00003495-198734040-00003

21. Vieira, A. V., Schneider, W. J., & Vieira, P. M. (1995). Retinoids: transport, metabolism, and mechanisms of action. *Journal of endocrinology, 146*(2), 201–207. https://doi.org/10.1677/joe.0.1460201

22. Reichrath, J., Lehmann, B., Carlberg, C., Varani, J., & Zouboulis, C. C. (2007). Vitamins as hormones. *Hormone and metabolic research = Hormon- und Stoffwechselforschung = Hormones et metabolisme, 39*(2), 71–84. https://doi.org/10.1055/s-2007-958715

23. Darlenski, R., Surber, C., & Fluhr, J. W. (2010). Topical retinoids in the management of photodamaged skin: from theory to evidence-based practical approach. *British journal of dermatology, 163*(6), 1157–1165. https://doi.org/10.1111/j.1365-2133.2010.09936.x

24. Fisher, G. J., & Voorhees, J. J. (1996). Molecular mechanisms of retinoid actions in skin. *FASEB journal: official publication of the Federation of American Societies for Experimental Biology, 10*(9), 1002–1013. https://doi.org/10.1096/fasebj.10.9.8801161

25. Napoli, J. L. (1996). Biochemical pathways of retinoid transport, metabolism, and signal transduction. *Clinical immunology and immunopathology, 80*(3 Pt 2), S52–S62. https://doi.org/10.1006/clin.1996.0142

26. Favennec, L., & Cals, M. J. (1988). The biological effects of retinoids on cell differentiation and proliferation. *Journal of clinical chemistry and clinical biochemistry. Zeitschrift fur klinische Chemie und klinische Biochemie, 26*(8), 479–489. https://doi.org/10.1515/cclm.1988.26.8.479

27. Bastien, J., & Rochette-Egly, C. (2004). Nuclear retinoid receptors and the transcription of retinoid-target genes. *Gene, 328*, 1–16. https://doi.org/10.1016/j.gene.2003.12.005

28. Griffiths, C. E., Russman, A. N., Majmudar, G., Singer, R. S., Hamilton, T. A., & Voorhees, J. J. (1993). Restoration of collagen formation in photodamaged human skin by tretinoin (retinoic acid). *New England journal of medicine, 329*(8), 530–535. https://doi.org/10.1056/NEJM199308193290803

29. Torras, H. (1996). Retinoids in aging. *Clinics in dermatology, 14*(2), 207–215. https://doi.org/10.1016/0738-081x(95)00156-a

30. Xiao, J. H., Feng, X., Di, W., Peng, Z. H., Li, L. A., Chambon, P., & Voorhees, J. J. (1999). Identification of heparin-binding EGF-like growth factor as a target in intercellular regulation of epidermal basal cell growth by suprabasal retinoic acid receptors. *EMBO journal, 18*(6), 1539–1548. https://doi.org/10.1093/emboj/18.6.1539

31. Kuenzli, S., & Saurat, J. H. (2001). Retinoids for the treatment of psoriasis: outlook for the future. *Current opinion in investigational drugs (London, England: 2000), 2*(5), 625–630.

32. Blomhoff, R., & Blomhoff, H. K. (2006). Overview of retinoid metabolism and function. *Journal of neurobiology, 66*(7), 606–630. https://doi.org/10.1002/neu.20242

33. Zaenglein, A. L., Pathy, A. L., Schlosser, B. J., Alikhan, A., Baldwin, H. E., Berson, D. S., Bowe, W. P., Graber, E. M., Harper, J. C., Kang, S., Keri, J. E., Leyden, J. J., Reynolds, R. V., Silverberg, N. B., Stein Gold, L. F., Tollefson, M. M., Weiss, J. S., Dolan, N. C., Sagan, A. A., … Bhushan, R. (2016). Guidelines of care for the management of acne vulgaris. *Journal of the American Academy of Dermatology, 74*(5), 945–973.e33. https://doi.org/10.1016/j.jaad.2015.12.037

34. Tolaymat, L., Dearborn, H., & Zito, P. M. Adapalene. [Updated July 20, 2021]. In: StatPearls [Internet]. Treasure Island (FL): StatPearls Publishing; 2021 January. https://www.ncbi.nlm.nih.gov/books/NBK482509/

35. Chivot, M. (2005). Retinoid therapy for acne. A comparative review. *American journal of clinical dermatology*, *6*(1), 13–19. https://doi.org/10.2165/00128071-200506010-00002

36. Talpur, R., Cox, K., & Duvic, M. (2009). Efficacy and safety of topical tazarotene: a review. *Expert opinion on drug metabolism & toxicology*, *5*(2), 195–210. https://doi.org/10.1517/17425250902721250

37. Commissioner, O. of the. (2020, March 24). *FDA approves Differin Gel 0.1% for over-the-counter use to treat acne.* FDA; FDA. https://www.fda.gov/news-events/press-announcements/fda-approves-differin-gel-01-over-counter-use-treat-acne

38. Shroot, B. (1998). Pharmacodynamics and pharmacokinetics of topical adapalene. *Journal of the American Academy of Dermatology*, *39*(2 Pt 3), S17–S24. https://doi.org/10.1016/s0190-9622(98)70440-2

39. Valins, W., Amini, S., & Berman, B. (2010). The expression of toll-like receptors in dermatological diseases and the therapeutic effect of current and newer topical toll-like receptor modulators. *Journal of clinical and aesthetic dermatology*, *3*(9), 20–29.

40. Leyden, J. (2001). Adapalene in clinical practice. *Cutis*, *68*(4 Suppl), 7–9.

41. Kang, S., Goldfarb, M. T., Weiss, J. S., Metz, R. D., Hamilton, T. A., Voorhees, J. J., & Griffiths, C. E. (2003). Assessment of adapalene gel for the treatment of actinic keratoses and lentigines: a randomized trial. *Journal of the American Academy of Dermatology*, *49*(1), 83–90. https://doi.org/10.1067/mjd.2003.451

42. Bagatin, E., Gonçalves, H. S., Sato, M., Almeida, L., & Miot, H. A. (2018). Comparable efficacy of adapalene 0.3% gel and tretinoin 0.05% cream as treatment for cutaneous photoaging. *European journal of dermatology: EJD*, *28*(3), 343–350. https://doi.org/10.1684/ejd.2018.3320

43. Herane, M. I., Orlandi, C., Zegpi, E., Valdés, P., & Ancić, X. (2012). Clinical efficacy of adapalene (differin®) 0.3% gel in Chilean women with cutaneous photoaging. *Journal of dermatological treatment*, *23*(1), 57–64. https://doi.org/10.3109/09546634.2011.631981

44. Jacyk, W. K., & Mpofu, P. (2001). Adapalene gel 0.1% for topical treatment of acne vulgaris in African patients. *Cutis*, *68*(4 Suppl), 48–54.

45. Verschoore, M., Bouclier, M., Czernielewski, J., & Hensby, C. (1993). Topical retinoids: their uses in dermatology. *Dermatologic clinics*, *11*(1), 107–115. https://doi.org/10.1016/S0733-8635(18)30287-0

46. Cunliffe, W. J. et al. (1997). Clinical efficacy and safety comparison of adapalene gel and tretinoin gel in the treatment of acne vulgaris: Europe and U.S. multicenter trials. *Journal of the American Academy of Dermatology*, *36*(6 Pt 2), S126–34. https://doi.org/10.1016/s0190-9622(97)70056-2

47. Thiboutot, D., Arsonnaud, S., & Soto, P. (2008 June). Efficacy and tolerability of adapalene 0.3% gel compared to tazarotene 0.1% gel in the treatment of acne vulgaris. *Journal of drugs in dermatology: JDD*, *7*(6 Suppl), s3–s10. [PubMed]

48. Pariser, D., Colón, L. E., Johnson, L. A., & Gottschalk, R. W. (2008 June). Adapalene 0.1% gel compared to tazarotene 0.1% cream in the treatment of acne vulgaris. *Journal of drugs in dermatology: JDD*, *7*(6 Suppl), s18–s23. [PubMed]

49. Sardana, K., & Sehgal, V. N. (2003 May). Retinoids: fascinating up-and-coming scenario. *Journal of dermatology*, *30*(5), 355–380. [PubMed]

50. Dosik, J. S., & Arsonnaud, S. (2007). Tolerability comparison of adapalene gel, 0.3% versus tazarotene cream, 0.05% in subjects with healthy skin. *Journal of drugs in dermatology: JDD*, *6*(6), 632–638.

51. Tu, P. et al. (2001). A comparison of adapalene gel 0.1% vs. tretinoin gel 0.025% in the treatment of acne vulgaris in China. *Journal of the European Academy of Dermatology and Venereology: JEADV*, *15*(Suppl 3), 31–36. https://doi.org/10.1046/j.0926-9959.2001.00010.x

52. Stein Gold, L. et al. (2017). Management of severe acne vulgaris with topical therapy. *Journal of drugs in dermatology: JDD*, *16*(11), 1134–1138.

53. Weiss, J. S., Thiboutot, D. M., Hwa, J., Liu, Y., & Graeber, M. (2008 June). Long-term safety and efficacy study of adapalene 0.3% gel. *Journal of drugs in dermatology: JDD*, *7*(6 Suppl), s24–s28. [PubMed]

54. https://www.accessdata.fda.gov/drugsatfda_docs/label/2018/020600s010lbl.pdf

55. https://www.accessdata.fda.gov/drugsatfda_docs/label/2017/208258Orig1s000lbl.pdf

56. Chandraratna, R. A. (1996). Tazarotene–first of a new generation of receptor-selective retinoids. *British journal of dermatology*, *135*(Suppl 49), 18–25. https://doi.org/10.1111/j.1365-2133.1996.tb15662.x

57. Phillips, T. J., Gottlieb, A. B., Leyden, J. J., Lowe, N. J., Lew-Kaya, D. A., Sefton, J., Walker, P. S., Gibson, J. R., & Tazarotene Cream Photodamage Clinical Study Group. (2002). Efficacy of 0.1% tazarotene cream for the treatment of photodamage: a 12-month multicenter, randomized trial. *Archives of dermatology, 138*(11), 1486–1493. https://doi.org/10.1001/archderm.138.11.1486

58. Machtinger, L. A., Kaidbey, K., Lim, J., Loven, K. H., Rist, T. E., Wilson, D. C., Parizadeh, D. D., Sefton, J., Holland, J. M., & Walker, P. S. (2004). Histological effects of tazarotene 0.1% cream vs. vehicle on photodamaged skin: a 6-month, multicentre, double-blind, randomized, vehicle-controlled study in patients with photodamaged facial skin. *British journal of dermatology, 151*(6), 1245–1252. https://doi.org/10.1111/j.1365-2133.2004.06186.x

59. Kang, S., Krueger, G. G., Tanghetti, E. A., Lew-Kaya, D., Sefton, J., Walker, P. S., Gibson, J. R., & Tazarotene Cream in Photodamage Study Group. (2005). A multicenter, randomized, double-blind trial of tazarotene 0.1% cream in the treatment of photodamage. *Journal of the American Academy of Dermatology, 52*(2), 268–274. https://doi.org/10.1016/j.jaad.2004.06.021

60. Kang, S., Leyden, J. J., Lowe, N. J., Ortonne, J. P., Phillips, T. J., Weinstein, G. D., Bhawan, J., Lew-Kaya, D. A., Matsumoto, R. M., Sefton, J., Walker, P. S., & Gibson, J. R. (2001). Tazarotene cream for the treatment of facial photodamage: a multicenter, investigator-masked, randomized, vehicle-controlled, parallel comparison of 0.01%, 0.025%, 0.05%, and 0.1% tazarotene creams with 0.05% tretinoin emollient cream applied once daily for 24 weeks. *Archives of dermatology, 137*(12), 1597–1604. https://doi.org/10.1001/archderm.137.12.1597

61. Lowe, N., Gifford, M., Tanghetti, E., Poulin, Y., Goldman, M., Tse, Y., Yamauchi, P., Rosenzweig, H., & Kang, S. (2004). Tazarotene 0.1% cream versus tretinoin 0.05% emollient cream in the treatment of photodamaged facial skin: a multicenter, double-blind, randomized, parallel-group study. *Journal of cosmetic and laser therapy: official publication of the European Society for Laser Dermatology, 6*(2), 79–85. https://doi.org/10.1080/14764170410032406

62. Grimes, P., & Callender, V. (2006). Tazarotene cream for postinflammatory hyperpigmentation and acne vulgaris in darker skin: a double-blind, randomized, vehicle-controlled study. *Cutis, 77*(1), 45–50.

63. Koo, J., Behnam, S. E., & Behnam, S. M. (2003). The efficacy of topical tazarotene monotherapy and combination therapies in psoriasis. *Expert opinion on pharmacotherapy, 4*(12), 2347–2354. https://doi.org/10.1517/14656566.4.12.2347

64. Cosio, T., Di Prete, M., Gaziano, R., Lanna, C., Orlandi, A., Di Francesco, P., Bianchi, L., & Campione, E. (2021). Trifarotene: a current review and perspectives in dermatology. *Biomedicines, 9*(3), 237. https://doi.org/10.3390/biomedicines9030237

65. Kassir, M., Karagaiah, P., Sonthalia, S., Katsambas, A., Galadari, H., Gupta, M., Lotti, T., Wollina, U., Abdelmaksoud, A., Grabbe, S., & Goldust, M. (2020). Selective RAR agonists for acne vulgaris: a narrative review. *Journal of cosmetic dermatology, 19*(6), 1278–1283. https://doi.org/10.1111/jocd.13340

66. Zhang, C., Hazarika, P., Ni, X., Weidner, D. A., & Duvic, M. (2002). Induction of apoptosis by bexarotene in cutaneous T-cell lymphoma cells: relevance to mechanism of therapeutic action. *Clinical cancer research: an official journal of the American Association for Cancer Research, 8*(5), 1234–1240.

67. Fu, P. P., Cheng, S. H., Coop, L., Xia, Q., Culp, S. J., Tolleson, W. H., Wamer, W. G., & Howard, P. C. (2003). Photoreaction, phototoxicity, and photocarcinogenicity of retinoids. *Journal of environmental science and health. Part C, environmental carcinogenesis & ecotoxicology reviews, 21*(2), 165–197. https://doi.org/10.1081/GNC-120026235

68. Fu, P. P., Xia, Q., Yin, J. J., Cherng, S. H., Yan, J., Mei, N., Chen, T., Boudreau, M. D., Howard, P. C., & Wamer, W. G. (2007). Photodecomposition of vitamin A and photobiological implications for the skin. *Photochemistry and photobiology, 83*(2), 409–424. https://doi.org/10.1562/2006-10-23-IR-1065

69. Lupo, M. P. (2001). Antioxidants and vitamins in cosmetics. *Clinics in dermatology, 19*(4), 467–473. https://doi.org/10.1016/s0738-081x(01)00188-2

70. Watson, R. E., Long, S. P., Bowden, J. J., Bastrilles, J. Y., Barton, S. P., & Griffiths, C. E. (2008). Repair of photoaged dermal matrix by topical application of a cosmetic 'antiageing' product. *British journal of dermatology, 158*(3), 472–477. https://doi.org/10.1111/j.1365-2133.2007.08364.x

71. Grimes, P. E. et al. (2004). The use of polyhydroxy acids (PHAs) in photoaged skin. *Cutis, 73*(2 Suppl), 3–13.

72. Serri, R., & Iorizzo, M. (2008). Cosmeceuticals: focus on topical retinoids in photoaging. *Clinics in dermatology, 26*(6), 633–635. https://doi.org/10.1016/j.clindermatol.2007.09.016

73. Green, C. et al. (1998). A clinicopathological study of the effects of topical retinyl propionate cream in skin photoageing. *Clinical and experimental dermatology, 23*(4), 162–167. https://doi.org/10.1046/j.1365-2230.1998.00331.x

74. Duell, E. A., Kang, S., & Voorhees, J. J. (1997). Unoccluded retinol penetrates human skin in vivo more effectively than unoccluded retinyl palmitate or retinoic acid. *Journal of investigative dermatology, 109*(3), 301–305. https://doi.org/10.1111/1523-1747.ep12335788

75. Duell, E. A., Derguini, F., Kang, S., Elder, J. T., & Voorhees, J. J. (1996). Extraction of human epidermis treated with retinol yields retro-retinoids in addition to free retinol and retinyl esters. *Journal of investigative dermatology, 107*(2), 178–182. https://doi.org/10.1111/1523-1747.ep12329576

76. Kang, S., Duell, E. A., Fisher, G. J., Datta, S. C., Wang, Z. Q., Reddy, A. P., Tavakkol, A., Yi, J. Y., Griffiths, C. E., & Elder, J. T. (1995). Application of retinol to human skin in vivo induces epidermal hyperplasia and cellular retinoid binding proteins characteristic of retinoic acid but without measurable retinoic acid levels or irritation. *Journal of investigative dermatology, 105*(4), 549–556. https://doi.org/10.1111/1523-1747.ep12323445

77. Kurlandsky, S. B., Xiao, J. H., Duell, E. A., Voorhees, J. J., & Fisher, G. J. (1994). Biological activity of all-trans retinol requires metabolic conversion to all-trans retinoic acid and is mediated through activation of nuclear retinoid receptors in human keratinocytes. *Journal of biological chemistry, 269*(52), 32821–32827.

78. Fluhr, J. W., Vienne, M. P., Lauze, C., Dupuy, P., Gehring, W., & Gloor, M. (1999). Tolerance profile of retinol, retinaldehyde and retinoic acid under maximized and long-term clinical conditions. *Dermatology (Basel, Switzerland), 199*(Suppl 1), 57–60. https://doi.org/10.1159/000051381

79. Piérard-Franchimont, C., Castelli, D., Cromphaut, I. V., Bertin, C., Ries, G., Cauwenbergh, G., & Piérard, G. E. (1998). Tensile properties and contours of aging facial skin. A controlled double-blind comparative study of the effects of retinol, melibiose-lactose and their association. *Skin research and technology: official journal of International Society for Bioengineering and the Skin (ISBS) [and] International Society for Digital Imaging of Skin (ISDIS) [and] International Society for Skin Imaging (ISSI), 4*(4), 237–243. https://doi.org/10.1111/j.1600-0846.1998.tb00116.x

80. Draelos, Z. D., & Peterson, R. S. (2020). A double-blind, comparative clinical study of newly formulated retinol serums vs tretinoin cream in escalating doses: a method for rapid retinization with minimized irritation. *Journal of drugs in dermatology: JDD, 19*(6), 625–631.

81. Varani, J., Warner, R. L., Gharaee-Kermani, M., Phan, S. H., Kang, S., Chung, J. H., Wang, Z. Q., Datta, S. C., Fisher, G. J., & Voorhees, J. J. (2000). Vitamin A antagonizes decreased cell growth and elevated collagen-degrading matrix metalloproteinases and stimulates collagen accumulation in naturally aged human skin. *Journal of investigative dermatology, 114*(3), 480–486. https://doi.org/10.1046/j.1523-1747.2000.00902.x

82. Kafi, R., Kwak, H. S., Schumacher, W. E., Cho, S., Hanft, V. N., Hamilton, T. A., King, A. L., Neal, J. D., Varani, J., Fisher, G. J., Voorhees, J. J., & Kang, S. (2007). Improvement of naturally aged skin with vitamin A (retinol). *Archives of dermatology, 143*(5), 606–612. https://doi.org/10.1001/archderm.143.5.606

83. Kikuchi, K., Suetake, T., Kumasaka, N., & Tagami, H. (2009). Improvement of photoaged facial skin in middle-aged Japanese females by topical retinol (vitamin A alcohol): a vehicle-controlled, double-blind study. *Journal of dermatological treatment, 20*(5), 276–281. https://doi.org/10.1080/09546630902973987

84. Tucker-Samaras, S., Zedayko, T., Cole, C., Miller, D., Wallo, W., & Leyden, J. J. (2009). A stabilized 0.1% retinol facial moisturizer improves the appearance of photodamaged skin in an eight-week, double-blind, vehicle-controlled study. *Journal of drugs in dermatology: JDD, 8*(10), 932–936.

85. Gold, M. H., Kircik, L. H., Bucay, V. W., Kiripolsky, M. G., & Biron, J. A. (2013). Treatment of facial photodamage using a novel retinol formulation. *Journal of drugs in dermatology: JDD, 12*(5), 533–540.

86. Reich, H., Wallander, I., Schulte, L., Goodier, M., & Zelickson, B. (2016). Comparative study of professional vs mass market topical products for treatment of facial photodamage. *Journal of drugs in dermatology: JDD, 15*(1), 37–44.

87. Randhawa, M., Rossetti, D., Leyden, J. J., Fantasia, J., Zeichner, J., Cula, G. O., Southall, M., & Tucker-Samaras, S. (2015). One-year topical stabilized retinol treatment improves photodamaged skin in a double-blind, vehicle-controlled trial. *Journal of drugs in dermatology: JDD, 14*(3), 271–280.

88. Bailly, J., Crettaz, M., Schifflers, M. H., & Marty, J. P. (1998). In vitro metabolism by human skin and fibroblasts of retinol, retinal and retinoic acid. *Experimental dermatology, 7*(1), 27–34. https://doi.org/10.1111/j.1600-0625.1998.tb00299.x

89. Creidi, P., & Humbert, P. (1999). Clinical use of topical retinaldehyde on photoaged skin. *Dermatology (Basel, Switzerland), 199*(Suppl 1), 49–52. https://doi.org/10.1159/000051379

90. Creidi, P., Vienne, M. P., Ochonisky, S., Lauze, C., Turlier, V., Lagarde, J. M., & Dupuy, P. (1998). Profilometric evaluation of photodamage after topical retinaldehyde and retinoic acid treatment. *Journal of the American Academy of Dermatology, 39*(6), 960–965. https://doi.org/10.1016/s0190-9622(98)70270-1

91. Diridollou, S., Vienne, M. P., Alibert, M., Aquilina, C., Briant, A., Dahan, S., Denis, P., Launais, B., Turlier, V., & Dupuy, P. (1999). Efficacy of topical 0.05% retinaldehyde in skin aging by ultrasound and rheological techniques. *Dermatology (Basel, Switzerland), 199*(Suppl 1), 37–41. https://doi.org/10.1159/000051377

92. Kwon, H. S., Lee, J. H., Kim, G. M., & Bae, J. M. (2018). Efficacy and safety of retinaldehyde 0.1% and 0.05% creams used to treat photoaged skin: a randomized double-blind controlled trial. *Journal of cosmetic dermatology, 17*(3), 471–476. https://doi.org/10.1111/jocd.12551

93. Kim, J., Kim, J., Jongudomsombat, T., Kim BS, E., Suk, J., Lee, D., & Lee, J. H. (2021). The efficacy and safety of multilamellar vesicle containing retinaldehyde: a double-blinded, randomized, split-face controlled study. *Journal of cosmetic dermatology, 20*(9), 2874–2879. https://doi.org/10.1111/jocd.13993

94. Yoham, A. L., & Casadesus, D. Tretinoin. [Updated December 5, 2020]. In: StatPearls [Internet]. Treasure Island, FL: StatPearls Publishing; 2021 January. https://www.ncbi.nlm.nih.gov/books/NBK557478/

95. Babcock, M., Mehta, R. C., & Makino, E. T. (2015). A randomized, double-blind, split-face study comparing the efficacy and tolerability of three retinol-based products vs. three tretinoin-based products in subjects with moderate to severe facial photodamage. *Journal of drugs in dermatology: JDD, 14*(1), 24–30.

96. Ellis, C. N., Weiss, J. S., Hamilton, T. A., Headington, J. T., Zelickson, A. S., & Voorhees, J. J. (1990). Sustained improvement with prolonged topical tretinoin (retinoic acid) for photoaged skin. *Journal of the American Academy of Dermatology, 23*(4 Pt 1), 629–637. https://doi.org/10.1016/0190-9622(90)70265-j

97. Griffiths, C. E., Goldfarb, M. T., Finkel, L. J., Roulia, V., Bonawitz, M., Hamilton, T. A., Ellis, C. N., & Voorhees, J. J. (1994). Topical tretinoin (retinoic acid) treatment of hyperpigmented lesions associated with photoaging in Chinese and Japanese patients: a vehicle-controlled trial. *Journal of the American Academy of Dermatology, 30*(1), 76–84. https://doi.org/10.1016/s0190-9622(94)70011-7

98. Griffiths, C. E., Kang, S., Ellis, C. N., Kim, K. J., Finkel, L. J., Ortiz-Ferrer, L. C., White, G. M., Hamilton, T. A., & Voorhees, J. J. (1995). Two concentrations of topical tretinoin (retinoic acid) cause similar improvement of photoaging but different degrees of irritation. A double-blind, vehicle-controlled comparison of 0.1% and 0.025% tretinoin creams. *Archives of dermatology, 131*(9), 1037–1044.

99. Ho, E. T., Trookman, N. S., Sperber, B. R., Rizer, R. L., Spindler, R., Sonti, S., Gotz, V., & Mehta, R. (2012). A randomized, double-blind, controlled comparative trial of the anti-aging properties of non-prescription tri-retinol 1.1% vs. prescription tretinoin 0.025%. *Journal of drugs in dermatology: JDD, 11*(1), 64–69.

100. Kligman, A. M., Grove, G. L., Hirose, R., & Leyden, J. J. (1986). Topical tretinoin for photoaged skin. *Journal of the American Academy of Dermatology, 15*(4 Pt 2), 836–859. https://doi.org/10.1016/s0190-9622(86)70242-9

101. Kligman, A. M., Dogadkina, D., & Lavker, R. M. (1993). Effects of topical tretinoin on non-sun-exposed protected skin of the elderly. *Journal of the American Academy of Dermatology, 29*(1), 25–33. https://doi.org/10.1016/0190-9622(93)70147-l

102. Kligman, D. E., & Draelos, Z. D. (2004). High-strength tretinoin for rapid retinization of photoaged facial skin. *Dermatologic surgery: official publication for American Society for Dermatologic Surgery [et al.], 30*(6), 864–866.

103. Leyden, J. J., Grove, G. L., Grove, M. J., Thorne, E. G., & Lufrano, L. (1989). Treatment of photodamaged facial skin with topical tretinoin. *Journal of the American Academy of Dermatology, 21*(3 Pt 2), 638–644. https://doi.org/10.1016/s0190-9622(89)70231-0

104. Olsen, E. A., Katz, H. I., Levine, N., Shupack, J., Billys, M. M., Prawer, S., Gold, J., Stiller, M., Lufrano, L., & Thorne, E. G. (1992). Tretinoin emollient cream: a new therapy for photodamaged skin. *Journal of the American Academy of Dermatology, 26*(2 Pt 1), 215–224. https://doi.org/10.1016/0190-9622(92)70030-j

105. Olsen, E. A., Katz, H. I., Levine, N., Nigra, T. P., Pochi, P. E., Savin, R. C., Shupack, J., Weinstein, G. D., Lufrano, L., & Perry, B. H. (1997). Tretinoin emollient cream for photodamaged skin: results of 48-week, multicenter, double-blind studies. *Journal of the American Academy of Dermatology, 37*(2 Pt 1), 217–226. https://doi.org/10.1016/s0190-9622(97)80128-4

106. Rafal, E. S., Griffiths, C. E., Ditre, C. M., Finkel, L. J., Hamilton, T. A., Ellis, C. N., & Voorhees, J. J. (1992). Topical tretinoin (retinoic acid) treatment for liver spots associated with photodamage. *New England journal of medicine, 326*(6), 368–374. https://doi.org/10.1056/NEJM199202063260603

107. Weiss, J. S., Ellis, C. N., Headington, J. T., Tincoff, T., Hamilton, T. A., & Voorhees, J. J. (1988). Topical tretinoin improves photoaged skin. A double-blind vehicle-controlled study. *JAMA, 259*(4), 527–532.

108. Weinstein, G. D., Nigra, T. P., Pochi, P. E., Savin, R. C., Allan, A., Benik, K., Jeffes, E., Lufrano, L., & Thorne, E. G. (1991). Topical tretinoin for treatment of photodamaged skin. A multicenter study. *Archives of dermatology, 127*(5), 659–665.

109. Woodley, D. T., Zelickson, A. S., Briggaman, R. A., Hamilton, T. A., Weiss, J. S., Ellis, C. N., & Voorhees, J. J. (1990). Treatment of photoaged skin with topical tretinoin increases epidermal-dermal anchoring fibrils. A preliminary report. *JAMA, 263*(22), 3057–3059.

110. https://www.accessdata.fda.gov/drugsatfda_docs/label/1999/20886lbl.pdf

111. Bubna, A. K. (2015). Alitretinoin in dermatology-an update. *Indian journal of dermatology, 60*(5), 520. https://doi.org/10.4103/0019-5154.164426

112. Baumann, L., Vujevich, J., Halem, M., Martin, L. K., Kerdel, F., Lazarus, M., Pacheco, H., Black, L., & Bryde, J. (2005). Open-label pilot study of alitretinoin gel 0.1% in the treatment of photoaging. *Cutis, 76*(1), 69–73.

113. Paterson, E. K., Ho, H., Kapadia, R., & Ganesan, A. K. (2013). 9-cis retinoic acid is the ALDH1A1 product that stimulates melanogenesis. *Experimental dermatology, 22*(3), 202–209. https://doi.org/10.1111/exd.12099

114. *Retinoids, topical—American Osteopathic College of Dermatology (AOCD).* (n.d.). Retrieved October 15, 2021, from https://www.aocd.org/page/Retinoidstopical

115. Del Rosso, J. Q. (2008). Retinoid-induced flaring in patients with acne vulgaris: does it really exist? *Journal of clinical and aesthetic dermatology, 1*(1), 41–43.

116. Williams, A. L., Pace, N. D., & DeSesso, J. M. (2020). Teratogen update: topical use and third-generation retinoids. *Birth defects research, 112*(15), 1105–1114. https://doi.org/10.1002/bdr2.1745

117. https://www.accessdata.fda.gov/drugsatfda_docs/label/2000/21056lbl.pdf

118. *Skin Conditions during Pregnancy.* (n.d.). Retrieved October 15, 2021, from https://www.acog.org/en/womens-health/faqs/skin-conditions-during-pregnancy

8

Neurotransmitter-Affecting Peptides

Rachel Maiman

Introduction

Perhaps the most fundamental method of utilizing cosmeceuticals is to deliver proteins and cytokines to the skin which are responsible for intercellular communication. This cellular "cross-talk" activates molecular signaling cascades on which regenerative processes such as neocollagenesis and epidermal turnover are dependent. Unfortunately, the cytokines and peptides integral to these processes wane with increasing age. Through topical delivery, however, depleted stores are restocked, resulting in skin rejuvenation.

Skin rejuvenation is the result of multiple cellular processes. To activate them requires multiple targets throughout the skin, all of which require different stimuli. For instance, the cytokines and peptides that act on the extracellular matrix to convince a senescent fibroblast to produce new collagen are different than those capable of inducing an atrophic epithelial cell to hypertrophy.

Peptides are short-chain sequences of amino acids and are a rapidly expanding category of cosmeceuticals. Tiny peptides, in particular, have revolutionized the field of cosmetic dermatology. At five to ten amino acids in size, these tiny peptides are highly specific and thus can uniquely stimulate or inhibit cellular processes by binding to a receptor like a "lock" and "key" (1). There are three main categories of cosmeceutical peptides: "signal" peptides, neurotransmitter-affecting peptides, and carrier peptides. This chapter focuses on neurotransmitter-affecting peptides, published studies on their theoretical effect, and their practical use in dermatology. Existing methods of utilizing these peptides as cosmeceuticals and potential means of doing so in the future will also be discussed.

The Science of Neurotransmitter-Affecting Peptides

As their name suggests, neurotransmitter-affecting peptides are those that stimulate or inhibit the release of one or several neurotransmitters upon receptor binding. There has been significantly less research on their use to date when compared to signal and carrier peptides; however, neurotransmitter-affecting peptides are being increasingly investigated in the cosmeceutical industry. They are particularly exciting when one considers that no other cosmeceutical ingredient, from antioxidant to hydroxy acid to peptide of another class, is capable of directly affecting one of the driving forces behind wrinkles – muscular contraction.

Several neurotransmitter-affecting peptides are incorporated into topical cosmetic formulations. While they vary in their specific mechanism of action, all were developed as topical mimics of botulinum toxin (2). Botulinum toxin is a neurotoxin of which there are several serotypes (BTXA-G). All of these serotypes are single-chain polypeptides which inhibit the release of acetylcholine from motor neurons into the neuromuscular junction. This prevents transmission of the signal required to induce muscular contraction. To do this requires a multi-step process. First, single-chain botulinum toxin polypeptides are cleaved by proteases into a double chain consisting of heavy- and light-chain moieties. Upon cleavage, the heavy chain binds to a high-affinity receptor on the presynaptic nerve terminal, which promotes uptake of bound toxin. The light chain acts on one of several possible targets depending on the

DOI: 10.1201/9781315165905-8

serological subtype of the neurotoxin. For instance, the intracellular target of BTX-A is synaptosome-associated protein of molecular weight 25 kDa (SNAP-25). This protein is required to dock acetylcho-line-containing vesicles on the presynaptic neuronal membrane, a necessary step before release into the neuromuscular junction. BTX-B, however, cleaves vesicle-associated membrane protein (VAMP). VAMP, also known as synaptobrevin, is also essential for the docking and fusion of acetylcholine-con-taining vesicles to the presynaptic membrane (3). Thus, by inhibiting signal transduction pathways at the neuromuscular junction, both BTX-A and BTX-B inhibit repetitive contractions of the intrinsic muscles of facial expression. The end result is attenuation of the hyperkinetic facial lines that form over time (4).

Neurotransmitter-Affecting Peptides as Cosmeceuticals

The biochemical research surrounding the use of botulinum toxins has greatly expanded our knowledge of how these molecules work and the mechanisms of action for the various subtypes of botulinum toxin are now well-categorized. More recently, it has been demonstrated that the entire botulinum toxin mol-ecule is not necessary to exert its effects. Rather, small peptide fragments have been shown to inhibit the release of neurotransmitters in a manner similar to the botulinum toxins (5). This discovery has led to the incorporation of these small peptides into cosmeceutical products in an effort to produce the same effects as injectable botulinum toxin in a less-invasive, more cost-effective manner.

All of the neurotransmitter-affecting cosmeceutical peptides currently in the market share similar but distinct mechanisms of action that, like botulinum toxin, impair signal transduction across the neu-romuscular junction. This is done through one of several targets, which disrupt acetylcholine vesicle docking or receptor binding. As a larger signal is required to overcome this inhibition, the threshold for minimal muscle activity required to induce movement is raised. Long-term, subconscious muscle move-ments are thus reduced over time (2). Each of these peptides and their mechanisms of action are outlined in Table 8.1.

Acetyl Hexapeptide-3

The most commonly used neurotransmitter-affecting peptide in cosmeceuticals is acetyl hexapeptide-3 (AC-gly glu-met-gln-arg-arg-NH$_2$). Presently, it is currently marketed as Argireline (McEit [Tianjin] International Trade Co., Ltd.) and is marketed most heavily as a component of eye care products (6). The acetyl hexapeptide-3 has been shown to mimic the N-terminal end of SNAP-25. As a result of this struc-tural similarity, acetyl hexapeptide-3 competes with SNAP-25 for a position in the SNARE complex, which is essential for synaptic vesicle exocystosis and acetylcholine release (7).

In topical formulations, acetyl hexapeptide-3 has been shown to penetrate the skin in vitro (8). With respect to efficacy as an anti-wrinkle treatment, studies to date have shown improvement with daily use. Skin topography analysis of an oil/water (O/W) emulsion containing 10% of acetyl hexapeptide-3 on ten healthy women volunteers reduced wrinkle depth in the lateral orbit up to 30% after 30 days of twice-daily application. These findings were drawn from evaluation of silicone imprints obtained from

TABLE 8.1

Currently Available Neurotransmitter-Affecting Cosmeceutical Peptides

Generic Name	Trade Name	Mechanism of Action
Acetyl hexapeptide-3	Argireline®	Prevents ACh vesicle docking by competing with SNAP-25 for SNARE complex binding
Pentapeptide-3	Vialox®	Blocks signal transduction across NMJ by competitively antagonizing the postsynaptic ACh receptor
Pentapeptide-18	Leuphasyl®	Prevents ACh vesicle fusion by coupling with enkephalin receptor
Tripeptide-3	SYN®-AKE	Blocks signal transduction across NMJ by reversibly antagonizing postsynaptic ACh receptors

Abbreviations: ACh = acetylcholine, NMJ = neuromuscular junction.

all patients at baseline and after treatment, which were analyzed by confocal laser scanning microscopy to assess the skin surface (8).

Pentapeptide-3

Pentapeptide-3 (Gly-Pro-Arg-Pro-Ala), currently marketed as Vialox® (Cellular Skin, Rx), is a peptide derived from snake venom. It is reported to act similarly to tubocurarine, the main active ingredient of curare, a highly toxic and potentially fatal paralytic poison isolated from several plant species (9). Like tubocurarine, pentapeptide-3 is a competitive antagonist of the acetylcholine receptor on the postsynaptic membrane. In the absence of acetylcholine binding, sodium channels fail to open and there is no influx of sodium ions to depolarize the cell and lead to muscle contraction.

Company-led studies have been performed and confirm efficacy in reducing muscle contraction and reducing wrinkle size both in vitro and in vivo. In vitro, muscle contractions were reduced 71% within one minute after treatment and 58% two hours later. In vivo, wrinkle depth was noted to reduce by 49% after 28 days of twice-daily application (10).

Pentapeptide-18

Pentapeptide-18 (Tyr-D-Ala-Gly-Phe-Leu), marketed as Leuphasyl® (Lipotec S.A.), is a lesser known peptide with an anti-wrinkle activity recently introduced into cosmeceuticals. Its mechanism of action is analogous to that of enkephalins, endogenous opioids that inhibit neuronal activity and neurotransmitter release (2). Enkephalin receptors, located on the extracellular neuronal membrane, are coupled to inhibitory G-proteins (Gi). On substrate binding, a signal cascade is activated which ultimately closes calcium ion channels and opens potassium ion channels. In the absence of calcium influx, vesicle fusion and acetylcholine release are inhibited (11). Pentapeptide-18 initiates the same downstream cascade by coupling to the enkephalin receptor and inducing an activating conformational change (2, 11). In vivo and in vitro placebo-controlled cosmeceutical studies performed by the company report efficacy of pentapeptide-18 at reducing neurotransmitter release and decreasing wrinkle depth as assessed by a skin topography analysis of silicon imprints. The studies also showed a synergistic effect when both Leuphasyl® and Argireline were applied together (12).

The efficacy and safety of topical pentapeptide-18 formulations have been studied in recent years. A 2014 study by Drogomirescu et al. evaluated three Leuphasyl emulsions at varying concentrations (0.5%, 1%, and 2%) applied on 20 volunteers for two months, at the level of the eyebrows zone (above the *corrugator supercilii* muscle) and at the periorbital zone (above the *orbicularis oculi* muscle). Wrinkle regression was evaluated using an optical imaging device. The investigators found improvement only with the 2% emulsion, which produced an average reduction in wrinkle trajectory by 34.7% for the eyebrows zone and 28.4% for the periorbital zone (13). A separate, company-supported trial of 43 women evaluated a cream with pentapeptide-18 (0.05%) compared to a cream with acetylhexapeptide-3 (0.05%) and a combination cream of both peptides. Average wrinkle reductions for creams containing pentapeptide-18, acetylhexapeptide-3, and both peptides were 11.64%, 16.26%, and 24.62%, respectively (12). The investigators proposed a synergistic effect for pentapeptide-18 in association with acetylhexapeptide-3.

Tripeptide-3

Tripeptide-3 (β-Ala-Pro-Dab-NHBn-2-Acetate), also named dipeptide diaminobutyroyl benzylamide diacetate, is an anti-aging peptide currently marketed as Syn-Ake (Pentapharm Ltd.) (2). Like other neurotransmitter-affecting cosmeceutical peptides, tripeptide-3 inhibits muscle contraction via blockade of acetylcholine-mediated signal transduction. Its proposed mechanism of action is analogous to waglerin-1, a neurotoxin found in the venom of the temple viper, *Tropidolaemus wagleri*. This neurotoxin serves as a reversible antagonist of nicotinic acetylcholine receptors (mnAChR) on the postsynaptic membrane of muscle fibers (14). In binding the epsilon subunit of mnAChR, acetylcholine is unable to interact with and open the receptor. This prevents sodium influx across the postsynaptic membrane such that depolarization does not occur and the muscle fibers remain relaxed (2, 9).

To date, all trials examining the efficacy of tripeptide-3 have been company-supported. Pentapharm Ltd. first performed an in vitro study, which showed that, at a concentration of 0.5 mM, Syn-Ake reduced the contraction frequency of innervated muscle cells by 82% (p < 0.05) after 2 hours (15). A subsequent study of 45 volunteers compared a cream containing 4% Syn-Ake against a cream containing 10% acetyl hexapeptide-3 and placebo. All participants applied the cream twice-daily for 28 days. The investigators used PRIMOS® (Phaseshift Rapid In-vivo Measurement Of Skin), an optical 3D in vivo skin measurement device, to generate qualitative and quantitative measurements of height profile between the highest peaks and deepest furrows on the forehead. A decrease in the maximum difference between the highest peak and the deepest furrow from baseline suggested an overall decrease in wrinkle depth. The mean difference for tripeptide-3 was found to be −20% compared to 2% for acetyl hexapeptide-3 (p < 0.05). Best results were seen in one participant who demonstrated wrinkle reduction of 52% with tripeptide-3 cream (15).

Conclusion

Despite comparisons to botulinum toxin, no neurotransmitter-affecting cosmeceutical peptide to date has been shown to have the same activity in a published clinical trial.

Overall, research into these peptides is lacking and most available data on efficacy and safety has been drawn from company-led, small-scale trials for which results have not yet been replicated. Consequently, the clinical significance of these data is uncertain and the consistency of these results in different anatomic areas and in patients of variable severity is unclear. As further studies on these peptides are undertaken, entirely new sequences are being investigated. These include SNAP-8, an octapeptide that acts similarly to acetyl hexapeptide-3 and acetyl hexapeptide-30. The latter has been reported to activate muscle-specific kinase (MuSK) by blocking the agrin-binding site and thereby disrupting acetylcholine receptor clustering (1).

Neurotransmitter-affecting peptides as cosmeceuticals is a relatively new market with potential to revolutionize the field of cosmetic dermatology. As our understanding of these peptides and epidermal barrier delivery increase, so will our ability to optimize their effects. In doing so, we may someday be able to offer our patients meaningful anti-aging skin care capable of resolving fine lines and wrinkles to a sufficient degree such that injections of botulinum toxin and their associated side effects are no longer a necessity.

REFERENCES

1) Draelos ZD. *Cosmetics in Dermatology*. 2nd ed. New York: Churchill Livingstone, 1995.
2) Lupo M. Cosmeceutical peptides. Dermatol Surg 2005;31:832–836.
3) Gart MS, Gutowski KA. Overview of botulinum toxins for aesthetic uses. Clin Plast Surg 2016;43(3): 459–471.
4) Yamauchi PS. Selection and preference for botulinum toxins in the management of photoaging and facial lines: Patient and physician considerations. Patient Prefer Adherence 2010;4:345–354.
5) Lima TN, Pedriali Moraes CA. Bioactive peptides: Applications and relevance for cosmeceuticals. Cosmetics 2018;5(1):21
6) Burgess CM. *Cosmetic Dermatology*. Berlin, Heidelberg: Springer-Verlag Berlin Heidelberg, 2005.
7) Gutierrez LM, Viniegra S, Reuda J, et al. A peptide that mimics the C-terminal sequence of SNAP-25 inhibits secretory vesicle docking in chromaffin cells. J Biol Chem 1997;272:2634–2639.
8) Blanes-Mira C, Clemente J, Jodas G, et al. A synthetic hexapeptide (Argireline) with anti-wrinkle activity. Int J Cosmet Sci 2002;24:303–310.
9) Schagen, S.K. Topical peptide treatments with effective anti-aging results. Cosmetics 2017;4:16.
10) Centerchem: Vialox®. http://www.centerchem.com/PDFs/VIALOX20Fact20Sheet.pdf, Basel, Switzerland. Accessed February 20, 2019.
11) Hughes J, Smith TW, Kosterlitz HW, et al. Identification of two related pentapeptides from the brain with potent opiate agonist activity. Nature 1975;258:577–580.

12) Centerchem: Leuphasyl®. http://www.centerchem.com/PDFs/D-Leuphasyl%20w%20stamp.pdf, Barcelona, Spain. Accessed November 08, 2019.

13) Dragomirescu AO, Andoni M, Ionescu D, Andrei F. The efficiency and safety of Leuphasyl—A Botox-like peptide. Cosmetics 2014;1:75–81.

14) McArdle JJ, Lentz TL, Witzemann V, Schwarz H, Weinstein SA, Schmidt JJ. Walglerin-1 selectively blocks the epsilon form of the muscle nicotinic acetylcholine receptor. J Pharm Exp Ther 1999; 289:543–550.

15) Centerchem: Syn®-Ake. http://www.centerchem.com/PDFs/SYN-AKE%20Fact%20Sheet.pdf, Basel, Switzerland. Accessed September 4, 2006.

9

Hyperpigmentation

Hayley Leight and Susan Bard

Introduction

Because hyperpigmentation may have significant psychosocial effects on patients, it is a frequently presented complaint in medical and cosmetic dermatology offices. While many physicians consider hyperpigmentation to be a purely aesthetic complication, there are many dermatologic and systemic conditions that are presented as facial or body dyschromia and it is prudent for the physician to complete a thorough evaluation of cause prior to prescribing treatment agents.

The melanogenesis pathway, while genetically predetermined, is complex and can be affected and upregulated by varying endogenous and exogenous factors, including age, hormones, systemic or local inflammation, and sun exposure [1–3]. Melanogenesis proceeds with the conversion of L-tyrosine to L-DOPA to L-dopaquinone and finally melanin via the action of the key enzyme tyrosinase. Once the melanin is made in melanocytes, it must be packed and processed into melanosomes and transferred to the keratinocytes, a process aided by the G-protein-coupled-receptor, protease-activated receptor 2 (PAR 2) [2]. At any phase in the melanogenesis pathway, upregulation, downregulation, or inhibition can lead to clinical changes in pigmentation. Treatments targeting these steps can thus influence melanin production and clinical outcomes [1, 3–5]. Among the mechanisms used to reduce pigmentation are tyrosinase inhibition (e.g., hydroquinone [HQ], kojic acid [KA], licorice extract, and mulberry) [1, 3–5]; inhibition of melanin/melanosome transport into keratinocytes (e.g., soy and niacinamide) [1, 3–5]; increased epidermal turnover (e.g., α-hydroxyacids and retinoids) [1, 3–5]; anti-inflammatory therapy (CoffeeBerry) [1, 3–5]; and a combination of multiple mechanisms (e.g., retinoids) [4]. Table 9.1 displays common medications/cosmeceuticals by the mechanism of action.

There are many agents to treat hyperpigmentation currently in the market. However, unknown safety profiles, lack of long-term data, and a relative paucity of clinical trials in ethnic patients has led to confusion and discrepancies about best treatments options for differing skin types. While HQ, corticosteroids, and retinoids have long been used as the standard of care in treatment, each of these products is limited by long-term safety concerns and application site irritation or intolerance in some patients. As will be discussed in the chapter, some agents in the market such as the antioxidants, botanical extracts, and synthetic medications have provided early promising results as monotherapies or adjunctive treatments to existing hyperpigmentation regimens. To achieve greater treatment success, recent clinical studies have begun evaluating combination products which target multiple steps in the melanogenesis pathway.

Hyperpigmentation can be a challenging medical complaint, often complicated by relapse and treatment failure. Having strong foundational knowledge in natural and synthetic treatment options will benefit an astute practitioner in managing this frequently occurring clinical problem.

Tyrosinase Inhibition

Hydroquinone

HQ, considered to be the gold standard treatment for melasma, is one of the most widely used prescription medications for treating pigmentation disorders. HQ competes with tyrosine for the catalytic

DOI: 10.1201/9781315165905-9

TABLE 9.1

Prescription/Cosmeceutical Agent by the Mechanism of Action

Tyrosinase Inhibition	Inhibition of Melanin/ Melanosome Transport	Increased Epidermal Turnover	Anti-Inflammatory Agents	Other
Aloesin	Niacinamide	Alpha hydroxy acids	CoffeeBerry	Tranexamic acid
Arbutin	Soy	Lactic acid	Ferulic acid	Linoleic acid
Ascorbic acid		Retinol		N-Acetyl-4-S-
Azelaic acid				cysteaminylphenol
Ellagic acid				
Glabridin				
Hydroquinone				
Kojic acid				
Mg Ascorbic phosphate				
N-Acetyl glucosamine				
Mulberry				
Hexylresorcinol				
Cinnamic acid				
Coumaric acid				
Gentisic acid				
Mequinol				
Glutathione				

enzyme tyrosinase, preventing the conversion step from L-tyrosine to L-Dopa and thus decreasing melanin production [6].

An early study by Amer and Metwalli demonstrated the efficacy of HQ as monotherapy [7]. Seventy patients with combinations of melasma, freckles, and post-inflammatory hyperpigmentation (PIH) were instructed to use 4% HQ and sunscreen twice daily for 12 weeks. While the sample size was moderate, findings noted that 89% and 75% of patients had good to excellent responses with melasma and PIH, respectively [7]. Importantly, most patients had local irritation from the HQ, but no ochronosis was seen. Haddad et al. performed a double-blind, randomized prospective clinical study comparing 4% HQ to placebo in one group and a skin-whitening complex (SWC) to placebo in the second [8]. Using a qualitative analysis of skin-whitening effects with independent investigator evaluations and patient questionnaire, findings noted a 76.9% improvement in the treatment group using HQ as a skin bleaching agent. However, an itchy eruption was noted in 25% of the HQ group [8].

The tolerability of HQ and the long-term safety concerns remain a few of the disadvantages of this medication. The most common adverse effects include mild skin irritation, erythema, pruritus, and burning; these are more common with the 4% prescription HQ than the over-the-counter 2% HQ concentrations [6]. Exogenous ochronosis which presents as a bluish/black macules and patches, erythema, or small papules, most commonly found on the face, is another complication of long-term use of HQ containing skin-lightening creams [9]. A pivotal six-year clinical study on a sample of more than 800 patients was conducted by Bentley-Phillips and Bayles [10] to determine an optimal and safe concentration for HQ. Their study found that 3% HQ or less produced negligible adverse effects irrespective of skin type [10].

Other chronic use adverse effects that are attributed to HQ include pigmented colloid milium, sclera and nail pigmentation, decreased elasticity, and impaired wound healing [11]. Perhaps the most concerning to the public, however, is the association of HQ with DNA damage and subsequent carcinogenesis. The studies on carcinogenicity were performed with parenteral and oral HQ administration however, and similar carcinogenesis has not been seen with topical preparations [11]. Because of the potential for adverse effects, careful medical supervision and limited duration of use are important in using HQ-based treatments. Some physicians propose taking "drug free" holidays – either stopping treatment completely for a short duration of time or using a non-HQ-containing cosmeceutical in the interim.

The above-noted adverse effects notwithstanding, HQ has continued to demonstrate efficacy in treating hyperpigmentation. More recent clinical studies compare botanical or synthetic agents directly with HQ to assess skin-lightening effectiveness; additionally, researchers are exploring synergistic responses of HQ with newer agents.

Aloesin

Aloesin, derived from the aloe plant, provides a topical skin-depigmenting agent that acts via inhibition of tyrosinase in murine, mushroom, and human sources [12, 13]. Additionally, tyrosine hydroxylase and 3,4-dihydroxyphenylalanine (DOPA) oxidase are also inhibited by aloesin in a dose-dependent manner giving the product multiple mechanisms for decreasing pigment production [12, 13].

Few studies have been performed that demonstrate the depigmenting ability of aloesin. Choi et al. [14] applied aloesin and arbutin independently as well as together against a control group on previously UV-irradiated volar forearm skin [14]. When compared against controls, findings noted pigment suppression with both aloesin and arbutin and a synergistic response when the two products were combined [14]. Jin et al. [15] hypothesized this synergy as likely derived from the differing mechanisms of action: aloesin as a non-competitive tyrosinase inhibitor and arbutin as a competitive inhibitor [15].

Arbutin

Arbutin represents another effective over-the-counter botanical agent acting via inhibition of the tyrosinase pathway and melanosome maturation [16]. Arbutin is a glycosylated derivative of HQ and can be found readily in bearberry flora (*Arctostaphylos uva-ursi*) and in the dried foliage of cranberry and blueberry plants, wheat, and pears [3, 4, 16]. Small clinical studies have shown efficacy of arbutin in treating hyperpigmentation. Among these was an investigation by Ertam et al. [17] in which ten patients with melasma had their pigmentation measured using a Mexameter®. After using 1% arbutin gel for six months, all ten patients showed significant improvement from baseline melanin level [17].

Deoxyarbutin (dA), a synthetic form of arbutin, represents a newer, more potent OTC treatment with an enhanced tyrosinase activity [18]. Boissy et al. [18] demonstrated the product's efficacy in a clinical trial with 34 Caucasian and 16 mixed ethnicity (dark skin subset) individuals, using 3% dA for a 12-week time frame. The study showed significant overall skin lightening and resolution of solar lentigenes in the Caucasian study group but modest, insignificant results in ethnic subjects [18].

Serratulae quinquefolia, a β-anomer of arbutin, was evaluated in a double-blind randomized control trial on 102 women with melasma and solar lentigenes [19]. Women in the treatment group applied cream compounded with the aqueous extract from the leaves of the five-leaf Serratula (active ingredient of 2.51% arbutin) twice a day for eight weeks; those in the control group applied the same cream without the active ingredient. Skin was assessed with a video dermatoscope and a probe Mexameter. Findings showed that for both clinical conditions, a significant decrease in the mean levels of melanin was demonstrated in the treatment group compared to placebo [19].

Ascorbic Acid

Ascorbic acid (AsA), also known as vitamin C, is another common agent used in cosmeceuticals. While a poor choice for skin-lightening monotherapy, AsA is often combined with other agents, such as soy or licorice extracts in multi-targeted skin therapeutics [16].

AsA plays multiple roles mechanistically to inhibit hyperpigmentation. AsA can interact with copper ions to reduce o-quinones, rendering tyrosinase and the melanogenesis process halted until all AsA is oxidized. Additionally, AsA reduces pre-oxidized melanin, changing the color from black to tan [20, 21]. Other properties of AsA include photoprotection, antioxidant production, drug metabolizing, and collagen synthesis [20, 21].

The downfall of AsA is instability—it rapidly oxidizes and decomposes in aqueous solutions [21, 22]. Hence, it leads to the creation of magnesium-l-ascorbyl-2-phosphate (MAP) [21, 22].

Magnesium-l-Ascorbyl-2-Phosphate

While both AsA and MAP have demonstrated clinical utility in multiple research studies, unlike AsA, MAP is stable in aqueous solutions. When acted upon by skin phosphatases to release L-ascorbic acid, the above-noted skin-lightening and protecting benefits may be realized [21].

In a split-face study with 16 female patients, a comparison was made of 4% HQ versus 5% AsA cream nightly for 16 weeks. While AsA led to improvement in over half of the participants, it was significantly less effective than HQ. However, unlike HQ, AsA was extremely well tolerated by patients with minimal side effects [20].

Kameyama et al. [21] studied the effects of MAP on hyperpigmentation as judged by a color difference meter. Results showed an effective or fairly effective improvement in 19 of 34 patients tested with hyperpigmented skin disease and similar improvement parameters in 3 of 25 patients with healthy skin [21].

Recent studies have used topical AsA as a supplement to other regimens. For example, multiple clinical trials have shown a benefit in skin pigmentation when AsA or MAP were used as adjuvant treatment modalities with trichloroacetic acid peels in melasma patients [23, 24]. While the skin-lightening results with AsA monotherapy may be modest, they do represent a promising and safe adjuvant therapy to other hyperpigmentation treatment regimens.

Azelaic Acid

Azelaic acid (AzA) has been shown to have multiple effects that can influence hyperpigmentation. AzA is anti-inflammatory, anti-bacterial, and anti-keratinizing, antioxidant, as well as a competitive inhibitor of tyrosinase [6, 25]. Multiple studies have noted the positive effects of AzA on skin hyperpigmentation and the treatment of melasma [26–28]. AzA has been shown to be an effective agent in the treatment of hyperpigmentation, comparing favorably with HQ in decreasing pigmentation and minimizing side effects. An early, double-blind study by Verallo-Rowell et al. compared 20% AzA and 2% HQ creams in more than 150 patients with melasma [29]. AzA outperformed the HQ cream in decreasing pigment intensity scores, reducing lesion size, and having a favorable therapeutic response [6, 29].

In a split-face clinical trial of 42 women aged 18–65, a comparison of 50% glycolic acid (GA) peel with a combination peeling agent which comprised 20% AzA, 10% resorcinol, and 6% phytic acid showed similar clinical efficacy in treating hyperpigmentation [30]. Importantly, the glycolic peel was statistically more likely to cause side effects (burning sensation that lasted for a few days and dyspigmentation) than the combination agent with AzA [30]. In a more recent clinical study on melasma, the addition of glycolic peels to a 20% topical AzA cream enhanced the therapeutic efficacy of the AzA cream and improved patient quality of life indices [31].

Ellagic Acid

Ellagic acid (EA) is a powerful botanical antioxidant that can be found in strawberries, blackberries, pomegranates, grapes, eucalyptus, and walnuts [3, 17, 32, 33]. Yoshimura's research on EA's rich pomegranate extract demonstrated that oral EA has the potential to result in skin whitening [33]. The lightening effects were hypothesized to occur via the inhibition of proliferating melanocytes and EA's copper-dependent inhibition of the tyrosinase enzyme, a theory advanced by others as well [32, 33].

Unique to EA is its non-melanotoxic effect rendering reversibility to the skin-whitening effect when the medication is stopped; this is in comparison to HQ, which is known to be melanotoxic and can lead to permanent depigmentation [32]. Studies on the brownish guinea pig demonstrated the efficacy of EA on skin whitening to be superior to that of arbutin and KA at the same 1% dose [32].

In a small 30-person sample comparing topical arbutin to synthetic EA and natural EA in the treatment of melasma, post-treatment levels of melanin as measured by the Mexameter were significantly decreased across all groups. Natural EA's whitening ability was found to be equally efficacious to that of the more well-known arbutin [17].

A double-blind clinical study with 54 multi-ethnic participants showed comparable skin depigmentation using a topical combination of 0.5% EA/0.1% salicylic acid compared to twice daily 4% HQ in early treatment; however, HQ was found to be more consistent in continuing to decrease hyperpigmentation at the two- and three-month treatment phase [34]. Of note, the EA topical combination was found to be superior aesthetically by subjective patient data [34]. This antioxidative, non-melanotoxic compound provides another safe alternative for the hyperpigmentation treatment toolbox.

Glabridin

Licorice extract from the root of the *Glycyrrhiza glabra* (*G. glabra*) has been touted throughout history as a folktale treatment for numerous medical ailments with antiviral, anti-inflammatory, and even anti-tumor and anti-ulcer properties [35]. While the hydrophilic constituents, glycyrrhizin and glycyrrhetic acids, are known to be anti-inflammatory, licorice's role in reducing hyperpigmentation relies heavily on the hydrophobic portion of the licorice extract, which comprised primarily the component, glabridin. In vitro studies performed by Yokota et al. [36] noted that glabridin works by inhibiting a tyrosinase activity, specifically the activity of the T1 and T3 tyrosinase isozymes. Their work also showed improvement in UVB-induced skin hyperpigmentation on the backs of brown guinea pigs after topical application of 0.5% glabridin for a period of three weeks. Additional results noted a significant inhibition of superoxide anion production and cyclooxygenase activity (COX) with the use of glabridin [36]. This finding was later supported by the work of Chandrasekaran et al. [35] who showed that the dual inhibitory effect of *G. glabra* on both cyclooxygenase and lipoxygenase activities is largely dependent on the constituent glabridin as compared to the other components present in *G. glabra* extract [35].

Kojic Acid

KA, a metabolic derivative produced by multiple fungi, including Acetoacetic, Aspergillus, and Penicillium, plays its role in reducing hyperpigmentation via copper chelation and subsequent direct tyrosinase inhibition [37–39]. Distinct from this mechanism of action however, newer research has also shown KA to act independently at the level of the keratinocyte/melanocyte paracrine regulation to influence melanogenic activity [40].

KA preparations, ranging in concentration from 1% to 4%, have been shown to have irritating and cytotoxic side effects, including erythema and contact dermatitis [39, 41]. Few relatively small clinical studies have shown efficacy of KA both in combination with other preparations and in monotherapy. An earlier clinical study by Garcia and Fulton [42], utilizing a split-face comparison of 39 patients, compared 2% KA/5% GA with 2% HQ/5% GA. Findings showed comparable efficacy of the two preparations without significant differences in outcome [42]. Another small 40 person split-face study by Lim [41] showed an improvement, albeit lacking statistical significance, when KA was added to a preparation of 10% GA and 2% HQ compared to the control group lacking the KA additive [41].

However, not all available data on KA are promising. In a more recent comparison, Monteiro et al. [43] report a small clinical trial of 60 patients comparing traditional 4% HQ with 0.75% KA cream (combination of 0.75% KA + 2.5% vitamin C) for the treatment of facial melasma. Results showed that the KA preparation was statistically inferior in treating hyperpigmentation as compared to HQ [43]. Because GA is commonly used to increase the penetration potential of the KA, this is an area of research interest [1].

N-Acetylglucosamine (NAG)

NAG is an amino sugar occurring in all human tissues which is a stable derivative of glucosamine. Glucosamine has been shown to inhibit the enzymatic glycosylation that converts pro-tyrosinase to the active tyrosinase enzyme, the key player in the melanogenesis pathway [44]. Glucosamines are also known to be antioxidative and anti-inflammatory. Perhaps even more interesting, works by Bissett [44] and others have now shown that NAG has the ability to alter (upregulate or downregulate) different pigment-related genes. A combination of these mechanisms likely underlies NAG's influence on skin pigmentation [44].

Bissett [45] has reported multiple clinical trials demonstrating clinical utility of NAG, both as monotherapy and in combination. In an eight-week, double-blind, placebo-controlled, split-face study on Japanese female subjects, 2% NAG outperformed the control in reducing hyperpigmentation [45]. Using a similar research design, the investigators examined the effect of combining 2% NAG with 4% niacinamide in a sample of healthy Caucasian females. Findings noted that the combined effect on hyperpigmentation was even more substantial [45]. Recently, a ten-week, double-blind, placebo-controlled, full-face, parallel-group clinical study conducted in women aged 40–60 years compared a moisturizing cream containing 4% niacinamide and 2% NAG versus control and showed statistically significant reduction in facial spots and appearance of pigmentation [46].

Mulberry

A member of the Moraceae family, mulberry leaves (*Morus alba*) contain many nutritional and medicinal components, including an anti-hyperglycemic effect in diabetic mice. In vitro research of the active ingredient Mulberroside F has demonstrated an ability to inhibit tyrosinase, provide superoxide scavenging activity, and inhibit melanin production in cultured Melan-A cells [47], making mulberry extract an excellent skin-lightening agent. Alvin et al. [48] conducted one randomized, single-blind, placebo-controlled trial of 50 patients with melasma and demonstrated improvement in MASI score, Mexameter reading, and melasma quality of life scores (MelasQOL) when using a 75% mulberry extract oil compared to placebo over an eight-week treatment course [48, 49].

Hexylresorcinol

Hexylresorcinol, used in shrimp processing to prevent "black spot" shrimp melanosis [50], is a well-known antiseptic and anesthetic [50, 51]. It is also a competitive tyrosinase inhibitor, making it an ideal primary or adjuvant treatment when considering hyperpigmentation [52]. While no clinical trials evaluate hexylresorcinol as a single agent for hyperpigmentation, its use in novel combination lightening creams has been noted. Multiple small-scale studies have used hexylresorcinol-containing skin-lightening products in the treatment of hyperpigmentation with reassuring results [51, 52]. However, given that the treatment arm in both studies contained combinations of multiple well-known lightening agents, it is impossible to delineate the contribution of hexylresorcinol alone.

Cinnamic Acid and Coumaric Acid

Cinnamic acid and derivatives, major components of the *Cinnamomum cassia* BLUME, are touted to be potent antioxidant, anti-inflammatory, and anticancer agents. Moreover, it was determined that cinnamic acid and its derivatives are potent mixed-type inhibitors of tyrosinase in early research studies and could be helpful agents for treating hyperpigmentation [53]. More recent clinical research has expanded and confirmed earlier studies showing both a dose-dependent inhibition of tyrosinase activity and a reduced expression of tyrosinase in cinnamic acid-treated Melan-A cells. Further, when tested on UVB-induced hyperpigmentation of brown guinea pig skin, the agent showed a skin-depigmenting effect [54].

Cinnamic acid has many derivatives that also benefit from melanogenesis inhibitory properties. Among these derivatives, P-Coumaric acid (PCA) and feurilic acid (discussed later in this chapter) are the more commonly used and discussed cosmeceuticals [55]. PCA, a hydroxy derivative of cinnamic acid, is made from tyrosine and phenylalanine and can be found in fruits, vegetables, cereals, and mushrooms [55]. Multiple studies have shown that PCA can effectively inhibit melanogenesis in murine melanoma cells [56, 57]. This led to further research by Song et al. [58] in a head-to-head skin permeation study comparing PCA to methyl p-coumarate (MPC) in a cream base. Authors reported superior permeability of the amphiphilic PCA when compared to the hydrophobic MPC, rendering it a more suitable agent for transdermal drug delivery. Additionally, PCA was superior to MPC in attenuating UVB-induced erythema and pigmentation on mouse models [58].

PCA efficacy was further tested in a small human clinical trial with 21 patients, Fitzpatrick skin types III and IV, on its effects when applied before and after UV-exposed human skin. The authors reported that the application of PCA was able to reduce UV-induced erythema and subsequent pigmentation in the skin [59]. While these results promise good potential for these agents, there remains a paucity of human clinical data testing the true efficacy of cinnamic acid and its derivatives in treating hyperpigmentation.

Gentisic Acid

Gentisic acid (GA), a competitive tyrosinase inhibitor, found in the root of *Gentiana*, is another safe agent for treating skin hyperpigmentation [60, 61]. In a study examining GA and its alkyl esters, methyl gentisate (MG) proved superior to other GA esters, retaining its tyrosinase inhibitory activity, with relatively less cytogenic and mutagenic properties [62].

Further comparative evaluation studies of GA ester derivatives by Ma et al. [60] reported MG to have the highest skin permeation rate in mouse models; however, GA was reported to have the least cytotoxicity and the greatest effect on tyrosinase inhibition [60]. Both data for GA and MG have rendered them potential candidates for skin-lightening agents, but no head-to-head clinical studies on patients have been performed to date.

Mequinol

An alternative to the more traditional HQ for treating hyperpigmentation is the product 4-hydroxyanisole, better known as mequinol. While the mechanism of action of mequinol is not well understood, it is thought to be a competitive inhibitor of tyrosinase [63]. Much of the clinical data on mequinol combines the product into a topical solution with 2% mequinol and 0.01% tretinoin. Multiple clinical trials have shown efficacy of this combination in treating solar lentigenes and one case series showed positive treatment outcomes in male patients with melasma [64–67]. In a large, randomized parallel-group study of 216 patients comparing a 2% mequinol/0.01% tretinoin solution with topical 3% HQ applied twice daily for 16 weeks, the combination product showed superior efficacy when treating solar lentigenes on the arms and similar efficacy for facial lesions [68].

Glutathione

Glutathione has been touted as a "wonder drug" for skin lightening and treatment of hyperpigmentation in the media. Among its many postulated mechanisms of action, inhibition of tyrosinase and potent-free radical scavenging activity support its efficacy in treating hyperpigmentation disorders [69]. Glutathione is currently being dispensed topically, orally as well as parenterally for these conditions—although few studies and small numbers of patient cohorts support this use. Based on clinical data, the reduced form of glutathione, GSH, seems to be more critical for skin-lightening properties than the oxidized form, GSSG [69].

Arjinpathana and Asawanonda [70] performed a double-blind placebo-controlled study on 60 healthy students with oral glutathione 500 mg daily in two divided doses for four weeks. Results were substantial with melanin index scoring improved in the GSH group as compared to placebo in all sites studied as well as remarkable tolerability of the medication [69, 70]. A similar trial by Handog et al. [71] gave a 500 mg buccal lozenge daily for eight weeks to 30 healthy women, with Fitzpatrick skin type IV or V. Lozenge delivery of the medication also showed statistically significant melanin index reduction in the treatment group over placebo and good patient tolerability of the lozenge [69, 71].

Watanabe et al. [72] performed a split-face study with 30 Filipino women, comparing a topical 2% GSSG lotion versus placebo with twice daily application over ten weeks. Results showed a significant Mexameter MX 18 melanin index reduction in the GSSG group as well as high patient tolerability of the product [69, 72].

Zubair et al. [73] evaluated the efficacy of intravenous GSH, in a small placebo-controlled study of 50 Pakistani female patients; those in the GSH treatment group received 1,200 mg IV GSH biweekly for six weeks compared to normal saline administration in the placebo group [73]. All patients had adverse outcomes – unspecified liver dysfunction developed in eight patients and anaphylactic shock in one patient. No data were provided on the patient's renal or thyroid function pre- or post-treatment [69, 73]. Analysis of the research by outside authors has pointed out multiple study design flaws and questions whether this data should be used as a basis for recommending intravenous glutathione to treat hyperpigmentation [69].

While the use of oral and topical glutathione seems to be promising, there are no data to support long-term efficacy of these medications. Parenteral administration of glutathione has minimal supporting clinical evidence and can be associated with severe and life-altering adverse effects. In addition to liver dysfunction noted in Zubair's [73] study above, other potential side effects from intravenous glutathione include cutaneous skin rashes, abdominal pain, thyroid and kidney dysfunction, and any complications from IV injections of medications [69]. More evidence and longer clinical studies are needed to determine if glutathione should be used in patients with hyperpigmentation and the best route and dose to achieve maximal clinical treatment success with a minimal risk.

Inhibition of Melanin/Melanosome Transport into Keratinocytes

The next section of botanical agents works via a different mechanism of action: inhibiting transport of the pigment-containing melanosomes to the epidermal keratinocytes [74].

Soy

Filled with biologically active isoflavones, flavonoids, tannins, vitamin E and serine proteinase inhibitors, soy and soy extracts have become a mainstay in the cosmetic industry [75, 76]. While the soy plant's existence in the United States dates back to the early 18th century, soybeans were actually first domesticated by Chinese farmers in 1100 BC [75]. Recent advances in science have identified the mechanism of action for its numerous medical benefits, including improving skin tone, photoaging, and skin lightening [76]. Soy protein has been shown to provide potent anti-inflammatory and antioxidant effects, protection from UV irradiation, increased elastin and collagen production, and clinically improved skin lightening [76]. The value of soy products in cosmetic moisturizers and whitening products is likely the result of an amalgamation of these numerous biologic processes.

Regarding skin coloration, keratinocytes derive their pigmentation from the phagocytosis of melanosomes from melanocytes, a process regulated in part by the proteinase activated receptor-2 (PAR-2) pathway. Soybean is rich in protease inhibitors, such as the Bowman-Birk inhibitor or the soybean trypsin inhibitor, which can interfere with the PAR-2 pathway [74]. Decreasing the keratinocyte's melanosome concentration via pathway interruption yields a clinical skin-whitening effect and the cosmetic pharmaceutical target [3, 74, 75]. Work by Huang et al. [77] has also shown that non-denatured soymilk can be used preventatively to decrease the deleterious effects of UVB irradiation and decrease UVB-induced skin carcinogenesis [75, 77].

Multiple double-blind controlled trials have shown soy's impact on hyperpigmentation. Serving as their own controls, Pierard et al. [78] examined the effect of soy extract on 16 Hispanic women with melasma. All but two of the subjects showed improvement with the average reduction of 12% in hyperpigmentation [3, 75, 78]. In a somewhat larger study of 63 women, soy bean moisturizer containing serine protease inhibitors was shown to improve pigmentation, fine lines, dullness, skin texture, blotchiness, and overall skin tone when compared to vehicle-only controls after a 12-week application period [79]. Almost all patients in the soy moisturizer group (28 of 31) had decreased pigmentation compared to approximately half in the vehicle control group (17 of 32). Decreased pigmentation in the latter group was attributed to seasonal changes [75, 79]. While other studies [80–82] have noted similar findings regarding the utility of soy for skin lightening, and the evidence to date has indicated that these produces are safe alternatives for treating hyperpigmentation, larger clinical studies comparing soy to other prescription depigmenting agents are currently unavailable.

Niacinamide

Niacinamide is a natural botanical compound found in many fruits, vegetables, and seeds and is the active form of vitamin B3. Niacinamide is well tolerated by the skin unlike other members of this vitamin family. Multiple studies have shown that niacinamide works by reversible inhibition of the transfer of melanosomes to keratinocytes and decreases melanogenesis by interfering in the communication between keratinocytes and melanocytes [4, 83, 84]. Niacinamide has little inhibitory effects on tyrosinase itself [83, 84].

Multiple clinical trials have demonstrated the effects of niacinamide on skin lightening. Hakozaki et al. [84] performed a double-blind split-face study on 18 Japanese women with hyperpigmentation. Results showed that the 5% niacinamide moisturizer was significantly better than vehicle in decreasing hyperpigmentation after four weeks of clinical use [84]. In a recent ten-week study, 207 Indian women were randomized into the use of test lotion with 4% niacinamide, 0.5% panthenol, and 0.5% tocopheryl acetate versus a control lotion. The test lotion group experienced significantly reduced appearance of hyperpigmentation, and improved skin tone evenness and texture [85]. Similarly, Navarrete-Solis et al. [82] found that niacinamide had similar colorimetric measurements, decreased inflammation and improved solar elastosis, and had fewer side effects in a split-face study comparing 4% HQ to 4% niacinamide. More recent clinical trials are adding niacinamide to other known brightening agents; positive effects on skin lightening and hyperpigmentation are being documented [51, 86, 87]. To date, evidence supports the use of niacinamide as a safe and effective treatment for hyperpigmentation either as monotherapy or in combination with other agents.

Increased Epidermal Turnover

Alpha Hydroxy Acids

Alpha hydroxy acids, such as GA or lactic acid (LA), are commonly used monotherapies in skin care as well as additives to many cosmeceutical products. These products affect pigmentation by increasing the rate of epidermal turnover, thus causing the pigment to disperse more evenly [3]. In addition, Usuki et al. [88] demonstrated that GA and LA can also cause a direct inhibition of tyrosinase enzyme activity, independent of the acidic nature of the products [3, 88].

While often used as components of cream-based treatments, the alpha hydroxy acids are also common peeling agents. Multiple studies have shown efficacy of alpha hydroxy acids in treating melasma and other pigmentary disorders [27, 42, 89, 90].

In a recent study on periorbital melanosis, repetitive GA peels were found to be more effective than repetitive LA peels and both were more effective than daily 20% topical vitamin C [91]. The occurrence of adverse effects corresponded to relative product efficacy; the highest incidence of undesirable outcomes was noted in subjects receiving GA peels [91].

Recent clinical trials are showing the efficacy of the alpha hydroxy acids when used with other agents. Thirty Indian patients with Fitzpatrick skin types III–V and facial PIH demonstrated improvement in an objective hyperpigmentation scoring system among those receiving both serial GA peels and a topical regimen containing HQ 2%, tretinoin 0.05%, and hydrocortisone 1% versus those receiving the topical regimen alone [92]. This study supports the data from other clinical research that alpha hydroxy acids are safe and efficacious additions to other pigment treatments regimens [92].

Retinoids

Derivatives of vitamin A, the retinoids such as retinol and retinoic acid, have a long and successful history in treating hyperpigmentation. The mechanism of action of retinoids on melanogenesis and pigment production is multi-faceted. Retinoids cause tyrosinase inhibition, decrease melanosome transfer to keratinocytes, and increase epidermal turnover, melanin dispersion, and pigment loss [3, 6, 11].

A 40-week study on Caucasian melasma patients by Griffiths et al. [93] comparing topical 0.1% tretinoin versus vehicle resulted in significantly lightened areas of melasma and a histological decrease in epidermal pigmentation in the tretinoin-treated patients [93]. Similarly, in a ten-month clinical trial by Kimbrough-Green et al. [94], African American patients with moderate-to-severe melasma showed similar colorimetric lightening toward normal skin color and decreased epidermal pigmentation on histology with tretinoin treatment versus vehicle [94].

The most common side effects of retinoids include application site erythema, stinging, desquamation, xerosis, and a paradoxical hyperpigmentation in a subset of patients [6, 11]. Retinoids have been successfully used in treatment combinations with topical steroids and HQ, where the retinoic acid works synergistically to decrease steroid-induced atrophy risk and enhance the penetration of HQ [11].

Anti-Inflammatory Agents

CoffeeBerry

CoffeeBerry™ extract (CBE) is a trade name, referring to a number of antioxidants that are harvested from the coffee plant fruit, from *Coffea arabica*. Among the antioxidants harvested for CBE from the coffee plant fruit prior to ripening (when the levels of antioxidants are highest) are chlorogenic acid, quinic acid, proanthrocyanidins, and ferulic acid [95, 96]. Clinical and scientific research into CBE has shown the extract to potentiate gene expression for collagen proteins and downregulate gene expression for matrix metalloproteinases and other inflammatory mediators, all key processes in the photoaging process [97].

In the pilot test study on 30 female patients (20 full-face and 10 split-face), CBE extract was applied topically for six weeks [0.1% cleanser; a 1% day cream (also containing 7.5% octinate and 4% oxybenzone); and a 1% night cream]. Findings noted that the topical treatments led to improvement in wrinkles and fine lines, hyperpigmentation, and an overall total improvement. Specifically, for hyperpigmentation (as graded by blinded experts), the full-face patients had a mean of 25% improvement in pigmentation; in the split-face patients, the CBE side showed greater improvement in pigmentation from baseline as compared to the vehicle side (15% to 5%) [11, 97].

Ferulic Acid

Ferulic acid (4-hydroxy-3-methoxycinnamic acid) is ubiquitous in botany and can be found in seeds, fruits, vegetables, and wheats such as barley and oats. Ferulic acid is a potent antioxidant with a radical scavenging ability. It is also a strong UV absorber, lending a photoprotective effect and inhibiting damaging free radical reactions. For these reasons, it is often used as an active ingredient in cosmeceuticals [98]. Ferulic acid can also act synergistically with other antioxidants such as α-tocopherol, β-carotene, and AsA to protect cells from damaging free radicals [99]. Clinically, when added to a topical solution of 15% L-ascorbic acid and 1% α-tocopherol, ferulic acid was able to lend increased chemical stability to the solution and improve photoprotection from solar irradiation superior to that of vitamins C and E in combination or ferulic acid solution as monotherapy [100]. While human clinical trials are presently lacking, utilizing the synergy of these products would likely provide clinically apparent advantages in photoaging, UV-induced skin carcinogenesis, and pigmentary appearance of the skin.

Other Mechanism of Action

Tranexamic Acid

Tranexamic acid (TXA), a plasmin inhibitor, has recently emerged as a new pharmaceutical for melasma—in both oral and topical preparations. Basic science research by Maeda and Tomita [101] has shown that TXA can inhibit melanin synthesis by interfering with the melanin stimulatory signal from the keratinocytes via the plasminogen/plasmin system [101, 102]. Additionally, TXA can inhibit the UV-induced plasmin activity in keratinocytes by preventing the binding of the plasminogen to keratinocytes. This, in turn, decreases the conversion of arachidonic acid to prostaglandins, a potent melanogenesis-promoting byproduct [102, 103].

Comprehensive reviews on the literature using TXA for melasma have shown that even low doses (i.e., 500 mg oral daily) over a period of two to three months can show efficacy in treating melasma resistant to gold standard treatments [102]. Clinical studies that have evaluated the efficacy of oral TXA have ranged from 500 mg to 1.5 g daily dosing and a time period of one month to six months [102, 104]. Gastrointestinal discomfort and menstrual irregularities were some of the more common side effects overall, though rare embolic or thrombotic events have occurred [104]. It is imperative to do a comprehensive evaluation to rule out any contraindications a patient may have prior to using oral TXA for melasma or hyperpigmentation treatment. While small clinical studies with topical TXA have shown improvement [105–107], there are not currently direct comparison studies of oral versus topical preparations of TXE.

Linoleic Acid

Unsaturated fatty acids, such as linoleic acid (LA) and α-linolenic acid, are useful in the treatment of hyperpigmentation. LA combats hyperpigmentation by suppressing melanin production from melanocytes independent of its ability to increase epidermal desquamation, making it a useful botanical treatment adjuvant [108]. Further biochemical research suggests that LA accelerates the degradation of tyrosinase enzyme likely via regulating proteasomal degradation [109]. Importantly, LA works best when delivered in a liposomal formulation to increase transdermal penetration and efficacy [110].

In a six-week double-blind randomized controlled clinical trial for melasma, nightly topical application of a combined product with lincomycin (LM), LA, and betamethasone valerate (BV) proved superior to a topical combination of LM and BV alone [111]. In another more recent study on Asian females, LA was used in a brightening complex cream, along with other agents discussed in this chapter—niacinamide, TXA, oxyresveratrol, and glutathione disulfide. The novel brightening cream was applied twice per day for 12 weeks to 26 Korean female patients. Results showed a statistically significant decrease in melanin index by eight weeks and an improvement in erythema index by 12 weeks, as well as favorable subjective improvement from patients and investigators alike [87]. While more clinical comparison trials are needed, preliminary data would suggest that LA is a useful adjunct for treating hyperpigmentation.

N-acetyl-4-S-Cysteaminylphenol

In the early 1990s, *N*-acetyl-4-S-cysteaminylphenol was studied as a novel depigmenting agent. Working as a substrate for the enzyme tyrosinase, *N*-acetyl-4-S-cysteaminylphenol only affects active melanin synthesizing melanocytes [112]. One retrospective case series of 12 patients applied a topical 4% *N*-acetyl-4-S-cysteaminylphenol in oil-in-water emulsion twice daily for up to six months. All patients showed improvement—eight patients with marked improvement, three patients with moderate improvement, and one patient had complete clearance. Side effects were minimal; one patient developed acneiform eruptions [112]. To our knowledge, no further studies have been performed with this agent in treating hyperpigmentation.

In conclusion, today's consumer increasingly demands skin care products derived from natural ingredients with less toxic properties than their synthetic counterparts. This trend has cultivated interest in identifying bioactive compounds derived from natural sources for use as cosmeceutical agents. In particular, significant attention has been given to topical formulations with skin-depigmenting effects, in large part because hyperpigmentation disorders are common afflictions among adults of all races.

This chapter has reviewed both frequently used prescription depigmenting agents as well as newer cosmeceutical agents for their mechanism of action and utility in treating pigmentary disorders. This area of inquiry holds much promise for the future.

REFERENCES

1. Alexis AF and P. Blackcloud, *Natural ingredients for darker skin types: growing options for hyperpigmentation.* J Drugs Dermatol, 2013. **12**(9 Suppl): p. s123–7.
2. Dadzie, O.E., A. Petit, and A.F. Alexis, *Ethnic Dermatology: Principles and Practice.* 2013, Wiley-Blackwell: Chichester, West Sussex, U.K.
3. Gonzalez, N. and M. Perez, *Natural cosmeceutical ingredients for hyperpigmentation.* J Drugs Dermatol, 2016. **15**(1): p. 26–34.
4. Leyden, J.J., et al., *Natural options for the management of hyperpigmentation.* J Eur Acad Dermatol Venereol, 2011. **25**(10): p. 1140–5.
5. Thornfeldt, C., R.L. Rizer, and N.S. Trookman, *Blockade of melanin synthesis, activation and distribution pathway by a nonprescription natural regimen is equally effective to a multiple prescription-based therapeutic regimen.* J Drugs Dermatol, 2013. **12**(12): p. 1449–54.

6. Gupta, A.K., et al., *The treatment of melasma: a review of clinical trials.* J Am Acad Dermatol, 2006. **55**(6): p. 1048–65.

7. Amer, M. and M. Metwalli, *Topical hydroquinone in the treatment of some hyperpigmentary disorders.* Int J Dermatol, 1998. **37**(6): p. 449–50.

8. Haddad, A.L., et al., *A clinical, prospective, randomized, double-blind trial comparing skin whitening complex with hydroquinone versus. placebo in the treatment of melasma.* Int J Dermatol, 2003. **42**(2): p. 153–6.

9. Bhattar, P.A., et al., *Exogenous ochronosis.* Indian J Dermatol, 2015. **60**(6): p. 537–43.

10. Bentley-Phillips, B. and M.A. Bayles, *Cutaneous reactions to topical application of hydroquinone. Results of a 6-year investigation.* S Afr Med J, 1975. **49**(34): p. 1391–5.

11. Sarkar, R., P. Arora, and K.V. Garg, *Cosmeceuticals for hyperpigmentation: what is available?* J Cutan Aesthet Surg, 2013. **6**(1): p. 4–11.

12. Jones, K., et al., *Modulation of melanogenesis by aloesin: a competitive inhibitor of tyrosinase.* Pigment Cell Res, 2002. **15**(5): p. 335–40.

13. Zhu, W. and J. Gao, *The use of botanical extracts as topical skin-lightening agents for the improvement of skin pigmentation disorders.* J Investig Dermatol Symp Proc, 2008. **13**(1): p. 20–4.

14. Choi, S., et al., *Aloesin inhibits hyperpigmentation induced by UV radiation.* Clin Exp Dermatol, 2002. **27**(6): p. 513–5.

15. Jin, Y.H., et al., *Aloesin and arbutin inhibit tyrosinase activity in a synergistic manner via a different action mechanism.* Arch Pharm Res, 1999. **22**(3): p. 232–6.

16. Draelos, Z.D., *Skin lightening preparations and the hydroquinone controversy.* Dermatol Ther, 2007. **20**(5): p. 308–13.

17. Ertam, I., et al., *Efficiency of ellagic acid and arbutin in melasma: a randomized, prospective, open-label study.* J Dermatol, 2008. **35**(9): p. 570–4.

18. Boissy, R.E., M. Visscher, and M.A. DeLong, *DeoxyArbutin: a novel reversible tyrosinase inhibitor with effective in vivo skin lightening potency.* Exp Dermatol, 2005. **14**(8): p. 601–8.

19. Morag, M., et al., *A double-blind, placebo-controlled randomized trial of Serratulae quinquefoliae folium, a new source of beta-arbutin, in selected skin hyperpigmentations.* J Cosmet Dermatol, 2015. **14**(3): p. 185–90.

20. Espinal-Perez, L.E., B. Moncada, and J.P. Castanedo-Cazares, *A double-blind randomized trial of 5% ascorbic acid versus. 4% hydroquinone in melasma.* Int J Dermatol, 2004. **43**(8): p. 604–7.

21. Kameyama, K., et al., *Inhibitory effect of magnesium L-ascorbyl-2-phosphate (VC-PMG) on melanogenesis in vitro and in vivo.* J Am Acad Dermatol, 1996. **34**(1): p. 29–33.

22. Petit, L. and G.E. Pierard, *Skin-lightening products revisited.* Int J Cosmet Sci, 2003. **25**(4): p. 169–81.

23. Dayal, S., et al., *Clinical efficacy and safety on combining 20% trichloroacetic acid peel with topical 5% ascorbic acid for melasma.* J Clin Diagn Res, 2017. **11**(9): p. Wc08–11.

24. Murtaza, F., et al., *Efficacy of trichloro-acetic acid peel alone versus combined topical magnesium ascorbyl phosphate for epidermal melasma.* J Coll Physicians Surg Pak, 2016. **26**(7): p. 557–61.

25. Nazzaro-Porro, M. and S. Passi, *Identification of tyrosinase inhibitors in cultures of Pityrosporum.* J Invest Dermatol, 1978. **71**(3): p. 205–8.

26. Balina, L.M. and K. Graupe, *The treatment of melasma. 20% azelaic acid versus 4% hydroquinone cream.* Int J Dermatol, 1991. **30**(12): p. 893–5.

27. Kakita, L.S. and N.J. Lowe, *Azelaic acid and glycolic acid combination therapy for facial hyperpigmentation in darker-skinned patients: a clinical comparison with hydroquinone.* Clin Ther, 1998. **20**(5): p. 960–70.

28. Lowe, N.J., et al., *Azelaic acid 20% cream in the treatment of facial hyperpigmentation in darker-skinned patients.* Clin Ther, 1998. **20**(5): p. 945–59.

29. Verallo-Rowell, V.M., et al., *Double-blind comparison of azelaic acid and hydroquinone in the treatment of melasma.* Acta Derm Venereol Suppl (Stockh), 1989. **143**: p. 58–61.

30. Faghihi, G., et al., *Solution of azelaic acid (20%), resorcinol (10%) and phytic acid (6%) versus glycolic acid (50%) peeling agent in the treatment of female patients with facial melasma.* Adv Biomed Res, 2017. **6**: p. 9.

31. Dayal, S., P. Sahu, and R. Dua, *Combination of glycolic acid peel and topical 20% azelaic acid cream in melasma patients: efficacy and improvement in quality of life.* J Cosmet Dermatol, 2017. **16**(1): p. 35–42.

32. Shimogaki, H., et al., *In vitro and in vivo evaluation of ellagic acid on melanogenesis inhibition.* Int J Cosmet Sci, 2000. **22**(4): p. 291–303.

33. Yoshimura, M., et al., *Inhibitory effect of an ellagic acid-rich pomegranate extract on tyrosinase activity and ultraviolet-induced pigmentation.* Biosci Biotechnol Biochem, 2005. **69**(12): p. 2368–73.

34. Dahl, A., et al., *Tolerance and efficacy of a product containing ellagic and salicylic acids in reducing hyperpigmentation and dark spots in comparison with 4% hydroquinone.* J Drugs Dermatol, 2013. **12**(1): p. 52–8.

35. Chandrasekaran, C.V., et al., *Dual inhibitory effect of Glycyrrhiza glabra (GutGard) on COX and LOX products.* Phytomedicine, 2011. **18**(4): p. 278–84.

36. Yokota, T., et al., *The inhibitory effect of glabridin from licorice extracts on melanogenesis and inflammation.* Pigment Cell Res, 1998. **11**(6): p. 355–61.

37. Asadzadeh, A., et al., *In vitro and in silico studies of the inhibitory effects of some novel kojic acid derivatives on tyrosinase enzyme.* Iran J Basic Med Sci, 2016. **19**(2): p. 132–44.

38. Cabanes, J., S. Chazarra, and F. Garcia-Carmona, *Kojic acid, a cosmetic skin whitening agent, is a slow-binding inhibitor of catecholase activity of tyrosinase.* J Pharm Pharmacol, 1994. **46**(12): p. 982–5.

39. Sarkar, R., et al., *Periorbital hyperpigmentation: a comprehensive review.* J Clin Aesthet Dermatol, 2016. **9**(1): p. 49–55.

40. Choi, H., et al., *Kojic acid-induced IL-6 production in human keratinocytes plays a role in its antimelanogenic activity in skin.* J Dermatol Sci, 2012. **66**(3): p. 207–15.

41. Lim, J.T., *Treatment of melasma using kojic acid in a gel containing hydroquinone and glycolic acid.* Dermatol Surg, 1999. **25**(4): p. 282–4.

42. Garcia, A. and J.E. Fulton, Jr., *The combination of glycolic acid and hydroquinone or kojic acid for the treatment of melasma and related conditions.* Dermatol Surg, 1996. **22**(5): p. 443–7.

43. Monteiro, R.C., et al., *A comparative study of the efficacy of 4% hydroquinone versus 0.75% kojic acid cream in the treatment of facial melasma.* Indian J Dermatol, 2013. **58**(2): p. 157.

44. Bissett, D.L., et al., *Genomic expression changes induced by topical N-acetyl glucosamine in skin equivalent cultures in vitro.* J Cosmet Dermatol, 2007. **6**(4): p. 232–8.

45. Bissett, D.L., et al., *Reduction in the appearance of facial hyperpigmentation by topical N-acetyl glucosamine.* J Cosmet Dermatol, 2007. **6**(1): p. 20–6.

46. Kimball, A.B., et al., *Reduction in the appearance of facial hyperpigmentation after use of moisturizers with a combination of topical niacinamide and N-acetyl glucosamine: results of a randomized, double-blind, vehicle-controlled trial.* Br J Dermatol, 2010. **162**(2): p. 435–41.

47. Lee, S.H., et al., *Mulberroside F isolated from the leaves of Morus alba inhibits melanin biosynthesis.* Biol Pharm Bull, 2002. **25**(8): p. 1045–8.

48. Alvin, G., et al., *A comparative study of the safety and efficacy of 75% mulberry (Morus alba) extract oil versus placebo as a topical treatment for melasma: a randomized, single-blind, placebo-controlled trial.* J Drugs Dermatol, 2011. **10**(9): p. 1025–31.

49. Hollinger, J.C., K. Angra, and R.M. Halder, *Are natural ingredients effective in the management of hyperpigmentation? A systematic review.* J Clin Aesthet Dermatol, 2018. **11**(2): p. 28–37.

50. Frankos, V.H., et al., *Generally recognized as safe (GRAS) evaluation of 4-hexylresorcinol for use as a processing aid for prevention of melanosis in shrimp.* Regul Toxicol Pharmacol, 1991. **14**(2): p. 202–12.

51. Farris, P., J. Zeichner, and D. Berson, *Efficacy and tolerability of a skin brightening/anti-aging cosmeceutical containing retinol 0.5%, niacinamide, hexylresorcinol, and resveratrol.* J Drugs Dermatol, 2016. **15**(7): p. 863–8.

52. Makino, E.T., et al., *Evaluation of a hydroquinone-free skin brightening product using in vitro inhibition of melanogenesis and clinical reduction of ultraviolet-induced hyperpigmentation.* J Drugs Dermatol, 2013. **12**(3): p. s16–20.

53. Tan, C., W. Zhu, and Y. Lu, *Aloin, cinnamic acid and sophorcarpidine are potent inhibitors of tyrosinase.* Chin Med J (Engl), 2002. **115**(12): p. 1859–62.

54. Kong, Y.H., et al., *Inhibitory effects of cinnamic acid on melanin biosynthesis in skin.* Biol Pharm Bull, 2008. **31**(5): p. 946–8.

55. Taofiq, O., et al., *Hydroxycinnamic acids and their derivatives: cosmeceutical significance, challenges and future perspectives, a review.* Molecules, 2017. **22**(2): p. 281.

56. An, S.M., et al., *p-Coumaric acid, a constituent of Sasa quelpaertensis Nakai, inhibits cellular melanogenesis stimulated by alpha-melanocyte stimulating hormone.* Br J Dermatol, 2008. **159**(2): p. 292–9.

57. Park, S.H., et al., *Inhibitory effect of p-coumaric acid by Rhodiola sachalinensis on melanin synthesis in B16F10 cells.* Pharmazie, 2008. **63**(4): p. 290–5.

58. Song, K., et al., *Comparison of the antimelanogenic effects of p-coumaric acid and its methyl ester and their skin permeabilities.* J Dermatol Sci, 2011. **63**(1): p. 17–22.

59. Seo, Y.K., et al., *Effects of p-coumaric acid on erythema and pigmentation of human skin exposed to ultraviolet radiation.* Clin Exp Dermatol, 2011. **36**(3): p. 260–6.

60. Ma, N.S., et al., *Skin permeation and comparative evaluation of gentisic acid ester derivatives as skin-lightening agents.* J Drug Deliv Sci Technol, 2014. **24**(2): p. 212–7.

61. Rigopoulos, D. and A.C. Katoulis, *Hyperpigmentation.* 2017, CRC Press: Boca Raton.

62. Curto, E.V., et al., *Inhibitors of mammalian melanocyte tyrosinase: in vitro comparisons of alkyl esters of gentisic acid with other putative inhibitors.* Biochem Pharmacol, 1999. **57**(6): p. 663–72.

63. Rossi, A.M. and M.I. Perez, *Treatment of hyperpigmentation.* Facial Plast Surg Clin North Am, 2011. **19**(2): p. 313–24.

64. Draelos, Z.D., *The combination of 2% 4-hydroxyanisole (mequinol) and 0.01% tretinoin effectively improves the appearance of solar lentigines in ethnic groups.* J Cosmet Dermatol, 2006. **5**(3): p. 239–44.

65. Fleischer, A.B., Jr., et al., *The combination of 2% 4-hydroxyanisole (mequinol) and 0.01% tretinoin is effective in improving the appearance of solar lentigines and related hyperpigmented lesions in two double-blind multicenter clinical studies.* J Am Acad Dermatol, 2000. **42**(3): p. 459–67.

66. Keeling, J., et al., *Mequinol 2%/tretinoin 0.01% topical solution for the treatment of melasma in men: a case series and review of the literature.* Cutis, 2008. **81**(2): p. 179–83.

67. Ortonne, J.P., et al., *Safety and efficacy of combined use of 4-hydroxyanisole (mequinol) 2%/tretinoin 0.01% solution and sunscreen in solar lentigines.* Cutis, 2004. **74**(4): p. 261–4.

68. Jarratt, M., *Mequinol 2%/tretinoin 0.01% solution: an effective and safe alternative to hydroquinone 3% in the treatment of solar lentigines.* Cutis, 2004. **74**(5): p. 319–22.

69. Sonthalia, S., et al., *Glutathione for skin lightening: a regnant myth or evidence-based verity?* Dermatol Pract Concept, 2018. **8**(1): p. 15–21.

70. Arjinpathana, N. and P. Asawanonda, *Glutathione as an oral whitening agent: a randomized, double-blind, placebo-controlled study.* J Dermatolog Treat, 2012. **23**(2): p. 97–102.

71. Handog, E.B., M.S. Datuin, and I.A. Singzon, *An open-label, single-arm trial of the safety and efficacy of a novel preparation of glutathione as a skin-lightening agent in Filipino women.* Int J Dermatol, 2016. **55**(2): p. 153–7.

72. Watanabe, F., et al., *Skin-whitening and skin-condition-improving effects of topical oxidized glutathione: a double-blind and placebo-controlled clinical trial in healthy women.* Clin Cosmet Investig Dermatol, 2014. **7**: p. 267–74.

73. Zubair, S., S. Hafeez, and G. Mujtaba, *Efficacy of intravenous glutathione versus. placebo for skin tone lightening.* J Pak Assoc Dermatol, 2016. **26**(3): p. 177–81.

74. Paine, C., et al., *An alternative approach to depigmentation by soybean extracts via inhibition of the PAR-2 pathway.* J Invest Dermatol, 2001. **116**(4): p. 587–95.

75. Leyden, J. and W. Wallo, *The mechanism of action and clinical benefits of soy for the treatment of hyperpigmentation.* Int J Dermatol, 2011. **50**(4): p. 470–7.

76. Waqas, M.K., et al., *Dermatological and cosmeceutical benefits of Glycine max (soybean) and its active components.* Acta Pol Pharm, 2015. **72**(1): p. 3–11.

77. Huang, M.T., et al., *Inhibitory effect of topical applications of nondenatured soymilk on the formation and growth of UVB-induced skin tumors.* Oncol Res, 2004. **14**(7–8): p. 387–97.

78. Pierard, G., et al. *Effects of soy on hyperpigmentation in Caucasian and Hispanic populations.* In *Poster presented at the 59th AAD meeting; March 2–7, 2001; Washington, DC.*

79. Wallo, W., J. Nebus, and J.J. Leyden, *Efficacy of a soy moisturizer in photoaging: a double-blind, vehicle-controlled, 12-week study.* J Drugs Dermatol, 2007. **6**(9): p. 917–22.

80. Hermanns, J.F., et al., *Unraveling the patterns of subclinical pheomelanin-enriched facial hyperpigmentation: effect of depigmenting agents.* Dermatology, 2000. **201**(2): p. 118–22.

81. Hermanns, J.F., et al., *Assessment of topical hypopigmenting agents on solar lentigines of Asian women.* Dermatology, 2002. **204**(4): p. 281–6.

82. Navarrete-Solis, J., et al., *A double-blind, randomized clinical trial of niacinamide 4% versus hydroquinone 4% in the treatment of melasma.* Dermatol Res Pract, 2011. **2011**: p. 379173.

83. Greatens, A., et al., *Effective inhibition of melanosome transfer to keratinocytes by lectins and niacinamide is reversible.* Exp Dermatol, 2005. **14**(7): p. 498–508.

84. Hakozaki, T., et al., *The effect of niacinamide on reducing cutaneous pigmentation and suppression of melanosome transfer.* Br J Dermatol, 2002. **147**(1): p. 20–31.

85. Jerajani, H.R., et al., *The effects of a daily facial lotion containing vitamins B3 and E and provitamin B5 on the facial skin of Indian women: a randomized, double-blind trial.* Indian J Dermatol Venereol Leprol, 2010. **76**(1): p. 20–6.

86. Crocco, E.I., et al., *A novel cream formulation containing nicotinamide 4%, arbutin 3%, bisabolol 1%, and retinaldehyde 0.05% for treatment of epidermal melasma.* Cutis, 2015. **96**(5): p. 337–42.

87. Jung, Y.S., et al., *Assessment of the efficacy and safety of a new complex skin cream in Asian women: a controlled clinical trial.* J Cosmet Dermatol, 2017. **16**(2): p. 253–7.

88. Usuki, A., et al., *The inhibitory effect of glycolic acid and lactic acid on melanin synthesis in melanoma cells.* Exp Dermatol, 2003. **12**(Suppl 2): p. 43–50.

89. Javaheri, S.M., et al., *Safety and efficacy of glycolic acid facial peel in Indian women with melasma.* Int J Dermatol, 2001. **40**(5): p. 354–7.

90. Lim, J.T. and S.N. Tham, *Glycolic acid peels in the treatment of melasma among Asian women.* Dermatol Surg, 1997. **23**(3): p. 177–9.

91. Dayal, S., et al., *Clinical efficacy and safety of 20% glycolic peel, 15% lactic peel, and topical 20% vitamin C in constitutional type of periorbital melanosis: a comparative study.* J Cosmet Dermatol, 2016. **15**(4): p. 367–73.

92. Sarkar, R., N.V. Parmar, and S. Kapoor, *Treatment of postinflammatory hyperpigmentation with a combination of glycolic acid peels and a topical regimen in dark-skinned patients: a comparative study.* Dermatol Surg, 2017. **43**(4): p. 566–73.

93. Griffiths, C.E., et al., *Topical tretinoin (retinoic acid) improves melasma. A vehicle-controlled, clinical trial.* Br J Dermatol, 1993. **129**(4): p. 415–21.

94. Kimbrough-Green, C.K., et al., *Topical retinoic acid (tretinoin) for melasma in black patients. A vehicle-controlled clinical trial.* Arch Dermatol, 1994. **130**(6): p. 727–33.

95. Charurin, P., J.M. Ames, and M.D. del Castillo, *Antioxidant activity of coffee model systems.* J Agric Food Chem, 2002. **50**(13): p. 3751–6.

96. Farris, P., *Idebenone, green tea, and Coffeeberry extract: new and innovative antioxidants.* Dermatol Ther, 2007. **20**(5): p. 322–9.

97. McDaniel, D., *Clinical safety and efficacy in photoaged skin with coffeeberry extract, a natural antioxidant.* Cosmet Dermatol, 2009. **22**: p. 610–6.

98. Graf, E., *Antioxidant potential of ferulic acid.* Free Radic Biol Med, 1992. **13**(4): p. 435–48.

99. Trombino, S., et al., *Antioxidant effect of ferulic acid in isolated membranes and intact cells: synergistic interactions with alpha-tocopherol, beta-carotene, and ascorbic acid.* J Agric Food Chem, 2004. **52**(8): p. 2411–20.

100. Lin, F.H., et al., *Ferulic acid stabilizes a solution of vitamins C and E and doubles its photoprotection of skin.* J Invest Dermatol, 2005. **125**(4): p. 826–32.

101. Maeda, K. and Y. Tomita, *Mechanism of the inhibitory effect of tranexamic acid on melanogenesis in cultured human melanocytes in the presence of keratinocyte-conditioned medium.* J Health Sci, 2007. **53**(4): p. 389–96.

102. Bala, H.R., et al., *Oral tranexamic acid for the treatment of melasma: a review.* Dermatol Surg, 2018. **44**(6): p. 814–25.

103. Maeda, K. and M. Naganuma, *Topical trans-4-aminomethylcyclohexanecarboxylic acid prevents ultraviolet radiation-induced pigmentation.* J Photochem Photobiol B, 1998. **47**(2–3): p. 136–41.

104. Taraz, M., S. Niknam, and A.H. Ehsani, *Tranexamic acid in treatment of melasma: a comprehensive review of clinical studies.* Dermatol Ther, 2017. **30**(3): e12465.

105. Banihashemi, M., et al., *Comparison of therapeutic effects of liposomal tranexamic acid and conventional hydroquinone on melasma.* J Cosmet Dermatol, 2015. **14**(3): p. 174–7.

106. Ebrahimi, B. and F.F. Naeini, *Topical tranexamic acid as a promising treatment for melasma.* J Res Med Sci, 2014. **19**(8): p. 753–7.

107. Kim, S.J., et al., *Efficacy and possible mechanisms of topical tranexamic acid in melasma.* Clin Exp Dermatol, 2016. **41**(5): p. 480–5.

108. Ando, H., et al., *Linoleic acid and alpha-linolenic acid lightens ultraviolet-induced hyperpigmentation of the skin.* Arch Dermatol Res, 1998. **290**(7): p. 375–81.

109. Ando, H., et al., *Fatty acids regulate pigmentation via proteasomal degradation of tyrosinase: a new aspect of ubiquitin-proteasome function.* J Biol Chem, 2004. **279**(15): p. 15427–33.

110. Shigeta, Y., et al., *Skin whitening effect of linoleic acid is enhanced by liposomal formulations.* Biol Pharm Bull, 2004. **27**(4): p. 591–4.

111. Lee, M.H., et al., *Therapeutic effect of topical application of linoleic acid and lincomycin in combination with betamethasone valerate in melasma patients.* J Korean Med Sci, 2002. **17**(4): p. 518–23.

112. Jimbow, K., *N-acetyl-4-S-cysteaminylphenol as a new type of depigmenting agent for the melanoderma of patients with melasma.* Arch Dermatol, 1991. **127**(10): p. 1528–34.

10

Cosmeceuticals for Hair and Nails

Rachel E. Maiman

Introduction

The interest in cosmeceuticals has exponentially increased over the last several decades. This movement directly parallels both an improved understanding of the science behind them and an ever-expanding emphasis on outward appearance in the age of technology and social media. In response to a demand for youth and beauty that transcends demographic, cosmeceutical formulations have become increasingly complex and effective. It behooves any medical professional in the practice of aesthetics to recognize that this demand is not limited solely to the skin; equally as important to self-esteem are hair and nails. Some of the most popular hashtags used on Instagram reflect this. #nails, #nailart, #nailsofinstagram, #manicure, #instanails, #hair, #hairstyle, #naturalhair, and #curlyhair are some of the most frequently tagged on the social media platform. A majority of posts that use these hashtags also use #beauty, #beautiful, and #pretty, thus exemplifying the inextricable tie between the appearance of one's hair and nails and a societal standard for attraction.

In the last decade, the range of cosmeceuticals available for hair and nail care has blossomed. Cosmeceutical formulations contain a number of active ingredients ranging from antioxidants, botanicals, minerals, vitamins, enzymes, or essential oils, as well as often necessary additives like moisturizers, fragrances, preservatives, emulsion stabilizers, surfactants, and viscosity controlling substances (1). The vast array of possible ingredients poses significant potential risks for adverse events, particularly considering that cosmeceuticals are not regulated to the same standard that pharmaceutical medications are (1). In contrast to the requirements that need to be met for a drug to be approved by the Food and Drug Administration (FDA), ingredients in cosmeceuticals need only be tested as safe and the beneficial claims of the active ingredient do not need to be proven (1). Likewise, there are few biological studies and even fewer randomized double-blind placebo-controlled trials on humans which test their efficacy and safety.

While laws and regulations impose more constraints on the cosmetic scientist and manufacturer now than ever before, it is important that practitioners be equipped to recommend or dissuade patients from incorporating a cosmeceutical into their regimen. This can only be done by weighing potential risks with a comprehensive and evidence-based evaluation of the data supporting or refuting its efficacy. Thus, this chapter aims to educate the reader on the relevant physiology of the hair and nail unit, the targets and mechanisms of action of existing hair and nail cosmeceuticals, their ingredients, safety, legal and regulatory considerations, vehicle, finished products, and delivery systems. It will also touch upon cosmeceuticals under development and theoretical targets under investigation.

Hair and Nail Cosmeceuticals

The same characteristics that make a cosmeceutical attractive for the skin are sought after in hair and nail formulations. These include safety, effectiveness, stability of formulation, cheap manufacturing, metabolism within the skin, novelty, and patent protection (2, 3). Cosmeceutical formulations for hair and nails are developed from a repository of familiar ingredients ranging from botanicals and natural plant extracts, essential oils, amino acids, vitamins, and others. Hair care products with cosmeceutical formulations include, but are not limited to, shampoos, conditioners, styling products, and hair color. Some cosmeceutical ingredients also have a therapeutic value in hair conditioning, growth promotion, and even the treatment of inflammatory conditions of the scalp, such as seborrheic dermatitis (1). Likewise, multiple nail cosmeceuticals exist which claim to have a value in nail strengthening and conditioning. Though the cosmetic industry has endeavored to follow the recommendations of the Cosmetic Ingredient Review (CIR) since its inception roughly 40 years ago in order to ensure the safety of these products, the lack of data on each individual ingredient makes this challenging (1). This is especially true with respect to botanicals, as plant biology is complex and differs with each species. The relevant chemistry is also specific to each plant part and can alter the final botanical extract (1).

Hair Cosmeceuticals

The most important interactions of hair cosmeceutical products occur at the hair fiber surface, in the first few layers of the cuticle, and in the cortex of damaged hair (6). Consequently, a thorough knowledge of hair anatomy, as well as the hair cycle, is fundamental. Without this, it is extremely difficult to understand the effects of various cosmeceuticals and nearly impossible to counsel a patient on the appropriate cosmeceutical product for their hair type and concern. An overview of the hair cycle and anatomy of the hair follicle is provided below.

Hair Anatomy

When we think of hair, we typically envision hair strands, the summation of which produces a distinctive appearance which can be styled in a variety of ways to improve cosmesis and optimize functionality or adorned to project a certain personality, mood, or culture. These strands, which come in a markedly diverse variety of hues and textures, develop as a downward extension of epithelial cells into the dermis referred to as the hair follicle. Although these follicles are surrounded by the dermis, the follicular epithelial cells are epidermal in origin and separated from the dermis by the basal lamina (4).

The hair consists of two main parts – the hair follicle and the hair shaft. The hair follicle is the essential unit for the generation of hair. The hair shaft is the cornified component of the follicle and is situated at its center. Much like the skin, hair is the product of rapid division and differentiation of stem cells into mature keratinocytes. This process begins at the lowermost portion of the mature hair follicle, called the hair bulb, which contains mitotically active germinative cells (Figure 10.1). It is also the location of functionally active melanocytes that produce melanin pigments which are the primary determinants of hair shaft color. Surrounded by the hair bulb is the hair papilla, made of connective tissue, a capillary plexus, and free nerve endings.

As mature keratinocytes migrate from the hair bulb, they migrate within the follicular epidermis from the stratum basale to the stratum corneum. During this process, the keratinocytes flatten and form the unit referred to as the hair shaft (4). The hair shaft itself is a unit consisting of three distinct cell layers which are visible in a longitudinal section of the hair follicle. These are the external cuticle, an inner cortex, and, in some hair types, a central medulla (Figure 10.1).

Made of very thin, flat cells reminiscent of fish scales, the cuticle's main function is protection of the underlying cortex and anchoring the follicle in place (Figure 10.2). Each cuticle cell has a complex composition consisting of an outer lipid monolayer connected to the underlying cuticle proteins via thioester bonds formed between a sulfur and carbonyl group. The importance of these bonds is highlighted in the pathophysiology of trichothiodystrophy, a genodermatosis characterized in part by brittle hair stemming from conformational abnormalities in disulfide bonds (5). Analogous to the stratum corneum, the cuticle also serves as a barrier to water loss.

The majority of hair fiber mass is attributable to the cortex. Unlike cells of the external cuticle, those of the cortex are thin, long, and longitudinally oriented parallel to the axis of the hair. Interdigitation of cortical cells confers mechanical strength to the hair shaft (4).

Found only in coarse hair, the medulla is located at the center of the hair fiber. The cells contained within the medulla are hollow, spherical, and loosely packed. The function of the medulla continues to remain unknown (4).

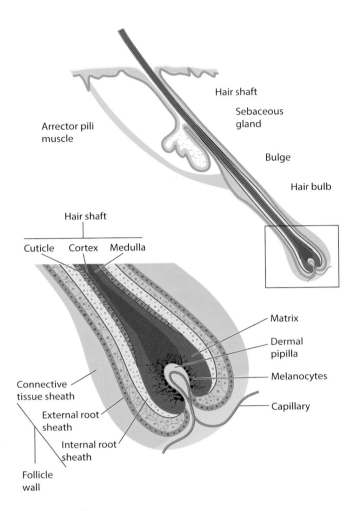

FIGURE 10.1   The hair shaft and bulb.

   Though distinct, all three layers of the hair shaft are permeated by a cell membrane complex (CMC), a lattice made of cell membrane lipids, free lipids, and lipoproteins. Continuous throughout the hair fiber, the CMC acts as a biological "glue" that fuses cortical cells together. The composition of the CMC imparts adaptability to hair. The ability of hair to change in response to external factors such as heat, water, and various products lies within the CMC. It also contributes to mechanical strength, cohesion, and hydrophobicity, as well as determines absorption and adsorption (6).

   Despite being the outermost portion of the hair shaft, the cuticle is not the outermost portion of the hair fiber. Rather, the hair shaft is enveloped by a structure referred to as the inner root sheath (IRS), a mechanically supportive tube that surrounds the fiber deep to the level of the isthmus (Figure 10.1). Superficial to this, the IRS is enzymatically degraded by proteolysis, which allows entry of the hair shaft into the hair canal to emerge from the follicular ostia at the skin surface. The IRS is composed of three concentric layers: the IRS cuticle, Huxley's layer, and Henle's layer (4).

   Along the entire length of hair, including that which is visible on the surface, the IRS is enclosed by the outer root sheath (ORS), a direct extension of the interfollicular epidermis (Figure 10.1). Contained within the ORS is the bulge, which serves as a reservoir for hair stem cells, and the sebaceous gland, responsible for hair lubrication. Along the length of the ORS is the glassy membrane, a thick, translucent, connective tissue sheath which connects the hair follicle to the dermis.

HAIR ANATOMY

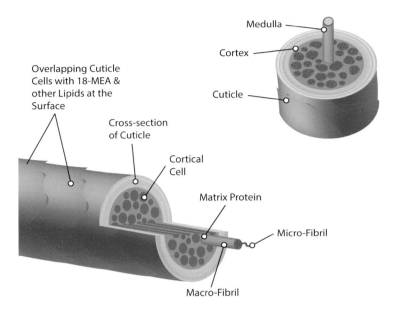

FIGURE 10.2   The shaft cuticle and cortex.

Properties of Hair

Various physical and cosmetic properties of hair have been identified, measured, and objectively quantified. They include response to factors like heat, water, bending, stretching, and twisting, as well as pH, hydrophobicity, electrostatic charge, volume, curl, deformability, elasticity, body, and feel (7). These properties have been analyzed with respect to hair condition (healthy, treated, damaged, etc.), allowing conclusions to be drawn about the relationship of various intrinsic and extrinsic factors and the quality of hair. Knowledge of this relationship is at the core of the hair cosmeceutical industry, which utilizes various ingredients to alter these properties in a way that produces an optimal cosmetic result.

Global Variations in Human Hair

It is important to remember that within human hair exists significant racial variation. Table 10.1 summarizes the characteristics of the three major ethnic groups – Caucasoid, African, and Asian. These inherent characteristics underscore many of the factors we consider in describing hair, from color to texture and curvature; they also impact how that hair interacts with products. Of course, limiting a discussion

TABLE 10.1

Racial Characteristics of Hair

Hair Type	Cross-Sectional Shape	Pigmentation	Cross-Sectional Diameter (μm^2)
Caucasoid	Round to oval	Brown/blond	**3857 ± 132**
Asian	Round	Black/brown	**4804 ± 159**
African	Elliptical or Flat	Black/brown	**4272 ± 215**

Source: See further 94.

SCIENCE OF HAIR
HAIR GROWTH CYCLE

VECTOR OBJECTS
EPS 10

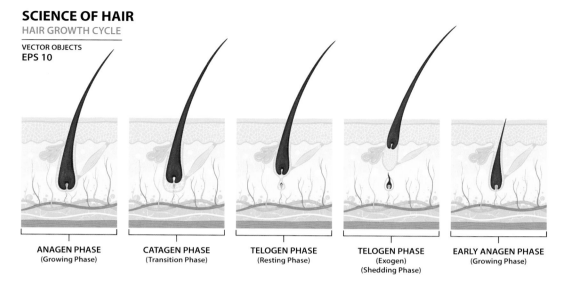

ANAGEN PHASE	CATAGEN PHASE	TELOGEN PHASE	TELOGEN PHASE	EARLY ANAGEN PHASE
(Growing Phase)	(Transition Phase)	(Resting Phase)	(Exogen) (Shedding Phase)	(Growing Phase)

FIGURE 10.3   The hair growth cycle.

to the three major ethnic groups grossly oversimplifies the picture. It fails to account for mixed race and also disregards the incalculable ethnic variation within each racial class (6).

The Hair Cycle

The hair follicle is a dynamic structure characterized by a process of rapid cycling that begins during embryogenesis and early postnatal life (4). The hair cycle contains three phases: anagen, catagen, and telogen. Anagen, the active growth phase of the hair cycle, lasts two to six years (8). After anagen, the cycle progresses through catagen, a transition phase, and ends with telogen, a resting phase that lasts two to three months (8) (Figure 10.3). Approximately 80–85% of scalp hair follicles are in anagen at any given time. The remaining 10–15% are in catagen and telogen (9). In a given day, loss of between 50 and 150 telogen hairs is average and considered to be physiologic (8).

The hair cycle is regulated in a complex fashion with the trigger for each phase predicated on the interaction of growth factors and hormones (8). Growth factors such as insulin-like growth factor-1 (IGF-1) are important in hair follicle cycling and have been shown to increase hair follicle growth in vitro (8). Transforming growth factor β3 (TGF-β3) and basic fibroblast growth factor (bFGF) are likely also important in stimulating follicle growth, as they have been shown to have much higher concentrations in anagen than in catagen (10). Hormones such as androgens, estrogens, and thyroxine are also influential in hair growth (8). At the level of the hair follicle, testosterone is converted into the more potent dihydrotestosterone (DHT) by type II 5-α-reductase (8). At the level of the dermal papillae, DHT stimulates the production of growth factors that, depending on the anatomic area, either induce or inhibit follicular growth (10). For example, in the axillary and pubic areas during pubertal adrenarche, vellus hairs enlarge to terminal pigmented hairs. Conversely, on the scalp, androgen-susceptible follicles miniaturize and revert to vellus hairs.

Hair Growth Promoters

Serenoa repens (*Saw Palmetto*)

Saw palmetto extract originates from the berries of a small evergreen palm tree native to Northeastern America. Also known as saw palmetto, its name is derived from its characteristic saw-shaped leaves (11). The combination of saw palmetto's liposterolic extract and beta sitosterol has been reported to induce hair growth in patients with androgenetic alopecia (AGA). This effect is attributed to its function as a competitive, nonselective inhibitor of 5-α-reductase types I and II, a property long exploited for its use in the management of prostatic conditions such as benign prostatic hyperplasia (10). In addition to its direct action on the synthesis of DHT, saw palmetto is also thought to inhibit DHT uptake and decrease binding of DHT to androgenetic receptors at the level of the hair follicle.

To date, significant evidence for advocating the use of saw palmetto in the treatment of AGA is lacking. This is the primary reason the National Center for Complementary and Integrative Health (NCCIH) presently does not support the use of saw palmetto for any health condition (12). Though studies have concluded saw palmetto to be of benefit in AGA, they are largely limited by small sample size and poor reproducibility of results.

A randomized double-blind placebo-controlled trial performed in 2002 using an oral liposterolic extract of *Serenoa repens* and β-sitosterol over five months concluded that six out of ten patients had demonstrable improvement in AGA on a seven-point investigator rating scale compared to only one out of nine patients in the placebo group (13). A 2016 study which evaluated the efficacy of topical *S. repens* in patients with AGA using no placebo controls concluded benefit, as well. In this prospective, open pilot study, 50 male patients between the ages of 20 and 50 years applied *S. repens* topically for 24 weeks. The primary endpoint for evaluation was hair count in an area of 2.54 cm^2 at week 24. The authors found an increase in both average and terminal hair counts at weeks 12 and 24 compared to baseline. However, these results were not universally sustained beyond week 24, a finding the authors attributed to stopping the *S. repens* extract after four weeks (14).

When analyzed head-to-head with finasteride, however, *S. repens* has not yielded comparable results in AGA. This is highlighted in a 2012 open-label study by A. 15 et al., which sought to compare the effectiveness of *S. repens* with finasteride in treating male AGA. One hundred male patients with clinically diagnosed mild-to-moderate AGA were enrolled. One group received *S. repens* 320 mg daily for 24 months and the other received finasteride 1 mg daily over the same time period. Treatment efficacy was assessed using score indices based on comparison of photographs taken at the beginning and end of treatment. The authors found an increase in hair growth in only 38% of patients treated with *S. repens,* compared to a 68% increase in those treated with finasteride (15). Interestingly, the authors also found differences in the location of results on the scalp. Based on clinical observations, they noted finasteride to act on hair loss in both the frontal and vertex scalp, whereas *S. repens* produced results predominantly in the vertex.

There are two types of herb palmetto supplements available in the market – dried saw palmetto berries and saw palmetto extract in tablet form. An article in the *Journal of Cutaneous and Aesthetic Surgery* recommends a dosage of 160 mg twice daily in tablet form, a dosage also used in clinical trial settings (16). As for all cosmeceuticals, saw palmetto is not approved, nor regulated, by the FDA. In addition to oral supplements, saw palmetto is also available in a variety of topical preparations and hair care products, such as shampoos and conditioners.

Ginkgo biloba

Ginkgo biloba has long been used in traditional Asian medicine. Derived from leaves of the *G. biloba* plant, the extract is a mixture that contains flavone glycosides such as quercetin, kaempferol, and terpenes (17). Though predominantly touted for its anti-inflammatory properties, a few studies suggest that *G. biloba* may promote hair growth in vitro by stimulating follicular proliferation and inhibiting apoptosis (17). Consequently, it is used commercially in several hair care products aimed at promoting hair growth (3).

Aloe (Aloe barbadensis, Aloe vera, Aloe capensis)

Aloe is a succulent plant found in the Southeastern United States and South Africa used as a traditional Asian therapy for its antibacterial, antiviral, and antifungal activities (11, 18). Apart from anti-inflammatory activities, it is believed to also promote hair growth (19). Aloe gel, specifically, is derived from pericyclic cells found beneath the plant's outer layer and in the inner central leaf region (3). Rich in nutrients, aloe gel contains mucopolysaccharides, allantoin, and anthracenes such as aloin, alkylchromone, flavenoids, amino acids, minerals, hydroxyquinine glycosides, and carboxypeptidases (18).

According to several studies evaluating the impact of *Aloe vera* on wound healing, topical application of the plant extract was shown to induce angiogenesis (20). Consequently, *A. vera* is thought to improve hair growth by promoting the delivery of oxygen and nutrients necessary for the replication and optimal functioning of hair follicle cells.

Recognition of these beneficial properties has made the *A. vera* plant a commonly employed base for studying various other topical herbal formulations on hair growth. A 2010 study in the *International Journal of Pharmacology* analyzed the hair growth activity of petroleum ether and ethanolic extracts from three plants (*Semecarpus anacardium*, *Trigonella foenumgraecum*, and *Trigonella corniculata*) based in Aloe vera gel compared to 2% minoxidil solution in albino rats over 30 days (21). The study concluded that *T. foenumgraecum* showed the best hair growth activity; however, postulated effects from the Aloe vera plant itself were also contributory (21). Proteolytic enzymes contained within Aloe vera were theorized to facilitate keratinocyte turnover, allowing for increased membrane fluidity and permeability as well as the outward flow of toxins and inward flow of nutrients (22, 23).

CIR safety data exist only for certain aloe species. Safety data on the extracts from other aloe species remain inadequate (3). Based on currently available data, the anthraquinone levels in *Aloe barbadensis* should be kept below an industry established level of 50 ppm in cosmetic formulations (24). The CIR has also recommended that the total polychlorinated biphenyl pesticide contamination of plant-derived cosmetic components be restricted (3, 24). Possible side effects of topical aloe include allergic contact dermatitis, phototoxic reactions, and mutagenicity (18). Owing to concerns for teratogenicity, it is contraindicated in pregnancy and lactation (18).

Ginseng radix

Ginseng has been used for years by China and Russia for its medicinal value and its extract is presently used in some hair care products (25). The major active constituents of ginseng are ginsenosides, which are touted as having anti-aging, anti-inflammatory, and antioxidant properties (17). Ginseng has been shown to promote hair growth in several recent studies. A study which evaluated the effect of a 70% methanol extract from both steamed and dry roots of red ginseng on cultured mice vibrissae hair follicles concluded hair growth-promoting activity when applied topically (26).

While data on the use of ginseng as a cosmeceutical in hair growth promotion are overall supportive, its mechanisms of action are still being elucidated. In 2015, a study published in the *Journal of Medicinal Food* investigated the effect of ginseng on human hair follicles (27). The authors treated cultured human hair follicles with red ginseng extract (RGE) and its ginsenosides and assessed cellular activity using Ki-67 immunostaining. The resulting effects on isolated human dermal papilla cells were evaluated using an immunoblot analysis of signaling proteins, cytotoxicity assays, and growth factors. The authors further analyzed the ability of RGE and ginsenosides to protect hair matrix keratinocyte proliferation against DHT-induced suppression and their effects on androgen receptor expression. Both RGE and its ginsenosides enhanced hair matrix keratinocyte proliferation. They were also found to prevent DHT-induced suppression of the hair matrix and DHT-induced upregulation of androgen receptor expression (27).

Vitis vinifera

Vitis vinifera, the common grape vine, is a well-known source of grape seed extract, a commonly incorporated nutraceutical in the cosmetic industry owing largely to its antioxidant activity. *V. vinifera* contains an abundance of anti-inflammatory ingredients such as flavenoids, stilbenes, fruit acids, tocopherols, essential fatty acids, and phenylacrylic acids (18). Its effect on hair growth, however, is most strongly correlated with the high concentration of proanthocyanidins found in *V. vinifera* seeds. A murine study performed by Takahashi et al. discovered proanthocyanidins extracted from *V. vinifera* seeds stimulated hair follicle cell proliferation by about 230% compared to 100% in controls (28). This was concluded to be the result of proanthocyanidin-induced alterations in the hair cycle noted by the same authors in vivo. They found that proanthocyanidins promoted hair follicle migration from the telogen phase to the anagen phase in C3H mice, likely by inhibition of TGF-β1 (28). Although proanthocyanidins are presently not listed in any topical hair care products, they are a frequent addition to nutritional supplements aimed at supporting hair growth (25).

Found predominantly in grape skin, resveratrol is another potent antioxidant and anti-inflammatory derived from *V. vinifera* which may have more specific benefit in treating AGA in women (17). Its potential use in the management of female pattern hair loss stems from its phytoestrogen activity (18). Phytoestrogens are naturally occurring plant-derived nonsteroidal compounds that are functionally and structurally similar to steroidal estrogens. They have attracted attention as safer alternatives to hormone replacement therapy (HRT) in the management of post-menopausal symptoms, including hormonally mediated alopecia, when ingested. A 2009 study in the *Journal of Nutritional Biochemistry* assessed the estrogen-like and anti-tumor effects of several phytoestrogens, namely resveratrol, genistein, and daidzein, as better tolerated alternatives to standard HRT (29). Although all three phytoestrogens conferred similar benefits, resveratrol was discovered to be the most promising candidate as a systemic HRT alternative (29). Oral forms of resveratrol and other phytoestrogens are expected to follow a similar trajectory of improvement in hair loss as synthetic HRT. This correlates with a minimum of two to four months for any discernible improvement in shedding and an even longer time to effect with respect to hair regrowth.

Resulting from its antioxidant and corollary anti-aging effects, the skin care industry has seen an exponential rise in cosmeceutical formulations containing resveratrol, from moisturizers to serums and toners. Similar topical formulations for hair care are lacking, but do exist, predominantly in the form of shampoos and conditioners. The efficacy of these products, however, is not yet clear, but some data exist to support their use. As an example, a solution of grape seed, jojoba, lavender, rosemary, and thyme was successfully used in patients with alopecia areata. In this study, statistically significant hair regrowth was seen after seven months of daily use compared to placebo (30).

Green Tea and Polyphenols

Among the fastest-growing cosmeceutical formulations are those that contain green tea extracts. Green tea, as well as black tea, is derived from the leaves of *Camellia sinensis* (31). Polyphenolic compounds in green tea have been shown to modulate biochemical pathways integral to cell proliferation, inflammatory responses, and tumor promoter responses (31, 32). Epigallocatechin gallate (EGCG) is the most potent antioxidant and the largest polyphenol catechin in green tea (18). EGCG has been shown to inhibit 5-α-reductase, with its most potent effect on type II 5-α-reductase (33). Other polyphenols contained within green tea, such as biochanin A, daidzein, and myricetin, have also been shown to have inhibitory effects on 5-α-reductase activity (33). This is hypothesized to allow for unopposed proliferation of cells in the dermal papilla and is the likely explanation for why topical application of EGCG in vitro has been correlated with increased hair growth (34). Kaempferol, found in green tea seed extract, has been shown to also inhibit types I and II 5-α-reductase enzyme activity in cell lines (31). Oral intake of green tea may also increase the concentration of sex hormone-binding globulin (SHBG), resulting in a decreased fraction of free and active testosterone and, consequently, a reduced androgen effect on hair follicles (35). Important to consider, however, is the knowledge that high intake of naturally occurring 5-α-reductase inhibitors by a pregnant woman may have adverse effects on the sexual development of a male fetus (33).

While the aforementioned properties suggest a possible role for green tea in the treatment of hair loss, most cosmeceutical products containing tea extracts or phenols have not been tested in controlled clinical trials (36). Currently, several hair care products exist which contain green tea extract. These include, but are not limited to, shampoos, conditioners, and conditioning masks. Unfortunately, the concentration of phenols is not standardized in these products; therefore, their therapeutic effects cannot be guaranteed, no matter how significant. In general, however, a 5% concentration of green tea extract or a 90% range concentration of polyphenols is thought to be effective (36).

Fatty Acids

Certain unsaturated fatty acids can inhibit 5-α-reductase in cultured cells and cell-free systems (37). Among them, γ-linolenic acid has been found to possess the most potent 5-α-reductase inhibitory activity. This is followed, in decreasing order of potency, by arachidonic acid and α-linolenic acid, linoleic acid, palmitoleic acid, oleic acid, and myristoleic acid (37). Other fatty acids, such as erucic acid and undecylenic acid, have not been shown to comparably inhibit 5-α-reductase (37). The CIR has examined the safety of fatty acids and approved their use in cosmetics at currently available concentrations and uses (38, 39).

The seeds of *Sesamum indicum*, a Chinese herb, are a natural reservoir of fatty acids. As such, *S. indicum* is used in Chinese medicine for hair growth. Its hair growth-promoting effect is thought to stem from the anti-androgen effects described above (40). Another botanical, *Boehmeria nipononivea*, also inhibits 5-α-reductase, as do other Boehmeria species, such as *B. longispica* and *B. plantanifolia* (41). Consequently, the use of acetone extracts derived from this plant has been investigated for the treatment of AGA. Fractionation of the leaves of *B. nipononivea* produced an extract containing six fatty acids, including α-linolenic acid, linoleic acid, palmitic acid, elaidic acid, stearic acid, and oleic acid (41). Hair regrowth in mice has been demonstrated with topical application of this extract. In one murine model, significant hair regrowth was noted on day 15 after topical application and continued until the 22nd day (41).

Lygodii spora

High concentrations of fatty acids are also thought to underscore improvement in hair growth seen following topical application of *Lygodii spora*, the spore of the Japanese fern known as *Lygodium japonicum*. The primary fatty acids contained within extracts from *L. spora* that possess anti-5-α-reductase activity are oleic, linoleic, and palmitic (42).

An extract derived from *L. spora* and 50% aqueous ethanol demonstrated 5-α-reductase inhibitory activity in vitro and in vivo anti-androgenic properties (42). In a study using shaved testosterone-treated mice, this extract stimulated hair regrowth (42).

Illicium anisatum

Because hair growth depends on a supportive vascular supply for anagen hair follicles, botanicals that induce angiogenesis or otherwise optimize the vascular environment have potential as hair care nutricosmeceuticals. An example is *Illicium anisatum*, also known as Japanese anise. A water-soluble extract derived from *I. anisatum* leaves, roots, and fruits added to an organ culture system of mouse vibrissae hair follicles demonstrated hair growth longer than controls (43). Although the exact compounds contained within the extract are not clearly known, a fractionation analysis showed the primary component to be shikimic acid. This cyclohexanecarboxylic acid is an important biochemical metabolite in plants and was shown to induce IGF-1, VEGF, and KGF by an analysis of mRNA expression in hair follicles (43). While these data suggests a potential for use in hair loss, *I. anisatum* has not yet been used in any hair products (44).

Bergamot

Bergamot extract, a citrus-derived oil with a pleasant fragrance derived from the rind of the bergamot orange, was found in many perfumes until a few years ago (45). In murine studies, bergamot extract applied topically for 42 days produced hair growth, a finding which has piqued the interest of the cosmeceutical industry for its potential use in hair growth formulations (46). Though bergamot oil is presently used in some hair care products, its application is largely limited by its ability to produce phototoxic reactions, a direct result of its high concentration of furocoumarins (25, 45).

Dabao

Dabao, a Chinese herb extract, has been used as a hair-restoring lotion (47). A standard dabao preparation contains water, ethanol, and extracts of mulberry leaves, saffron flowers, stemona root, sesame leaves, ginger root, fruits of the hawthorn and pepper plants, Chinese angelica root, bark of pseudolarix, and the skin of a Sichuan pepper fruit (47). In a randomized, placebo-controlled study, Dabao applied topically to the scalp twice daily for six months increased hair in men with AGA when compared to placebo (p < 0.03) (47). However, side effects of use included allergic contact dermatitis and folliculitis (47). A study performed much later in 2008 also reported positive results. This double-blind, six-month clinical trial of 396 patients produced a statistically significant increase in terminal vs vellus hairs in the Dabao-treated group when compared to the placebo-treated group (48).

Hair Growth Inhibitors

Soy Protein

Thioglycollate, the primary ingredients in chemical depilatory creams, removes hair at the level of the hair surface by breaking down disulfide bonds (49). Although generally considered painless and inexpensive, chemical depilatory creams can cause irritant contact dermatitis (49). Consequently, a focus of ongoing research is the creation of products capable of hair removal but which are not limited by the potential for such adverse events.

One ingredient with evidence supporting its ability to inhibit hair growth is soy. Topical skin care preparations of soy have been available for many years, where they are typically marketed for a variety of conditions, including, but not limited to, hyperpigmentation and photoaging (17). Soy contains phospholipids such as phosphatidylcholine and also contains small amounts of isoflavones, saponins, essential amino acids, phytosterols, calcium, and iron (18). The most active constituents in soy, however, are protease inhibitors. Both soybean trypsin inhibitor (STI) and Bowman-Birk protease inhibitor (BBI) have been shown to decrease the rate of hair growth and reduce hair shaft dimensions in mice and in a small human study when delivered in topical soy applications (50). Genistein, an isoflavone and phytoestrogen found in soy, also reduces hair growth on cultured hair follicles (51). The synergistic effects of these proteins suggest that soy may have a role as a cosmeceutical in the management of unwanted hair in patients with hirsutism. It should be noted, however, that patients with a family or personal history of breast or other estrogen-sensitive cancers should be counseled on the potential tumorigenic potential (17).

Hair Colorants

Henna

Henna is well known as a red-brown natural hair colorant/dye prepared from the plant *Lawsonia inermis*, also known as the henna tree, the mignonette tree, and the Egyptian privet (50). Found in many natural hair colorants, topical application of henna can produce a variety of hair colors ranging from red, neutral, brown, and black, an outcome dependent on the type of henna used (52). The chemical dye contained in henna is lawsone, a naphthoquinone (2-hydroxy-1,4-naphthoquinone) incapable of penetrating hair shafts, but which attaches to thiol groups of hair keratins to impart a vibrant color (52, 53). Other colors can be produced by adding other dye agents or by treating hair with another rinse from different plants. These include, but are not limited to, apigenin from Chamomile flowers to produce a yellow color, onion (*Allium cepa*) to give a copper color and curcumin to generate colors ranging from yellow to deep orange (3, 52, 54, 55). Adverse effects of natural henna include staining of the skin, nails, and clothes if accidental contact occurs (52) Although it is considered to be of low allergic potential, henna has been reported to cause both irritant and allergic contact dermatitis (52, 56, 57).

Annatto

Annatto is an orange-red colorant derived from the seeds of the achiote tree (*Bixa orellana*) (58). The reddish orange dye predominantly comes from the tarry outer covering of the plant's seeds. The yellow to orange color is produced by the carotenoids bixin and norbixin. Unlike β-carotene, however, annatto-based pigments are not vitamin A precursors. Although it is mainly used in food coloring, annatto has gained some traction as a natural and quick hair color rinse.

Brazilwood

Brazilwood is traditionally used as a food and beverage colorant in Indonesia. Owing to its high tannin content, it is also employed in the treatment of leather. When in contact with oxygen and light, brazilin, found in abundance in the trunk and larger branches of the tree, is readily converted to brazilein, a compound which possesses a strong coloring power (58). For this reason, brazilwood has been utilized as a natural source of brown hair dye (58).

Hair Shampoo and Conditioning Agents

Shampoos

Shampoos are formulated to cleanse the hair by eliminating sebum, sweat, yeast, scale, dirt, and styling products (59). As with all hair products, shampoos are not universal; rather, they are formulated variably with respect to target hair type. This includes variations that are not limited to dry vs oily, fine vs coarse, and straight vs curly. Other factors that dictate shampoo composition include the frequency with which the consumer shampoos and underlying conditions, such as seborrheic dermatitis (7, 58).

Water comprises about 70–80% of shampoo formulas. Its primary function is to dilute surfactants, improve spreadability, and lessen expense (6). The remaining 10–15% of the product is made up of surfactants (detergents), which are primarily derived from natural fatty acids or sulfates (lauryl and laureth sulfate). All synthetic surfactants used in shampoos are amphiphilic, meaning that they possess both hydrophilic and lipophilic moieties. The lipophilic moiety clings to dirt and oil, whereas the affinity of the hydrophilic moiety for water allows the surfactant to be rinsed away. Surfactants can, however, differ in their chemical properties. These variations underscore the four primary types of surfactants seen in shampoos – anionic, cationic, amphoteric, and nonionic (60).

Lauryl and laureth sulfates are the primary surfactants used in shampoos and are classified as anionic. They are popular as a result of their ability to produce a rich lather and work even in hard water; however, they are harsh and tend to leave hair dry, making them more optimal choices for oily hair compared to hair that is naturally coarse and dry, such as curly hair. Comparatively, laureth sulfate is slightly more gentle than lauryl sulfate. Other, less commonly incorporated anionic surfactants include sarcosines and sulfosuccinates.

Because they are more hydrophobic and thus do not produce as great of a lather, cationic surfactants are preferred for hair which necessitates only mild cleansing, such as hair that is chemically treated (60). Nonionic shampoos are infrequently used as a solitary surfactant and rather are used as an additive with other, charged surfactants. Amphoteric shampoos are unique in that they switch from anionic to cationic as a response to changing hair pH (60). They tend to be gentle on hair and so are commonly marketed for fine and chemically treated hair. They are also the primary surfactant used in "no cry" baby shampoos.

A typical shampoo formula contains multiple surfactants of varying types combined with additional additives. These additives may serve one or several functions, including, but not limited to, product stability, greater appeal, and improved ingredient delivery. Shampoos may contain up to 30 ingredients, including cleansing agents, stabilizers, preservatives, fragrances, conditioning agents, and special care ingredients with active properties to treat specific hair conditions such as oily hair or an inflamed scalp (7).

Practitioners should know that damage as a result of a particular shampoo is unlikely, given the short duration of contact. Similarly, hair loss attributed to shampoo is usually misguided and more often is the result of excessive traction and friction from wet combing chemically treated and fine hair, aggressive towel drying, and/or repeated heat styling. There are instances, however, in which repeat and frequent use of strong anionic surfactants on fine hair can produce damage by gradually dissolving the cuticular layer (60). In a similar vein, the short contact of shampoos with hair renders growth-promoting ingredients largely ineffective. This is also because their potency wanes significantly when they are diluted with water (7, 59).

Seborrheic dermatitis presents with scalp pruritus, erythema, and yellowish scale and is caused by commensal *Malassezia* species, previously known as *Pityrosporum* species (59, 60). Treatment consists of prescription and over-the-counter medications such as zinc pyrithione, ketoconazole, imidazoles, selenium sulfide, and tar (61). Botanical agents reported to be useful for seborrheic dermatitis are extracts of sage, rosemary, thyme, garlic, and walnut (3).

Hair Conditioning Agents

Hair conditioners supply the hair with the beneficial effects of sebum while avoiding the greasy appearance that occurs when too abundant. The fundamental action of all conditioners is sorption to the hair fiber so as to make the hair easier to comb while both wet and dry. Combing is made easier by repair of cuticular degeneration and damage to the hair cortex, which occurs due to weathering and exposure to hair grooming practices such as heated styling and chemical relaxers. By repairing these injuries and restoring cortical and cuticular function, hair conditioners restore glossiness, smoothness, and hydration to hair (57). Conditioners also help to improve manageability of hair and reduce frizz and fly-aways (5, 7, 59). Some conditioners deposit positive ions to reduce net negative charges on hair which produce static and frizz. Others, depending on size and other properties, fill gaps between cuticular cells in dehydrated strands, analogous to ceramides which repair the brick and mortar structure of the stratum corneum (60).

The type of conditioner required depends primarily on individual variations in hair curvature and the degree of hair shaft fragility (6). While all types of hair can benefit from conditioner, naturally coarse and dry hair as well as hair subject to frequent chemical treatments and heated styling are likely to derive the most benefit (59). Common conditioning agents include wax, lanolin compounds, vegetable oils, silicones, quaternary ammonium compounds, and protein hydrolysates (62).

Quaternary ammonium compounds such as stearalkonium chloride, cetrimonium chloride, and trimethylammonium chloride are conditioning agents that serve predominantly to neutralize negative charge, reducing static and intershaft repulsion. Cationic polymers such as polyquaternium 6, 7, 10, 11, and 16 are referred to as "film-forming" conditioners which reduce static electricity in a different way. These conditioners eliminate negative charges by forming polymers around the hair strands rather than by depositing neutralizing positive charges. Because they are cationic and thus inherently positively charged, they can be difficult to remove with shampooing once deposited. Consequently, over-conditioning with these agents can cause undesirable greasiness, especially when used on fine or chemically treated hair (60).

Protein-containing conditioners work by intercalating into fractured areas of the hair shaft resulting from chemicals and procedures. Panthenol is one of the most well-recognized ingredients used in protein-containing conditioners. Considered safe by the CIR, it is found in hundreds of hair care products at concentrations up to 6%. A potent humectant, it is well-absorbed into the hair shaft (58, 59, 61).

Silicones, such as dimethicones, are often found in "intensive" conditioners owing to their ability to condition the hair more deeply than cationic conditioners (62). They give the hair sheen by forming a thin film on the hair that reduces static electricity (60). More recently, it has been shown that conditioning efficacy can be increased when silicone conditioners are combined with cationic surfactants and cationic polymers (60).

Hair Fixatives

Fixatives are products used to ease styling and include gels, mousses, lotions, sprays, waxes, pomades, and aerosols. Their functions are variable and to meet the needs of various hair types, their compositions vary widely. Consumer needs include, but are not limited to, adding volume, preventing frizz, defining curls, and adding hold. Resins composed of bimodal copolymers are the most widely used fixative agents. Their appeal is largely related to their ability to hold hairstyles without producing a result that is too sticky or crunchy (6).

In recent years, modern consumers have become drawn to "natural" products owing in part to a misconception about their relative safety and tolerability compared to synthetic alternatives. Though the efficacy of these products is highly variable, as is their safety, they continue to surge in popularity.

Chitosan

Owing to being bio-adhesive and film-forming, chitosan adds stiffness to synthetic polymers and so is often used for its curl retention properties (60). Consequently, chitosan is often used as a hair care ingredient for hair gels, hair sprays, permanent wave agents, hair styling lotions, and hair tonics. In addition, since some derivatives of chitin and chitosan (e.g., glyceryl chitosan) form foam and have an emulsifying action, they can be used directly in shampoo.

Oligosaccharides

Oligosaccharides such as *Gossypium hirsutum* have been shown to be effective in softening the hair surface by smoothing the cuticle cells (63). The extract contains oligosaccharides such as fructose, glucose, inositol, melezitose, saccharose, trehalulose, and trehalose suggesting a role for them in hair conditioning (63).

Essential Oils

Essential oils, such as chamomile, rosemary, West Indian Bay, argan, coconut, sage, thyme, garlic, and tea tree oil are incorporated into hair care products for their fragrance and conditioning properties (64). They can be extracted from different parts of the plant, including the leaves, the flowers, and the root (64). There are few articles published about the effects of these oils on human hair and their mechanisms of action are not well-established (65). However, the main physical property of this class of ingredients is the hydrophobicity of the oil, and it is this property that appears to underlie benefits seen when used on hair (65). Because of their ability to penetrate the hair, some oils reduce the amount of water absorbed, hygral fatigue (repeated swelling and drying), a factor that can damage hair (7). By filling gaps between cuticle cells, they are also able to prevent penetration of aggressive substances, such as surfactants (7).

Coconut oil, which predominantly contains a triglyceride of lauric acid, was shown to reduce protein loss in damaged and undamaged human hair samples when incorporated into both pre- and post-wash grooming products (66). Using secondary ion mass spectrometry with time-of-flight mass spectrometry, coconut oil was found to be able to penetrate the hair cortex and reduce swelling of the hair fiber when exposed to water (67). The CIR completed a safety assessment of coconut oil in 2008 and found it to be safe in presently used concentrations (68).

In traditional folk medicine, rosemary is used as a hair rinse to promote hair growth, body, and shine (66). Rosemary extract, flower extract, flower/leaf/stem extract, and leaf extract are all currently found as ingredients in hair care products (3, 25). Its benefits are thought to derive from rosmarinic acid and caffeic acid, both of which are purported to have antioxidant properties (64). Rosemary is also used as a conditioner for oily hair and as a rinse for the treatment of dandruff (64). Its use as a hair growth promoter requires further study.

Salvia officinalis, also known as common sage or garden sage, is believed to condition hair, add shine, and promote hair growth (64). Sage extract, flower/leaf/stem extract, and leaf extract are all currently found in hair care products (3, 25). Incorporated into a massage oil for the scalp, sage extract is also used for dandruff (64). Thyme flower/leaf extract and leaf extract are also used in hair care products today for the same uses (3, 25).

Anti-Dandruff Agents

Allium sativum (*Garlic*)

Garlic bulb extract and garlic oil are presently listed as ingredients in hair care products (3, 25). Garlic lotion has been used as a dandruff treatment in folk medicine for centuries (64). Its popularity as a herbal remedy also stems from its antiseptic, antibacterial, and antioxidant properties (69, 70). Its use, however, can be limited by the development of irritant and allergic contact dermatitis when in contact with the skin (64).

Melaleuca alternifolia (*Tea Tree Oil*)

Tea tree oil (melaleuca oil), an essential oil extracted from the leaves of the Australian *M. alternifolia* tree, has long been used as an antiseptic and antimicrobial agent. These properties are attributed to hydrocarbons and terpinenes, such as cineol, contained within the plant (3, 17, 18). Its antimicrobial properties have been studied and are well-established. For example, one study found that a 5% tea tree oil shampoo was effective against *Pityrosporum ovale*. Its use resulted in a 41% improvement compared to placebo among patients with seborrheic dermatitis (73). Potentially limiting adverse effects include irritant and allergic contact dermatitis, for which terpinen, a monoterpene, is thought to be the significant sensitizing agent (1). Additionally, prepubertal gynecomastia has been reported in young boys receiving topical formulations of lavender and tea tree oils (71).

Moroccan Argan Oil

Moroccan argan oil has become increasingly popular as a main cosmetic ingredient in hair products because of its ability to keep hair moisturized and hydrophobic. The oil is derived from the argan tree (*Argania spinosa*), an endemic tree in Morocco (7). It is the kernels of argan fruits, specifically, from which the oil is harvested, which have been sun-dried for a few days to several weeks. Because argan oil is rich in tocopherols and polyphenols, powerful antioxidants, its potential in skin care is better described. Data on its benefits for hair care are lacking (72). One explanation for reduced efficacy of cosmetic formulations of argan oil compared to the edible oil is variations in moisture content. The moisture content is higher in cosmetic argan oil than in edible oil and its phospholipid content is lower (72). Consequently, the shelf life of cosmetic argan oil is much shorter, with a preservation time of around six months (72).

Emerging Concepts in Hair Cosmeceuticals

Owing largely to growing demand for products with greater efficacy, paired with constantly changing regulations to improve safety, the cosmeceutical industry faces an ever-present need for well-funded and groundbreaking research. The hair care market is no exception. Advances in everything from restorative and hair styling products, shampoos, and conditioners continue to emerge. A recently described, newly emerging trend never before seen includes the realm of "immunocosmeceuticals" aimed at revolutionizing formulations for hair repair.

New cationic conditioning polymers able with improved conditioning abilities and which can coexist in an anionic environment are under development (73). Performance ingredients such as silicones now benefit from improved delivery in chemical straighteners for Afro-ethnic hair (74). Also under investigation are effective technologies for deposition of 18-methyl eicosanoic acid onto the surface of alkaline-treated hair (6). Techniques to improve adsorption of silicone onto the hair fiber surface are being modified and recently developed silicone oil-in-water nanoemulsions are promising additions to the market for conditioning and straightening products (75).

Perhaps even more revolutionary are recent trends in hair restoration. For instance, human eye γD-crystallins are currently under investigation as strengthening agents owing to their ability to bind and penetrate the hair fiber. This has been shown to improve the mechanical properties of damaged hair, even when compared to virgin hair (76). Ceramides, which are incorporated with increasing frequency into skin care products for their ability to restore a damaged skin barrier, are now also being used to treat damaged hair. Ceramide-rich liposomes derived from internal wool lipids can restore the lipid composition of chemically treated hair fibers and reduce breakage (77). Trehalose, a disaccharide synthesized by some bacteria, fungi, plants, and invertebrate animals as an energy source able to withstand long periods of desiccation, has been shown to produce a durable straightening effect to heat-styled hair even in humid conditions (78).

In addition to ceramides, other ingredients typically associated with skin care are under investigation for their potential uses in hair products. One of these ingredients is glycolic acid. Chemours, the manufacturer of Glypure™, a cosmetic grade of glycolic acid, investigated the role glycolic acid could play in the formulation of hair care products in 2009. Initial results from those experiments were reported in a white paper published by DuPont. In these studies, hair treated with glycolic acid requires an increase in temperature by ~10°C to denature compared to untreated hair. Additionally, stiffness of hair fibers treated with glycolic acid was reduced compared to untreated hair when evaluated with tensile testing. Proof that glycolic acid penetrated the fibers to exert these effects was proven with radiolabel studies (79). Although the population in the initial experiments was Caucasian, these benefits were reproduced in subsequent studies on Asian hair (79). For instance, the amount of frictional force required to comb through Asian hair treated with Glypure was significantly less than that required to comb through the untreated hair. The study therefore concluded that the positive lubricity effect of the glycolic acid-based hair conditioning could be expected to transcend ethnicity (79). Analogous to its benefits in skin care, glycolic acid is postulated to increase the efficacy of other ingredients when incorporated into hair care products targeted toward a variety of consumers. The ability of glycolic acid to penetrate the hair shaft, for instance, suggests that it has the potential to augment the effects of various cosmeceutical ingredients, from hair conditioners to hair strengtheners, by improving their absorption. These effects underlie the incorporation of glycolic acid-based hair products in the market today.

The concept of "immunocosmeceuticals" is one of the most recent and innovative trends in hair care. Immunocosmeceuticals presently show the most promise in products aimed at hair restoration. The concept is best described in 2013 by Selvan et al. in *Chronicles of Young Scientists*. The immunocosmeceutical process involves immunizing hens with extracts of damaged human hair to provoke the formation of anti-hair antibodies. Able to be extracted from egg yolk, these anti-hair antibodies possess specificity for damaged hair. The authors found that the resulting interaction prevented and restored split ends, effects that were sustained despite repeated shampooing (80).

Hair nanocosmeceuticals are another developing sector which includes diverse classes of nanocarriers like liposomes, niosomes, solid lipid nanoparticles, nanostructured lipid carriers, and nanoemulsions (81). They are used in hair care preparations, such as in the treatment of hair loss, fade-resistant shampoos for colored hair, hair repairing shampoos, conditioners, and hair serums (81). These novel delivery systems control the release of active substances by taking advantage of intrinsic properties of the active ingredient as well as the unique size of nanoparticles.

A few examples of presently available nanocosmeceuticals in hair care include shampoo nanoparticles that seal moisture within the hair cuticle by forming a protective film that optimizes contact time with the scalp and hair follicle (82). Conditioning nanocosmeceuticals agents are better able to impart softness, shine, silkiness, and gloss and also enhance detangling.

Nail Cosmeceuticals

Though often considered to have primarily a cosmetic function, the normal nail is also important in touch, fine manipulation, and protection for the distal phalanx (83). Its mechanical functions also include dexterity, scratching, and manipulation of small objects. Despite these more functional properties, the appearance and quality of nails are considered to be of aesthetic importance and convey a picture of one's overall health and well-being. Accordingly, a large sector of the beauty industry is devoted to nail care.

Environmental factors such as water, soap, and detergents can damage the nail. Age and common nail disorders can also alter nail appearance in a cosmetically undesirable way. These alterations include findings such as discoloration, onycholysis, ridging, and loss of normal consistency, as with brittle nails. A broad array of vitamins, minerals, and topical lacquers exist as formulations aimed at correcting these irregularities and improving nail cosmesis. While data are limited on their efficacy, some evidence does exist to support their use.

Nail Biology

When references are made to the nail, the image that comes to mind is the nail plate. The nail plate is the free end of the nail unit, which is in and of itself composed of four epithelial structures. These structures are illustrated in Figure 10.4. They are the proximal nail fold (PNF), nail bed, nail matrix,

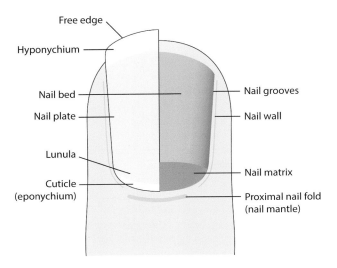

FIGURE 10.4   Structures of the nail.

and hyponychium (84). The nail matrix, which is bordered proximally by the PNF and distally by the proximal portion of the nail bed, houses the germinative layer that produces the mature cells that form the nail plate. The most distal portion of the nail matrix which abuts the nail bed is contained within the lunula, the white crescent or half-moon-shaped area from which it derives its name (84). In proximity to this is the eponychium, also known as the cuticle, a modified outer layer of the epidermis that protects the matrix (85). The nail bed extends distally beneath the nail plate to its endpoint at the hyponychium, a small zone of epidermis critical to protecting the nail unit from foreign bodies and microbes (85).

Nail Care Products

Cuticle Softeners

Cuticle emollients can be creams, lotions, oils, waxes, or ointments (83). They soften the keratin of the nail plate and surrounding skin. Emollients used in cuticle care preparations include lanolin, mineral oil, urea, and petroleum jelly (83). Plant oils such as safflower oil, wheat germ oil, tea tree oil, grapeseed oil, apricot kernel oil, and avocado oil are sometimes also incorporated (83). Several other ingredients, such as vitamin C (ascorbic acid), vitamin E (tocopherol acetate), Aloe vera, amino acids, collagen, wheat protein, and salicylic acid, can be added, as well (84). The efficacy of these additives, however, has not been evaluated in human randomized controlled trials.

Cuticle Removers

In manicures, the cuticle is softened by a cuticle remover and pushed proximally with a metal or wooden cuticle pusher (83). Occasionally, a cuticle trimmer is used to remove excess cuticle (86). If this manipulation of the cuticle is too forceful, injury to the cuticle and PNF can occur and lead to acute and chronic paronychia (83). Cuticle removers are placed over the cuticle and the proximal edge of the nail plate for a few minutes to soften the cuticle prior to removal (83). They typically contain substances such as 2–5% sodium hydroxide or potassium hydroxide in a liquid or cream base. Both of these substances soften the cuticle by breaking cysteine-rich disulfide bonds (83, 87). To decrease irritation and product evaporation, some cuticle removers also contain propylene glycol and glycerol (83). Organic bases, like trolamine, and inorganic salts, such as trisodium phosphate and tetrasodium pyrophosphate, are weaker cuticle removers and overall less effective (83). Irrespective of the specific formulation, irritant dermatitis can occur if a cuticle remover is left for too long. Allergic contact dermatitis, however, is rare (83).

Nail Hardeners

Nail hardeners aim to both harden and strengthen the existing nail and are typically applied like nail polish (83). Common formulations contain substances such as Teflon, polymers made of zirconium, silicon, or titanium, nylon, acrylic resins, and silk (83). Some formulations also add minerals and vitamins, such as biotin and calcium, which are claimed to further harden the nail when applied (83). In the United States, many nail hardeners contain 5% formaldehyde. Formaldehyde works by forming keratin cross-links, which increases the strength and hardness of the nail, but reduces its flexibility. Consequently, recurrent use of formaldehyde-based nail hardeners can cause brittle nails overall (83). Formaldehyde resins are for use on the free edge of the nail only, so as to keep the skin protected (83). Improper and/or excessive use is known to cause several possible side effects, including allergic contact dermatitis, painful onycholysis, subungual hyperkeratosis, hemorrhage, and nail plate discoloration (83).

More recently, a specially formulated nail lacquer containing a plant extract derived from *Equisetum arvense*, the common horsetail, was evaluated for improving nail strength and integrity in patients suffering from nail fragility and splitting. In addition to the *E. arvense* extract, which contains organic silica, the lacquer contains a sulfur donor group and a film-forming agent called hydroxyl-propyl chitosan (HPCH) (88). The purpose of the sulfur donor group is to support nail growth and integrity by strengthening the disulfide bonds that provide much of the foundation for the nail plate. The chitosan derivative (HPCH), a film-forming agent, is added to increase nail hydration and facilitate better delivery of the active ingredients (89). Two clinical studies using this lacquer showed significant reduction in longitudinal nail grooves, nail fragility, and lamellar splitting (90). A significant reduction was also noted in psoriasis-related nail onychodystrophy (90). These results were reproduced in a subsequently performed randomized, double-blind study (91).

Though the data are conflicting, evidence from several clinical studies suggest that oral biotin supplementation may improve the appearance of brittle nails (84). The mechanism of action by which biotin strengthens nails is still unclear; however, it is thought to do so by stimulating the differentiation of epidermal cells. The end result is an increased density of keratin matrix proteins which make up the structural foundation of the nail plate. Theoretically, and as suggested by some studies, this mechanism may also increase nail growth rate (92). Current therapeutic doses of biotin used in clinical studies to improve brittle nails range between 2.5 and 10 mg per day.

Conclusion

Cosmeceuticals continue to experience exponential market growth, popularity, and clinical applications. It behooves the clinician to be aware of botanical ingredients and other active ingredients frequently incorporated into these products in order to counsel patients on product safety and marketing claims of efficacy. This ability is equally important for hair and nail care as it is for skin care. Since cosmeceuticals are considered intermediate between an over-the-counter product and a drug, they often contain higher concentrations of active ingredients with greater potential for adverse events. Although the FDA does not directly monitor their use, claims of biological activity sometimes promote investigations which, on occasion, result in the withdrawal of a product from the market. Few available clinical studies support the use of active botanicals and chemical ingredients in hair and nail care products; however, safety and quality data reviewed by the CIR support the safety of some chemical ingredients and allows for the application of any necessary restrictions on present uses.

REFERENCES

1. Bergfeld WF, Andersen FA. Natural Products for Hair Care and Treatment. In: [eds.] U. Blume-Peytavi, A. Tosti, D.A. Whiting and R. Trueb. Hair Growth and Disorders. Berlin: Springer-Verlag, 2008, pp. 515–24.
2. Trueb RM, Swiss Trichology Study Group. The value of hair cosmetics and pharmaceuticals. Dermatology 2001; 202: 275–82.

3. Dooley TP. Is There Room for a Moderate Level Regulatory Oversight?. In: [ed.] W. Hori. Drug Discovery Approaches for Developing Cosmeceuticals: Advanced Skin Care and Cosmetic Products. Southborough: IBC Library Series, 1997, 1.4, pp. 1–16.
4. Bolognia J, Jorizzo JL, Schaffer JV, eds. Dermatology. Philadelphia: Elsevier Saunders, 2012.
5. Spitz, JL. Genodermatoses: A Clinical Guide to Genetic Skin Disorders. Philadelphia: Lippincott Williams & Wilkins, 2005. Print.
6. Sivamani RK, Jagdeo JR, Elsner P, Maibach HI, eds. Cosmeceuticals and Active Cosmetics. London: CRC Press, 2016.
7. Gavazzoni Dias MF. Hair cosmetics: An overview. Int J Trichol 2015; 7: 2–15.
8. Paus R, Cotsarelis G. The biology of hair follicles. N Eng J Med 1999; 341: 491–7.
9. Kligman AM. Pathologic dynamics of human hair loss. Arch Dermatol 1961; 83: 175–98
10. Messenger AG. The control of hair growth: An overview. J Invest Dermatol 1993; 101(Suppl): 4S–9S.
11. Hutchens AR. Indian Herbalogy of North America. Boston: Shambala Publications Inc., 1973.
12. Agbabiaka TB, Pittler MH, Wider B, et al. *Serenoa repens* (saw palmetto): A systematic review of adverse events. Drug Safety 2009; 32(8): 637–47.
13. Prager N, Bickett K, French N, et al. A randomized double blind placebo controlled trial to determine the effectiveness of botanically derived inhibitors of 5-alpha-reductase in the treatment of androgenetic alopecia. J Alternat Complem Med 2002; 8: 143–52.
14. Wessagowit et al. Treatment of male androgenetic alopecia with topical products containing *Serenoa repens* extract: AGA treatment with *Serenoa repens*. Aust. J. Dermatol 2015; 57: e76–82.
15. Rossi A, Mari E, Scarnò M, et al. Comparitive effectiveness and finasteride vs *Serenoa repens* in male androgenetic alopecia: A two-year study. Int J Immunopathol Pharmacol 2012; 25(4): 1167–73.
16. Murugusundram S. *Serenoa repens*: Does it have any role in the management of androgenetic alopecia? J Cutan Aesthet Surg 2009; 2: 31–2. doi: 10.4103/0974-2077.53097.
17. Baumann L. Botanical ingredients in cosmeceuticals. J Drugs Dermatol 2007; 6: 1084–8.
18. Thornfeldt C. Cosmeceuticals containing herbs: Fact, fiction, and future. Dermatol Surg 2005; 31: 873–80.
19. Grindley D, Reynolds T. The aloe vera phenomenon: A review of the properties and modern uses of the leaf parenchyma gel. J Ethnopharmacol 1986; 16: 117–51.
20. Heggers JP, Kucukcelebi A, Listengarten D, et al. Beneficial effect of aloe on wound healing in an excisional wound model. J Altern Complement Med 1996; 2(2): 271–7.
21. Semalty M, Semalty A, Joshi GP, Rawat MSM. Herbal hair growth promotion strategies for alopecia. Indian Drugs 2008; 45: 689–700.
22. Reynolds T, Dweck AC. Aloe vera leaf gel: A review update. J Ethnopharmacol 1999; 68: 3–37.
23. Moon EJ, Lee YM, Lee OH, Lee MJ, Lee SK, et al. A novel angiogenic factor derived from aloe vera gel: Beta-sitosterol, a plant sterol. Angiogenesis 1999; 3: 117–23.
24. Cosmetic Ingredient Review (CIR). Final Report on the Safety Assessment of *Aloe andongensis* extract, *Aloe andongensis* leaf juice, *Aloe arborescens* leaf extract, *Aloe arborescens* leaf juice, *Aloe arborescens* leaf protoplasts, *Aloe barbadensis* flower extract, *Aloe barbadensis* leaf, *Aloe barbadensis* leaf extract, *Aloe barbadensis* leaf juice, *Aloe barbadensis* leaf polysaccharides, *Aloe barbadensis* leaf water, *Aloe ferox* leaf extract, *Aloe ferox* leaf juice, and *Aloe ferox* leaf juice extract. Washington, DC: CIR, 2004.
25. Food and Drug Administration (FDA). Frequency of Use of Cosmetic Ingredients. FDA Database. Washington, DC: FDA, 2006.
26. Matsuda H, Yamazaki M, Asanuma Y, Kubo M. Promotion of hair growth by *Ginseng radix* on cultured mouse vibrissal hair follicles. Phytother Res 2003; 17: 7097–800.
27. Park, Gyeong-Hun et al. J Med Food 2003; 17(7): 797–800.
28. Kamimura A, Takahashi T. Procyanidin B-3, isolated from barley and identified as a hair growth stimulant, has the potential to counteract the inhibitory regulation of TGFβ. Exp Dermatol 2002; 11(6): 532–41.
29. Sakamoto T, Horiguchi H, Oguma E, Kayama F. Effects of diverse dietary phytoestrogens on cell growth, cell cycle and apoptosis in estrogen-receptor-positive breast cancer cells. J Nutr Biochem 2010; 21(9): 856–64.
30. Hey IC, Jamieson M, Ormerod AD. Randomized trial of aromatherapy. Arch Dermatol 1998; 143: 1356–60.

31. Park J-S, Yeom M-Y, Park W-S, et al. Enzymatic hydrolysis of green tea seed extract and its activity on 5-alpha-reductase inhibition. Biosci Biotechnol Biochem 2006; 70: 387–94.
32. Katiyar SK, Ahmad N, Mukhtar H. Green tea and skin. Arch Dermatol 2000; 136(8): 989–94.
33. Hiipakka RA, Zhang H-Z, Dai W, et al. Structure activity relationship for inhibition of human 5-alpha-reductase by polyphenols. Biochem Pharmacol 2002; 63: 1165–76.
34. Kwon OS, Han JH, Yoo HG, et al. Human hair growth enhancement in vitro by green tea epigallocatechin-3-gallate (EGCG). Phytomedicine 2007; 14: 551–5.
35. Nagata C, Kabuto M, Shimizu H. Association of coffee, green tea, and caffeine intakes with serum concentrations of estradiol and sex hormone binding globulin in premenopausal Japanese women. Nutr Cancer 1998; 30: 21–4.
36. Stallings AF, Lupo MP. Practical uses of botanicals in skin care. J Clin Aesthet Dermatol 2009; 2: 36.
37. Liang T, Liao S. Inhibition of steroid 5-alpha-reductase by aliphatic unsaturated fatty acids. Biochem J 1992; 285: 557–62.
38. Elder RL, ed. Final report on the safety assessment of oleic acid, lauric acid, palmitic acid, myristic acid, and stearic acid. J Am Coll Toxicol 1987; 6: 321–401.
39. Andersen FA, ed. Annual review of cosmetic ingredient safety assessments – 2004/2005. Int J Toxicol 2006; 25(Suppl 2): 40–7.
40. Matsuda H, Yamazaki M, Naruto S, et al. Anti-androgenic and hair growth promoting activity of *Lygodii spora* (spore of *Lygodium japonicum*) I. Active constituents inhibiting testosterone 5-alpha-reductase. Biol Pharm Bull 2002; 25: 622–6.
41. Shimizu K, Kondo R, Sakai K, et al. Steroid 5 alpha reductase inhibitory activity and hair regrowth effects of an extract from *Boehmeria nipononivea*. Biosci Biotechnol Biochem 2000; 64: 875–7.
42. Sakaguchi I, Ishimoto H, Matusuo M, et al. The water soluble extract of *Illicium anisatum* stimulates mouse bibrisse follicles in organ culture. Exp Dermatol 2004; 13: 499–504.
43. Gottschalck T, McEwen GN, Jr, eds. International Cosmetic Ingredient Dictionary and Handbook, 11th edn. Washington, DC: Cosmetic, Toiletry, and Fragrance Association, 2006.
44. Kaddu S, Kerl H, Wolf P. Accidental bullous phototoxic reactions to bergamot aromatherapy oil. J Am Acad Dermatol 2001; 45: 458–61.
45. Shao LX. Effects of the extracts from bergamot and boxthorn on the delay of skin aging and hair growth in mice. Responsible for promoting hair regrowth. Zhongtguuo Zhong Yao Za Zhi 2003; 28: 766–9.
46. Kessels AG, Cardynaals RL, Borger RI, et al. The effectiveness of the hair restorer "Dabao" in males with alopecia androgenetica. A clinical experiment. J Clin Epidemiol 1992; 44: 439–47.
47. Shenefelt Philip D. Herbal Treatment for Dermatologic Disorders. In: [eds.] Iris F.F. Benzie and Sissi Wachtel-Galor. Herbal Medicine: Biomolecular and Clinical Aspects. 2nd edn. Boca Raton: CRC Press/Taylor & Francis, 2011, 18, pp. 383–404.
48. Mofid A, Alinaghi SA, Zansieh S, Yazdani T. Hirsutism. Int J Clin Pract 2008; 62: 433–43.
49. Seiberg M, Liu JC, Babiarz L, et al. Soymilk reduces hair growth and hair follicle dimensions. Exp Dermatol 2001; 10: 405–13.
50. Hoffman R, Eicheler W, Wenzel E, et al. Interleukin-1-beta induced inhibition of hair growth in vitro is mediated by cyclic AMP. Invest Dermatol 1997; 108: 40–2.
51. Natow AJ. Henna. J Cosmetol 1986; 40(12): 754–6.
52. Ali R, Sayeed SA. Lawsone; phenolic of henna and its potential use in protein-rich foods and staining. ACE Symp Series 1997; 662: 223–44.
53. Tonnesen HH. Chemistry of curcumin and curcuminoids. ACS Symposium Series 506 (Phenolic Compounds Food Their Eff Health 1) 1992; 143–53.
54. Carle R, Gomaa K. Chamomile: A pharmacological and clinical profile. Drugs Today 1992; 28: 559–65.
55. Nour SA, Abd Elhady SE, Ghouraaab M. A natural coloring agent from *Hibiscus sabdariffa*. Bull Fac Pharm 1993; 31: 387–92.
56. Belhadjali H, Ghannouchi N, Amri CH, et al. Contact dermatitis to henna used as a hair dye. Contact Derm 2008; 58: 182.
57. Shahi Z et al. A review of the natural resources used to hair color and hair care products. Int J Pharm Sci Res 2017; 9: 1026–30.
58. Trueb, RM. Dermocosmetic aspects of hair and scalp. J Invest Dermatol Symp Proc 2005; 10: 289–92.
59. Sharad J. Cosmeceuticals, In: [eds.] K. França and T. Lotti. Advances in Integrative Dermatology. West Sussex: Wiley Blackwell, 2019, pp. 393–411.

60. Andersen FA, ed. Annual review of cosmetic ingredient safety assessments—2004/2005. Panthenol and Pantothenic Acid. Int J Toxicol 2006: 25(Suppl 1): 61–3.
61. Sinclair RD. Healthy hair: What is it? J Invest Dermatol Symp Proc 2007; 12: 2–5.
62. Oberto G, Berghi A, Portolan F, et al. Cotton honeydew (*Gossypium hirsutum* L.) extract offers very interesting properties for hair cosmetics and care products. Drugs Exp Clin Res 2005; 31: 131–40.
63. Aburjai T, Natsheh FM. Plants used in cosmetics. Phytother Res 2003; 17: 987–1000.
64. Meinert K, Springob C, Schmidt CU et al. Influence of antioxidants on the sun protection properties of hair care products. J Cosmet Sci 2004; 55(Suppl): S105–12.
65. Rele AS, Mohile RB. Effect of mineral oil, sunflower oil, and coconut oil on prevention of hair damage. J Cosmet Sci 2003; 54: 175–92.
66. Ruetsch SB, Kamath YK, Rele AS, et al. Secondary ion mass spectrometric investigation of penetration of coconut and mineral oils into human hair fibers: Relevance to hair damage. J Cosmet Sci 2001; 52: 169–84.
67. CIR. Final report on the safety of Cocos nucifera (coconut) oil, and ammonium coco monoglyceride sulfate, butylene glycol cocoate, caprylic/capric/coco glycerides, cocoglycerides, coconut acid, coconut alcohol, coconut oil decyl esters, decyl cocoate, ethylhexyl cocoate, hydrogenated cocoglycerides, hydrogenated coconut acid, hydrogenated coconut oil, isodecyl cocoate, lauryl cocoate, magnesium cocoate, methyl cocoate, octyldodecyl cocoate, pentaerythrityl cocoate, potassium cocoate, potassium hydrogenated cocoate, sodium cocoate, sodium coco monoglyceride sulfate, sodium hydrogenated cocoate, and tridecyl cocoate. 2008. Washington, DC: CIR.
68. Ariga T, Seki T. Antithrombotic and anticancer properties of garlic-derived sulfur compounds: A review. Biofactors 2006; 26: 93–103.
69. Bruneton J. Phamacognosy, Phytochemistry, Medicinal Plants. Paris: Lavoisier Publishing, 1999.
70. Henley DV, Lipson N, Korach KS, et al. Prepubertal gynecomastia linked to lavender and tea tree oils. N Eng J Med 2007; 356: 479–85.
71. El Abbassi A, Khalid N, Zbakh H, Ahmad A. Physicochemical characteristics, nutritional properties, and health benefits of argan oil: A review. Crit Rev Food Sci Nutr 2014; 54(11): 1401–14.
72. Hössel P, Dieing R, Nörenberg R, Pfau A, Sander R. Conditioning polymers in today's shampoo formulations—efficacy, mechanism and test methods. Int J Cosmetic Sci 2000; 22: 1–10.
73. deSá Dias TC, Baby AR, Kaneko TM, Robles Velasco MV. Relaxing/straightening of Afro-ethnic hair: Historical overview. J Cosmet Dermatol 2007; 6(1): 2–5.
74. Hu Z, Liao M, Chen Y, et al. A novel preparation method for silicone oil nanoemulsions and its application for coating hair with silicone. Int J Nanomedicine 2012; 7: 5719–24.
75. Ribeiro A, Matamá T, Cruz CF, Gomes AC, Cavaco-Paulo AM. Potential of human γ-D-crystallin for hair damage repair: Insights into the mechanical properties and biocompatibility. Int J Cosmet Sci 2013; 35: 458–66.
76. Méndez S, Manich AM, Martí M, Parra JL, Coderch L. Damaged hair retrieval with ceramide-rich liposomes. J Cosmet Sci 2011; 62(6): 565–77.
77. Pye S, Paul PK. Trehalose in hair care: Heat styling benefits at high humidity. J Cosmet Sci 2012; 63(4): 233–41.
78. Stasko JM. Determining the effect of using glycolic acid in hair care products. Cosmetic and Toiletries Magazine, September 2009.
79. Selvan Karthika, et al. Immunocosmeceuticals: An emerging trend in repairing human hair damage. Chron Young Sci 2013; 4(2): 81.
80. Kaul S, Gulati N, Verma D, Mukherjee S, Nagaich U. Role of nanotechnology in cosmeceuticals: A review of recent advances. J Pharm (Cairo) 2018; 2018: 3420204.
81. Rosen J, Landriscina A, Friedman AJ. Nanotechnology-based cosmetics for hair care. Cosmetics 2015; 2: 211–24.
82. Moosavi M, Scher RK. Nail care products. Clin Dermatol 2001; 19: 445–8.
83. Scheinfeld N, Dahdah MJ, Scher R. Vitamins and minerals: Their role in nail health and disease. J Drugs Dermatol 2007; 6: 782–7.
84. de Berker DAR, Andre J, Baran R. Nail biology and nail science. Int J Cosmet Sci 2007; 29: 241–75.
85. Brauer E, Baran R. Cosmetics—The Care and Adornment of the Nail. In: [eds.] R. Baran and R.P.R Dawber. Diseases of the Nails and their Management, 2nd edn. Oxford: Blackwell Science, 1994, pp. 285–96.

86. Baran R. Nail cosmetics: Allergies and irritations. Am J Clin Dermatol 2002; 3: 547–55.
87. Holzhüter G, Narayanan K, Gerber T. Structure of silica in *Equisetum arvense*. Anal Bioanal Chem 2003; 376: 512–7
88. Monti D, Tampucci S, Chetoni P, Burgalassi S, Mailland F. Ciclopirox vs amorolfine: In vitro penetration into and permeation through human healthy nails of commercial nail lacquers. J Drugs Dermatol 2014; 13: 143–7.
89. Sparavigna A, Setaro M, Frisenda L. Physical and microbiological properties of a new nail protective medical device. J Plastic Dermatol 2008; 4: 5–12.
90. Cantoresi F, Sorgi P, Arcese A, et al. Improvement of psoriatic onychodystrophy by a water-soluble nail lacquer. J Eur Acad Dermatol Venereol 2009; 23(7): 832–4.
91. Mali JWH, ed. Some Fundamental Approaches in Skin Research. Current Problems in Dermatology. Basel: Karger, 1981, 9, pp. 102–49.
92. Leerunyakul K, Suchonwanit P, Asian hair: A review of structures, properties, and distinctive disorders. Clin Cosmet Investig Dermatol 2020; 13: 309–18.

11

Photoprotection (Polypodium leucotomos, *UV, and IR Blockers*)

Bridget P. Kaufman, Ajay Kailas, and Andrew F. Alexis

Introduction

Electromagnetic radiation in the infrared, ultraviolet (UV), and visible spectra can produce deleterious and/or aesthetically undesirable effects in the skin, making adequate photoprotection of utmost importance. Many cosmeceuticals, particularly those marketed as "anti-aging," incorporate sunscreens and antioxidants that help mitigate light-induced damage to the skin. Under the FDA sunscreen monograph, only products containing broad-spectrum sunscreen with SPF >15 can claim to reduce the risks of skin cancer and premature aging (1). Nonetheless, the addition of vitamins, botanicals, and marine-derived antioxidants is thought to help prevent UV- and IR-induced sunburn and oxidative damage to DNA, thereby helping to reduce cutaneous photocarcinogenesis and photoaging (2–4). Oral supplementation with *Polypodium leucotomos* (PL) confers additional photoprotection and has been shown to be beneficial when used alone and in combination with sunscreen (5, 6).

Effects of Ultraviolet, Visible, and Infrared Radiation on the Skin

Two types of UV radiation are responsible for the majority of UV-induced damage to the skin, UVB (290–320 nm) and UVA (UVA-1:340–400 nm, UVA-2:320–340 nm). Due to its short wavelength and consequent superficial penetration of the skin, UVB directly damages DNA and cellular structures within epidermal keratinocytes and melanocytes. Acute UVB exposure leads to transient erythema, sunburn, immediate/delayed pigment darkening, and skin thickening (7, 8). Chronic effects include immune suppression, photoaging (dark spots, wrinkles), and skin cancer (7, 9, 10). UVA irradiation penetrates into the deeper dermal layers where it causes long-term skin damage via induction of reactive oxygen species (ROS), neutrophil infiltration, decreased collagen synthesis, and increased collagen degradation (7, 11, 12). Like UVB, UVA contributes to cutaneous erythema, immediate/delayed pigment darkening, immunosuppression, photoaging, and photocarcinogenesis, and it also plays a role in the development of photodermatoses and photosensitization (7, 10, 13).

VL and IR are a large component of sunlight, each representing about 40% of the sun's rays (14). VL has been shown to induce cutaneous erythema and hyperpigmentation, and contributes to worsening of melasma (and possibly post-inflammatory hyperpigmentation) following sun exposure (15). IR causes transient warmth and erythema of the skin. On a cellular level, it decreases collagen synthesis and stimulates the production of ROS and matrix metalloproteinases (MMPs), which results in decreased antioxidant levels and degradation of collagen within the skin (16).

Topical Cosmeceutical Agents for Ultraviolet Protection

The deleterious effects of UVA and UVB necessitate the development of cosmeceuticals with protection against wavelengths of light ranging from 290 to 400 nm. Typically, organic and inorganic filters are

DOI: 10.1201/9781315165905-11

TABLE 11.1

Electromagnetic Action Spectrum of FDA-Approved Organic and Inorganic Filters

Agent	UVB (290–320 nm)	UVA-2 (320–340 nm)	UVA-1 (340–400 nm)	Visible	IR
Avobenzone			X		
Cinoxate	X				
Dioxybenzone	X	X			
Ecamsule	X	X			
Ensulizole	X				
Methyl anthranilate		X			
Octocrylene	X	X			
Octyl methoxycinnamate	X				
Oxybenzone	X	X			
Padimate O	X				
Para-aminobenzoic acid	X				
Salicylates	X				
Sulisobenzone	X	X			
Zinc Oxide	X	X	X	X	
Titanium Dioxide	X	X		X	

combined to increase the sun protection factor (SPF) and broaden the coverage spectrum (Table 11.1). Topical antioxidants may be added to enhance the efficacy of sunscreens in the UV and IR ranges (2). However, the poor stability of antioxidants may limit their contribution to the photoprotective effect of many cosmeceuticals (17).

Current evidence suggests that sunscreens are effective in reducing the risk of UV-induced tumorigenesis, photoaging, and cutaneous immunosuppression (18–21). Numerous studies have demonstrated a reduction in the development of melanocytic nevi, actinic keratoses (AKs), nonmelanoma skin cancers (NMSCs), and malignant melanoma (MM) with the use of sunscreen, although results have been inconsistent (20–27). Inefficient or inadequate sunscreen application, longer durations of sun exposure in sunscreen-users, and use of products with low SPF (<15) and poor UVA protection may partially explain the increased risk of photocarcinogenesis observed in some studies (26–29). It is anticipated that an increasing use of broad-spectrum sunscreens with SPF >15 will be associated with a reduction in the incidence of skin cancer in the future (21, 29).

Organic Filters

Organic filters are benzene ring-containing compounds that absorb UV radiation, resulting in excitation of electrons to a higher energy state. The energy is then released in the form of heat or fluorescent radiation, which may inactivate or degrade the organic filter if it is not adequately photostabilized (30). The resulting photoproducts can exert toxic effects on the skin; combining organic filters to achieve maximal stability is important to minimize the incidence of phototoxic reactions (30–32).

Benzophenones are UV filters derived from the aromatic ketone 2-hydroxybenzophenone, three of which are FDA-approved sunscreens. Oxybenzone (OB, benzophenone-3 or 2-hydroxy-4-methoxybenzophenone) is a short-wave UVA and UVB filter with two absorption peaks seen at 290–300 nm and 325–340 nm (33). OB has been a common ingredient in the U.S. sunscreens since the 1970s, in part due to a lack of other FDA-approved filters with combined UVA/UVB protection. Sulisobenzone (benzophenone-4) and dioxybenzone (benzophenone-8) are currently not used as sunscreens; sulisobenzone is a common ingredient in hair care products.

Avobenzone (AVB, butyl methoxydibenzoylmethane) has one of the broadest UV absorption ranges (290–390 nm) and highest UVA protection factors as a stand-alone sunscreen (33). Given the paucity of FDA-approved UVA-1 blockers, AVB is frequently added to sunscreens to confer protection against higher wavelengths. Due to its poor photostability, AVB must be combined with sunscreen agents that help maintain its structure, including OB, octocrylene (OC), or salicylates (31).

Octyl methoxycinnamate (OMC), also known as octinoxate, is a potent UVB filter with peak absorption at 300–320 nm (33). Like other organic filters, OMC degrades or dimerizes into photoproducts that may trigger phototoxic reactions (32). This can be minimized by combining OMC with other sunscreens; the most effective stabilizers are OB and OC (30).

OC is a lipophilic chemical UV filter in the cinnamate family that protects against UVB and UVA-1 (33). It is used as a photostabilizer in combination with OMC, AVB, and OB (30).

Salicylates (octisalate, homosalate, trolamine salicylate) are among the oldest sunscreens still available in the U.S. They are weak UVB absorbers with maximal absorption at 310–320 nm and are often combined with OB and AVB to enhance UVB protection (33).

Ecamsule (EC), also known as terephthalylidene dicamphor sulfonic acid, is FDA approved as Mexoryl SX® (L'Oreal, France) for use in combination sunscreen products. With a peak absorbance of 345 nm, EC enhances photoprotection at short UVA wavelengths. It has been found to reduce UV-induced photocarcinogenesis and biochemical changes in collagen and elastin in mice, thus decreasing the appearance of sagging and wrinkling (34, 35). In humans, EC prevents the formation of photoaging-associated elastin deposits (36). A double-blind, randomized controlled study in PMLE found that a tetrad combination of EC, OC, AVB, and TiO_2 increased time to the onset of PMLE and reduced severity of flares compared to the triad product without EC (37).

Other FDA-approved organic filters include ensulizole, meradimate, Padimate O, para-aminobenzoic acid (PABA), and cinoxate. Ensulizole is a UVB absorber that is added to moisturizers and makeup products to increase the SPF. Methyl anthranilate (meradimate) is a weak UVA blocker that can be found in a few SPF-containing tinted moisturizers and lip balms. Padimate O (octyl dimethyl para-aminobenzoic acid) has been used in several lip balms and hair products. PABA is no longer used in the U.S. sunscreen products due to its risk of phototoxic and photoallergic reactions, cellular UV damage, and clothing discoloration. Cinoxate is also no longer used.

While organic filters are typically well tolerated, they are known to cause photoallergic reactions, which may limit their use in some patients. OB is the most common photoallergen in sunscreen products, implicated in 70.2% of positive patch tests to sunscreens from 2001 to 2010 (38, 39). Positive patch tests have also been reported with AVB, OMC, OC, and salicylates, albeit less frequently than with benzophenones (38–41).

Several studies have raised concern about possible neurotoxic, endocrine, and reproductive effects of organic filters, but these have not been observed in humans to date (42–46). Overall, organic filters are considered to be safe and effective sunscreens. They should be used with caution in young children who have not fully developed the enzymes responsible for metabolizing these compounds (46).

Inorganic Filters

Inorganic filters, zinc oxide (ZnO) and titanium dioxide (TiO_2), are commonly used in sunscreen-containing cosmeceuticals due to their broad-spectrum protection and good safety profile. ZnO attenuates throughout UVB and UVA wavelengths (up to 380 nm) and protects against UV-induced cellular damage and oxidative stress, primarily through its antioxidant properties (47). TiO_2 only confers protection against UVB and UVA-2 and, therefore, is often combined with ZnO or AVB to enhance UVA-1 protection (31, 48).

Early formulations of inorganic filters were thick white pastes, which were cosmetically unappealing and limited patient compliance. The development of micronized metal particles (10–200 nm) has allowed for a more cosmetically desirable product that is more translucent and easier to apply (48). These smaller particles shift the UV attenuation toward the UVB range (and eliminate VL protection), creating a delicate balance between photoprotective efficacy and cosmetic acceptability. Fortunately, the addition of pigments (i.e., iron oxide) further improves the suitability of these products for darker skin types while also enhancing photoprotection in the VL range (49). The use of a tinted broad-spectrum sunscreen has been shown to temper melasma worsening due to partial protection against VL (15).

The favorable tolerability and safety profile of inorganic filters, even in damaged skin, makes them frequent additions to sunscreens (50, 51). They are also recommended for use in children due to minimal systemic absorption after topical application.

Antioxidants

Vitamin C, Vitamin E, and Ferulic Acid

Vitamins C and E are potent antioxidants that are commonly incorporated into anti-aging cosmeceutical products. Formulations of vitamin C (i.e., L-ascorbic acid and magnesium ascorbyl phosphate) and vitamin E (i.e., α-tocopherol and tocopherol acetate) have been found to decrease UVB-induced erythema, sunburn cell formation, and immunosuppression and mitigate UVA-induced phototoxic reactions (52–55). Vitamin C also stimulates collagen production and helps regenerate vitamin E (55, 56).

The efficacy of vitamins C and E appears to be enhanced when used together and in combination with other antioxidants and commercial sunscreens. When added to a sunscreen regimen, vitamins C and E confer additive protection against UVB- and greater than additive protection against UVA-induced phototoxic damage (52). Ferulic acid stabilizes vitamins C and E and doubles the degree of protection against UV-mediated oxidative damage (57–59). When used alone, ferulic acid has been shown to block UVB-induced MMPs 2 and 9 in mouse skin, thereby decreasing collagen degradation, abnormal elastin deposition, and epidermal hyperplasia (60). In one study, an antioxidant preparation of ascorbyl phosphate, tocopherol acetate, *Echinacea pallida* extract, chamomile extract, and caffeine reduced UV-induced skin pigmentation, immune suppression, and epidermal hyperproliferation. Adding broad-spectrum sunscreen enhanced these effects and completely prevented induction of MMP-9 (2).

Tea Polyphenols

Green tea, derived from the plant *Camellia sinensis*, contains four major polyphenols with anti-aging, anti-inflammatory, and photoprotective properties (3, 61). In humans, topical application of green tea polyphenols has been shown to reduce the presence of erythema, sunburn cells, and UV-induced DNA damage (62). In mice, topical and oral administration prevents UV-induced carcinogenesis (3). Black tea extracts and polyphenols have also been shown to reduce erythema and inflammation after UVB exposure (63).

Although tea extracts and polyphenols are common ingredients in cosmeceuticals, controlled clinical trials demonstrating their efficacy are lacking. Further, there is a wide variability in concentrations used and products with less than 5% green tea extract or 90% polyphenols are unlikely to have a therapeutic effect (61).

Botanicals and Marine-Derived Products

Plant-derived botanicals, which are commonly added to cosmeceutical products, exhibit antioxidant properties that may reduce short- and long-term photodamage. Genistein, a soybean isoflavone, diminishes signs of photoaging in mice and humans and inhibits skin carcinogenesis in mice (64). Feverfew (*Tanacetum parthenium*) is a non-steroidal anti-inflammatory that reduces UVB-mediated erythema, DNA damage, and epidermal hyperplasia (65). A combination of feverfew, soy extract, γ-tocopherol, and sunscreen also mitigates the effects of VL on the skin compared to sunscreen alone, reducing ROS release and cytokine and MMP expression (66). Carotenoids, such as lycopene and β-carotene, decrease UV-induced erythema and oxidative damage to the skin but do not appear to prevent skin cancer (20, 67, 68). Pomegranate extract and other pomegranate-derived products have been found to prevent UV-mediated damage to human keratinocytes (69, 70).

Marine natural products are also widely used in photoprotective cosmeceuticals due to their antioxidant properties. Multicellular algae extracts have been found to reduce UV-induced sunburn cell formation, DNA damage, oxidative stress, and MMP expression (4). The blue-green algae, *Spirulina*, when combined with sunscreen and other antioxidants significantly reduces the formation of free radicals in response to UV, VL, and IR (71). Recent research has focused on the photoprotective effects of mycosporine-like amino acids synthesized by marine organisms. Although not currently incorporated into cosmeceutical products, these amino acids are promising due to their ability to absorb UV radiation and reduce UV-induced free radical formation and DNA damage (72).

Oral Supplements for Photoprotection

Polypodium leucotomos

PL is a tropical fern plant from Central America marketed as an oral supplement for protection against sun-related skin damage and premature aging. With a growing body of research suggesting its clinical benefits, dermatologists are increasingly recommending PL as a daily preventative therapy, both alone and in combination with sunscreen-containing products (Table 11.2).

The photoprotective effects of PL primarily derive from its antioxidant properties (73). Studies of PL *in vivo* and *in vitro* have demonstrated a decrease in UV-induced sunburn cells, cyclobutane pyrimidine dimers, and markers of cellular proliferation and inflammation (6, 74, 75). PL also reduces IR- and VL-stimulated MMP-1 expression (76). On histological examination, PL-treated skin is characterized by lower UV-induced erythema and preservation of immune cells compared to untreated skin (75, 77). These beneficial effects have primarily been demonstrated in Fitzpatrick Skin Types I–III, although research in darker skin (types III–IV) has found that PL increases minimal erythema, melanogenic, and phototoxic doses (6, 75, 77). Studies in human-reconstructed epidermis and mouse models suggest that oral PL significantly delays tumor development, but data in humans are currently lacking (73, 74, 78).

PL may be particularly beneficial in individuals who are more susceptible to the effects of solar radiation. In polymorphic light eruption (PMLE) and solar urticaria, treatment with oral PL for two weeks prior to sunlight exposure reduces the incidence of skin reactions and subjective symptoms in up to 80% of patients (79–81). A study of daily oral PL in 30 subjects with PMLE demonstrated no response to UVA in 30% of patients and no response to UVB in 28% after two weeks of PL, versus 100% and 60%, respectively, at baseline. The mean number of UVA and UVB irradiations required to elicit a light eruption also increased (79). Administration of PL in combination with sunscreen has also been shown to decrease melasma severity, although results have been inconsistent (5, 82, 83).

PL is safe and well tolerated when administered orally. No adverse events in humans have been reported at doses as high as 1,200 mg daily (6, 75, 77, 84). PL can be recommended for patients with photodermatoses and facial hyperpigmentation, as well those with frequent sun exposure and high risk of skin cancer.

Nicotinamide

Nicotinamide, also known as niacin, is an amide form of vitamin B3 that is required for the production of adenosine triphosphate (ATP). When administered prior to or following UV exposure, nicotinamide reduces UV-induced cellular energy loss, which may help preserve ATP needed for DNA repair (85). Administration of nicotinamide prior to UV exposure has been shown to reduce DNA damage, enhance DNA repair of photodamaged keratinocytes, and prevent immunosuppression (86, 87). Two double-blind, placebo-controlled trials of oral nicotinamide 500 mg given once and twice daily demonstrated a 29% and 35% relative reduction in the number of AKs, respectively, at four months (88). A subsequent study, in which 386 participants with at least two NMSCs were given nicotinamide 500 mg twice daily for 12 months, showed a 23% reduction in new NMSCs and 11% reduction in new AKs compared to placebo ($P = 0.02$) (89). Overall, nicotinamide is safe and well tolerated as an oral supplement and may be a useful adjunctive therapy in the prevention of UV-induced DNA damage (88, 89).

TABLE 11.2

A Summary of Clinical Studies Evaluating *Polypodium leucotomos* Extract

Reference	N	Underlying Condition	FST/ Race	Dose	Route	Frequency/ Duration	Comparator	Results
(Tanew et al., 2012)	35	PMLE	I–IV	≤55 kg: 730 mg 56–70 kg: 960 mg >70 kg: 1,200 mg	PO	Daily 3 weeks	None	After 2 weeks of PL treatment, 30% and 28% of patients did not react to repeated UVA and UVB exposure, respectively. The mean number of UVA exposures required to induce PMLE increased from 1.95 ± 1.07 to 2.62 ± 1.02 ($P = .005$). The mean number of UVB exposures required to elicit PMLE increased from 2.38 ± 1.19 to 2.92 ± 0.95 ($P = .047$).
(Caccialanza et al., 2007)	26 2	PMLE Solar urticaria	NR	240 mg	PO	BID > 2 weeks	None	80% of patients reported a reduction in cutaneous manifestations and symptoms of PMLE or solar urticaria during sunlight exposure.
(Caccialanza et al., 2011)	53 4	PMLE Solar urticaria	NR	240 mg	PO	BID > 2 weeks	None	73.68% of subjects reported decrease in skin reaction and symptoms during sunlight exposure ($P < 0.05$).
(Ahmed et al., 2013)	40	Melasma	Hispanic	240 mg	PO	TID 12 weeks	Placebo	There was 28.8% improvement in MI with PL versus 13.8% with placebo at week 12. No statistically significant difference in MI was found between PL and placebo ($P = 0.14$).
(Martin et al., 2012)	21	Melasma (epidermal)	NR	NR	PO	BID 12 weeks	Placebo	Significant decrease in mean MASI score in PL group (5.7 to 3.3, $P < 0.05$) but not the placebo group (4.7 to 5.7, $P > 0.05$).
(Gonzalez et al., 1997)	21	None	III–IV	1080 mg	PO	Once	Topical PL (10%, 35%, and 50%)	Oral and topical administration of PL increased the dose needed for IPD, MED, and MPD in psoralen-treated skin ($P < 0.01$). Oral PL increased MED by 2.8+/−0.59 and MPD by 2.75 +/- 0.5 (5-MOP) and 6.8 +/−1.3 (8-MOP). Depletion of Langerhans cells was prevented by both oral and topical PL.
(Middelkamp-Hup et al., 2004)	9	None	II–III	7.5 mg/kg	PO	Two doses separated by one day	None	Oral administration of PL was associated with a decrease in erythema ($P < .01$) and fewer sunburn cells ($P < .05$), cyclobutane pyrimidine dimers ($P < .001$), proliferating epidermal cells ($P < .001$), and dermal mast cell infiltration ($P < .05$) on biopsy.
(Kohli et al., 2017)	22	None	I–III	240 mg	PO	Two doses separated by one hour	None	Cutaneous erythema intensity after PL administration was 8% lower than that of pretreated skin ($P < .05$). Histological examination revealed a 76–100% reduction in proliferative markers (e.g., cyclin D1, Ki67), and inflammatory markers (COX-2) ($P < .05$).

Abbreviations:

N = number of subjects, FST = Fitzpatrick skin type. PO = by mouth, TID = three times daily, BID = twice daily, MI = melanin index, NR = not reported, MASI = melasma area and severity index, IPD = immediate pigment darkening, MOP = methoxy psoralen, MED = minimal erythema dose, MPD= minimal phototoxic dose, PMLE = polymorphic light eruption.

Infrared Radiation Blockers

Despite increasing evidence that IR contributes to sun-induced photodamage, commercially available UV filters are largely ineffective in blocking IR (90). Cosmetic products containing non-micronized titanium dioxide have been shown to reflect IR and minimize IR-induced erythema, but cosmetic dissatisfaction may limit their use (90, 91). Currently, topical antioxidants are the most promising agents for reducing IR-induced damage. Botanical and marine-derived products, including β-carotene and *Spirulina*, have been found to protect against IR-induced free radical formation (68, 71). Topical application of a vitamin C, vitamin E, grape seed extract, and ubiquinone-containing product has been shown to prevent IRA-induction of MMP-1 (16, 92). When used alone, vitamin C and green tea polyphenols also significantly reduce upregulation of MMP-1, whereas vitamin E has a minimal effect. Overall, more studies are needed to establish the efficacy of antioxidants in protecting against IR-induced skin damage. The development of IR-specific blockers will also be essential for reducing photodamage induced by these longer wavelengths of light.

Conclusion

Further research into products that mitigate the effects of UV, IR, and VL on the skin is needed. Cosmeceuticals that combine inorganic filters, organic filters, and antioxidants maximize protection against all wavelengths of UV radiation but offer limited protection against VL and IR. The development of dedicated VL- and IR-blockers is essential for enhancing the anti-aging, anti-hyperpigmentation, and skin cancer prevention efficacy of cosmeceutical products.

REFERENCES

1. Over-the-counter sunscreen drug products; required labeling based on effectiveness testing (2017). 21CFR201.327.
2. Wu Y, Matsui MS, Chen JZ, et al. Antioxidants add protection to a broad-spectrum sunscreen. Clin Exp Dermatol. 2011;36(2):178–87.
3. Yusuf N, Irby C, Katiyar SK, et al. Photoprotective effects of green tea polyphenols. Photodermatol Photoimmunol Photomed. 2007;23(1):48–56.
4. Saewan N, Jimtaisong A. Natural products as photoprotection. J Cosmet Dermatol. 2015;14(1):47–63.
5. Ahmed AM, Lopez I, Perese F, et al. A randomized, double-blinded, placebo-controlled trial of oral *Polypodium leucotomos* extract as an adjunct to sunscreen in the treatment of melasma. JAMA Dermatol. 2013;149(8):981–3.
6. Kohli I, Shafi R, Isedeh P, et al. The impact of oral *Polypodium leucotomos* extract on ultraviolet B response: a human clinical study. J Am Acad Dermatol. 2017;77(1):33–41.e1.
7. Jansen R, Wang SQ, Burnett M, et al. Photoprotection: part I. Photoprotection by naturally occurring, physical, and systemic agents. J Am Acad Dermatol. 2013;69(6):853.e1–12; quiz 65–6.
8. Kelly DA, Young AR, McGregor JM, et al. Sensitivity to sunburn is associated with susceptibility to ultraviolet radiation-induced suppression of cutaneous cell-mediated immunity. J Exp Med. 2000;191(3):561–6.
9. Dumaz N, van Kranen HJ, de Vries A, et al. The role of UV-B light in skin carcinogenesis through the analysis of p53 mutations in squamous cell carcinomas of hairless mice. Carcinogenesis. 1997;18(5):897–904.
10. Damian DL, Barnetson RS, Halliday GM. Low-dose UVA and UVB have different time courses for suppression of contact hypersensitivity to a recall antigen in humans. J Invest Dermatol. 1999;112(6):939–44.
11. Gilchrest BA, Soter NA, Hawk JL, et al. Histologic changes associated with ultraviolet A–induced erythema in normal human skin. J Am Acad Dermatol. 1983;9(2):213–9.
12. Lavker RM, Veres DA, Irwin CJ, et al. Quantitative assessment of cumulative damage from repetitive exposures to suberythemogenic doses of UVA in human skin. Photochem Photobiol. 1995;62(2):348–52.

13. Ortel B, Tanew A, Wolff K, et al. Polymorphous light eruption: action spectrum and photoprotection. J Am Acad Dermatol. 1986;14(5 Pt 1):748–53.
14. Sklar LR, Almutawa F, Lim HW, et al. Effects of ultraviolet radiation, visible light, and infrared radiation on erythema and pigmentation: a review. Photochem Photobiol Sci. 2013;12(1):54–64.
15. Boukari F, Jourdan E, Fontas E, et al. Prevention of melasma relapses with sunscreen combining protection against UV and short wavelengths of visible light: a prospective randomized comparative trial. J Am Acad Dermatol. 2015;72(1):189–90.e1.
16. Schroeder P, Lademann J, Darvin ME, et al. Infrared radiation-induced matrix metalloproteinase in human skin: implications for protection. J Invest Dermatol. 2008;128(10):2491–7.
17. Wang SQ, Osterwalder U, Jung K. Ex vivo evaluation of radical sun protection factor in popular sunscreens with antioxidants. J Am Acad Dermatol. 2011;65(3):525–30.
18. Seite S, Colige A, Piquemal-Vivenot P, et al. A full-UV spectrum absorbing daily use cream protects human skin against biological changes occurring in photoaging. Photodermatol Photoimmunol Photomed. 2000;16(4):147–55.
19. Moyal DD, Fourtanier AM. Broad-spectrum sunscreens provide better protection from solar ultraviolet-simulated radiation and natural sunlight-induced immunosuppression in human beings. J Am Acad Dermatol. 2008;58(5 Suppl 2):S149–54.
20. Green A, Williams G, Neale R, et al. Daily sunscreen application and betacarotene supplementation in prevention of basal-cell and squamous-cell carcinomas of the skin: a randomised controlled trial. Lancet. 1999;354(9180):723–9.
21. Ghiasvand R, Weiderpass E, Green AC, et al. Sunscreen use and subsequent melanoma risk: a population-based cohort study. J Clin Oncol. 2016;34(33):3976–83.
22. Naylor MF, Boyd A, Smith DW, et al. High sun protection factor sunscreens in the suppression of actinic neoplasia. Arch Dermatol. 1995;131(2):170–5.
23. Olsen CM, Wilson LF, Green AC, et al. Cancers in Australia attributable to exposure to solar ultraviolet radiation and prevented by regular sunscreen use. Aust N Z J Public Health. 2015;39(5):471–6.
24. Ley RD, Reeve VE. Chemoprevention of ultraviolet radiation-induced skin cancer. Environ Health Perspect. 1997;105(Suppl 4):981–4.
25. Gallagher RP, Rivers JK, Lee TK, et al. Broad-spectrum sunscreen use and the development of new nevi in white children: a randomized controlled trial. Jama. 2000;283(22):2955–60.
26. Autier P, Dore JF, Cattaruzza MS, et al. Sunscreen use, wearing clothes, and number of nevi in 6- to 7-year-old European children. European Organization for Research and Treatment of Cancer Melanoma Cooperative Group. J Natl Cancer Inst. 1998;90(24):1873–80.
27. Westerdahl J, Ingvar C, Masback A, et al. Sunscreen use and malignant melanoma. Int J Cancer. 2000;87(1):145–50.
28. Garland CF, Garland FC, Gorham ED. Could sunscreens increase melanoma risk? Am J Public Health. 1992;82(4):614–5.
29. Diffey BL. Sunscreens and melanoma: the future looks bright. Br J Dermatol. 2005;153(2):378–81.
30. Gaspar LR, Maia Campos PM. Evaluation of the photostability of different UV filter combinations in a sunscreen. Int J Pharm. 2006;307(2):123–8.
31. Beasley DG, Meyer TA. Characterization of the UVA protection provided by avobenzone, zinc oxide, and titanium dioxide in broad-spectrum sunscreen products. Am J Clin Dermatol. 2010;11(6):413–21.
32. Stein HV, Berg CJ, Maung JN, et al. Photolysis and cellular toxicities of the organic ultraviolet filter chemical octyl methoxycinnamate and its photoproducts. Environ Sci Process Impacts. 2017;19(6):851–60.
33. Diffey BL, Tanner PR, Matts PJ, et al. In vitro assessment of the broad-spectrum ultraviolet protection of sunscreen products. J Am Acad Dermatol. 2000;43(6):1024–35.
34. Fourtanier A, Labat-Robert J, Kern P, et al. In vivo evaluation of photoprotection against chronic ultraviolet-A irradiation by a new sunscreen Mexoryl SX. Photochem Photobiol. 1992;55(4):549–60.
35. Fourtanier A. Mexoryl SX protects against solar-simulated UVR-induced photocarcinogenesis in mice. Photochem Photobiol. 1996;64(4):688–93.
36. Seite S, Moyal D, Richard S, et al. Mexoryl SX: a broad absorption UVA filter protects human skin from the effects of repeated suberythemal doses of UVA. J Photochem Photobiol B. 1998;44(1):69–76.
37. DeLeo VA, Clark S, Fowler J, et al. A new ecamsule-containing SPF 40 sunscreen cream for the prevention of polymorphous light eruption: a double-blind, randomized, controlled study in maximized outdoor conditions. Cutis. 2009;83(2):95–103.

38. Warshaw EM, Wang MZ, Maibach HI, et al. Patch test reactions associated with sunscreen products and the importance of testing to an expanded series: retrospective analysis of North American Contact Dermatitis Group data, 2001 to 2010. Dermatitis. 2013;24(4):176–82.

39. Scalf LA, Davis MD, Rohlinger AL, et al. Photopatch testing of 182 patients: a 6-year experience at the Mayo Clinic. Dermatitis. 2009;20(1):44–52.

40. Beach RA, Pratt MD. Chronic actinic dermatitis: clinical cases, diagnostic workup, and therapeutic management. J Cutan Med Surg. 2009;13(3):121–8.

41. Karlsson I, Vanden Broecke K, Martensson J, et al. Clinical and experimental studies of octocrylene's allergenic potency. Contact Dermatitis. 2011;64(6):343–52.

42. Janjua NR, Mogensen B, Andersson AM, et al. Systemic absorption of the sunscreens benzophenone-3, octyl-methoxycinnamate, and 3-(4-methyl-benzylidene) camphor after whole-body topical application and reproductive hormone levels in humans. J Invest Dermatol. 2004;123(1):57–61.

43. Ruszkiewicz JA, Pinkas A, Ferrer B, et al. Neurotoxic effect of active ingredients in sunscreen products, a contemporary review. Toxicol Rep. 2017;4:245–59.

44. Alamer M, Darbre PD. Effects of exposure to six chemical ultraviolet filters commonly used in personal care products on motility of MCF-7 and MDA-MB-231 human breast cancer cells in vitro. J Appl Toxicol. 2018;38(2):148–59.

45. Axelstad M, Boberg J, Hougaard KS, et al. Effects of pre- and postnatal exposure to the UV-filter octyl methoxycinnamate (OMC) on the reproductive, auditory and neurological development of rat offspring. Toxicol Appl Pharmacol. 2011;250(3):278–90.

46. Jansen R, Osterwalder U, Wang SQ, et al. Photoprotection: part II. Sunscreen: development, efficacy, and controversies. J Am Acad Dermatol. 2013;69(6):867.e1–14; quiz 81–2.

47. Schwartz J, Mills K. Cosmeceutical Metals. In: Draelos Z, editor. Cosmeceuticals, 3rd edition. Canada: Elsevier Inc.; 2016.

48. Mitchnick MA, Fairhurst D, Pinnell SR. Microfine zinc oxide (Z-cote) as a photostable UVA/UVB sunblock agent. J Am Acad Dermatol. 1999;40(1):85–90.

49. Martini APM, Campos P. Influence of visible light on cutaneous hyperchromias: clinical efficacy of broad spectrum sunscreens. Photodermatol Photoimmunol Photomed. 2018;34(4):241–8.

50. Newman MD, Stotland M, Ellis JI. The safety of nanosized particles in titanium dioxide- and zinc oxide-based sunscreens. J Am Acad Dermatol. 2009;61(4):685–92.

51. Monteiro-Riviere NA, Wiench K, Landsiedel R, et al. Safety evaluation of sunscreen formulations containing titanium dioxide and zinc oxide nanoparticles in UVB sunburned skin: an in vitro and in vivo study. Toxicol Sci. 2011;123(1):264–80.

52. Darr D, Dunston S, Faust H, et al. Effectiveness of antioxidants (vitamin C and E) with and without sunscreens as topical photoprotectants. Acta Derm Venereol. 1996;76(4):264–8.

53. Trevithick JR, Xiong H, Lee S, et al. Topical tocopherol acetate reduces post-UVB, sunburn-associated erythema, edema, and skin sensitivity in hairless mice. Arch Biochem Biophys. 1992;296(2):575–82.

54. Yuen KS, Halliday GM. alpha-Tocopherol, an inhibitor of epidermal lipid peroxidation, prevents ultraviolet radiation from suppressing the skin immune system. Photochem Photobiol. 1997;65(3):587–92.

55. Darr D, Combs S, Dunston S, et al. Topical vitamin C protects porcine skin from ultraviolet radiation-induced damage. Br J Dermatol. 1992;127(3):247–53.

56. Pinnel SR, Murad S, Darr D. Induction of collagen synthesis by ascorbic acid. A possible mechanism. Arch Dermatol. 1987;123(12):1684–6.

57. Murray JC, Burch JA, Streilein RD, et al. A topical antioxidant solution containing vitamins C and E stabilized by ferulic acid provides protection for human skin against damage caused by ultraviolet irradiation. J Am Acad Dermatol. 2008;59(3):418–25.

58. Lin FH, Lin JY, Gupta RD, et al. Ferulic acid stabilizes a solution of vitamins C and E and doubles its photoprotection of skin. J Invest Dermatol. 2005;125(4):826–32.

59. Tournas JA, Lin FH, Burch JA, et al. Ubiquinone, idebenone, and kinetin provide ineffective photoprotection to skin when compared to a topical antioxidant combination of vitamins C and E with ferulic acid. J Invest Dermatol. 2006;126(5):1185–7.

60. Staniforth V, Huang WC, Aravindaram K, et al. Ferulic acid, a phenolic phytochemical, inhibits UVB-induced matrix metalloproteinases in mouse skin via posttranslational mechanisms. J Nutr Biochem. 2012;23(5):443–51.

61. Stallings AF, Lupo MP. Practical uses of botanicals in skin care. J Clin Aesthet Dermatol. 2009;2(1):36–40.

62. Camouse MM, Domingo DS, Swain FR, et al. Topical application of green and white tea extracts provides protection from solar-simulated ultraviolet light in human skin. Exp Dermatol. 2009;18(6):522–6.

63. Zhao J, Jin X, Yaping E, et al. Photoprotective effect of black tea extracts against UVB-induced phototoxicity in skin. Photochem Photobiol. 1999;70(4):637–44.

64. Wei H, Saladi R, Lu Y, et al. Isoflavone genistein: photoprotection and clinical implications in dermatology. J Nutr. 2003;133(11 Suppl 1):3811s–9s.

65. Martin K, Sur R, Liebel F, et al. Parthenolide-depleted feverfew (*Tanacetum parthenium*) protects skin from UV irradiation and external aggression. Arch Dermatol Res. 2008;300(2):69–80.

66. Liebel F, Kaur S, Ruvolo E, et al. Irradiation of skin with visible light induces reactive oxygen species and matrix-degrading enzymes. J Invest Dermatol. 2012;132(7):1901–7.

67. Stahl W, Heinrich U, Wiseman S, et al. Dietary tomato paste protects against ultraviolet light-induced erythema in humans. J Nutr. 2001;131(5):1449–51.

68. Darvin ME, Fluhr JW, Meinke MC, et al. Topical beta-carotene protects against infra-red light-induced free radicals. Exp Dermatol. 2011;20(2):125–9.

69. Syed DN, Malik A, Hadi N, et al. Photochemopreventive effect of pomegranate fruit extract on UVA-mediated activation of cellular pathways in normal human epidermal keratinocytes. Photochem Photobiol. 2006;82(2):398–405.

70. Afaq F, Zaid MA, Khan N, et al. Protective effect of pomegranate-derived products on UVB-mediated damage in human reconstituted skin. Exp Dermatol. 2009;18(6):553–61.

71. Souza C, Maia Campos P, Schanzer S, et al. Radical-scavenging activity of a sunscreen enriched by antioxidants providing protection in the whole solar spectral range. Skin Pharmacol Physiol. 2017;30(2):81–9.

72. Lawrence KP, Gacesa R, Long PF, et al. Molecular photoprotection of human keratinocytes in vitro by the naturally occurring mycosporine-like amino acid (MAA) palythine. Br J Dermatol. 2017;178(6):1353–63.

73. Bhatia N. *Polypodium leucotomos*: a potential new photoprotective agent. Am J Clin Dermatol. 2015;16(2):73–9.

74. Torricelli P, Fini M, Fanti PA, et al. Protective effects of *Polypodium leucotomos* extract against UVB-induced damage in a model of reconstructed human epidermis. Photodermatol Photoimmunol Photomed. 2017;33(3):156–63.

75. Middelkamp-Hup MA, Pathak MA, Parrado C, et al. Oral *Polypodium leucotomos* extract decreases ultraviolet-induced damage of human skin. J Am Acad Dermatol. 2004;51(6):910–8.

76. Truchuelo M, Jiménez N, Mascaraque M, et al. Pilot study to assess the effects of a new oral photoprotector against infrared-visible radiations (abstract). J Invest Dermatol. 2019;6(2):1–3.

77. Gonzalez S, Pathak MA, Cuevas J, et al. Topical or oral administration with an extract of *Polypodium leucotomos* prevents acute sunburn and psoralen-induced phototoxic reactions as well as depletion of Langerhans cells in human skin. Photodermatol Photoimmunol Photomed. 1997;13(1–2):50–60.

78. Rodriguez-Yanes E, Cuevas J, Gonzalez S, et al. Oral administration of *Polypodium leucotomos* delays skin tumor development and increases epidermal p53 expression and the anti-oxidant status of UV-irradiated hairless mice. Exp Dermatol. 2014;23(7):526–8.

79. Tanew A, Radakovic S, Gonzalez S, et al. Oral administration of a hydrophilic extract of *Polypodium leucotomos* for the prevention of polymorphic light eruption. J Am Acad Dermatol. 2012;66(1):58–62.

80. Caccialanza M, Percivalle S, Piccinno R, et al. Photoprotective activity of oral *Polypodium leucotomos* extract in 25 patients with idiopathic photodermatoses. Photodermatol Photoimmunol Photomed. 2007;23(1):46–7.

81. Caccialanza M, Recalcati S, Piccinno R. Oral *Polypodium leucotomos* extract photoprotective activity in 57 patients with idiopathic photodermatoses. G Ital Dermatol Venereol. 2011;146(2):85–7.

82. Nestor M, Bucay V, Callender V, et al. *Polypodium leucotomos* as an adjunct treatment of pigmentary disorders. J Clin Aesthet Dermatol. 2014;7(3):13–7.

83. Martin L, Woolery-LLoyd H, Avashia N. A randomized double-blind placebo controlled study evaluating the effectiveness and tolerability of oral *Polypodium leucotomos* in patients with melasma (abstract). J Am Acad Dermatol. 2012;66(4, Suppl. 1):AB21.

84. Nestor MS, Berman B, Swenson N. Safety and efficacy of oral *Polypodium leucotomos* extract in healthy adult subjects. J Clin Aesthet Dermatol. 2015;8(2):19–23.

85. Park J, Halliday GM, Surjana D, et al. Nicotinamide prevents ultraviolet radiation-induced cellular energy loss. Photochem Photobiol. 2010;86(4):942–8.

86. Surjana D, Halliday GM, Damian DL. Nicotinamide enhances repair of ultraviolet radiation-induced DNA damage in human keratinocytes and ex vivo skin. Carcinogenesis. 2013;34(5):1144–9.

87. Yiasemides E, Sivapirabu G, Halliday GM, et al. Oral nicotinamide protects against ultraviolet radiation-induced immunosuppression in humans. Carcinogenesis. 2009;30(1):101–5.

88. Surjana D, Halliday GM, Martin AJ, et al. Oral nicotinamide reduces actinic keratoses in phase II double-blinded randomized controlled trials. J Invest Dermatol. 2012;132(5):1497–500.

89. Chen AC, Martin AJ, Choy B, et al. A phase 3 randomized trial of nicotinamide for skin-cancer chemoprevention. N Engl J Med. 2015;373(17):1618–26.

90. Schroeder P, Calles C, Benesova T, et al. Photoprotection beyond ultraviolet radiation–effective sun protection has to include protection against infrared A radiation-induced skin damage. Skin Pharmacol Physiol. 2010;23(1):15–7.

91. Violin L, Girard F, Girard P, et al. Infrared photoprotection properties of cosmetic products: correlation between measurement of the anti-erythemic effect in vivo in man and the infrared reflection power in vitro. Int J Cosmet Sci. 1994;16(3):113–20.

92. Grether-Beck S, Marini A, Jaenicke T, et al. Effective photoprotection of human skin against infrared A radiation by topically applied antioxidants: results from a vehicle controlled, double-blind, randomized study. Photochem Photobiol. 2015;91(1):248–50.

12

Nutraceuticals

Radha Mikkilineni

Introduction

In recent years, the association between healthy skin, hair, nails, and nutrition has gained much attention. While it is well-known that a balanced diet is recommended for overall health, there has been an increasing emphasis on food and vitamins, minerals, and phytochemical components of food to enhance, prevent, or improve skin health. These are collectively known as "nutraceuticals" or "dietary supplements" that are a subset of food taken orally. Recent research predicted that the global market will reach $340 billion by 2024 at a compounded annual growth rate of 7.2% (1). Broadly, there is an increasing acceptance among people of the idea that "what goes inside is seen outside." A number of factors contribute to this growing focus on nutrition, wellness, and a holistic and preventative approach to healthcare, including patient's desire for autonomy in self-care and personal control of their health outcomes and decision-making processes (2). Moreover, there is a desire to treat or manage health conditions and promote beauty with less toxic or pharmaceutical-grade medicines to avoid side effects (3, 4). Unfortunately, the level of evidence for the use of supplements for the management of skin disease or improvement of skin health is either preliminary or equivocal in many cases, as large-scale studies are not required by the Food and Drug Administration (FDA) and are challenging to conduct due to time expense and a lack of uniformity among supplement components (4). This chapter will review the current state of the evidence for the most promising or predominant nutraceuticals used for skin health today.

Regulation of Dietary Supplements

The federal government regulates dietary supplements through the FDA and the Federal Trade Commission (FTC), which oversees interstate commerce. The seminal act passed in 1994, known as the Dietary Supplement Health and Education Act (DSHEA) of 1994, established regulations as primarily post-market, with only limited pre-market regulations. The latter means that manufacturers cannot make unsupported claims regarding disease-specific treatment but can claim general nutritional, physiologic structure, and functional support (5). Evidence to support these claims must also exist. In addition, manufacturers must place a disclaimer on labels stating that "The FDA has not reviewed these claims" (6–8).

Post-marketing audits and review of manufacturing procedures and protocols exist for the supplement to carry a label claiming Good Manufacturing Practice, or GMP. In addition, reporting adverse side effects is mandatory, as well as disclosure and notification to the FDA of the use of new ingredients. Of note, supplements are globally marketed, but there is no global consensus on what constitutes a dietary supplement, how they should be regulated, and what type of evidence should be required for their use. Quality manufacturers will often disclose the source of their products and will typically also be certified and vetted by independent organizations such as the United States Pharmacopeia (USP) and the National Sanitation Foundation now known as NSF International. The USP certification verifies that the product contains the ingredients listed on the label in the amount and potency declared, does not contain harmful levels of contaminants, that the product will break down and be released in the body in a specified amount of time, and has been made according to the FDA current GMPs under sanitary and well-controlled procedures. NSF certification is similar to USP but is also used to verify botanicals, extracts, amino acids, herbs, and sports supplements (9). Nevertheless, additional regulatory hurdles may be necessary to improve quality and surveillance for side effects of supplements as they increase in popular utilization, in particular, for the treatment or modulation of disease (8). Finally, a word about the strength of evidence. Many commonly used supplements have a long history over thousands of years of use in eastern Ayurvedic or Traditional Chinese Medicine and more recently Western Herbalism. When evaluating the strength of data, historical experience across thousands of years must be taken into consideration as this level of evidence is surely better than anecdote although not to the level of the gold standards of Western medicine (10). While a randomized clinical trial is the gold standard, and well-conducted randomized controlled trials (RCTs) should be evaluated first and foremost when available, there is much to be gleaned from in vitro and in vivo basic science research, observational and case studies, case series, and meta-analyses. The *Journal of the American Academy of Dermatology* has useful guidelines for evaluating levels of evidence as follows: Level IA evidence includes evidence from a meta-analysis of RCTs; level IB evidence includes evidence from ≥1 RCT; level IIA evidence includes evidence from ≥1 controlled study without randomization; level IIB evidence includes evidence from ≥1 other type of experimental study; level III evidence includes evidence from nonexperimental descriptive studies, such as comparative studies, correlation studies, and case-control studies; and level IV evidence includes evidence from expert committee reports or opinions, or clinical experience of respected authorities, or both. Much of the evidence for the use of nutraceuticals for skin health, anti-aging or to treat specific skin ailments is level IIA or lower (11). All treatment recommendations for patients need to adequately address the risks and benefits of a supplement protocol and the potential for drug interactions. Practitioners of standard, Western medicine should have an understanding for diversity in healing practices across cultures as we formulate our approach to the use of dietary supplements in our patients, particularly as we shall encounter more patients utilizing, requesting, and asking us about them. Trends have shown consistent increases in the use of supplements over time, although the types have varied with a decrease in the use of *Ginkgo biloba*, for example, and an increase in the use of vitamin D and omega-3 fatty acids (12, 13). This likely reflects additional research showing more consistent increased benefit with low risk of the latter nutrients. In particular, consumers and many practitioners are unfamiliar or have limited knowledge of the risks of supplement usage (14). We practitioners are in a unique position to offer guidance based on the best available evidence and our judgment as scientists and healers.

Dietary supplements or nutraceuticals are biologically active peptides and oligosaccharides, polyphenols, vitamins, polyunsaturated fatty acids (PUFAs), minerals, probiotics, and whole herb or plant supplements (Figure 12.1) (15).

In this chapter, we will discuss the health benefits of this class of products on skin aging and review the mechanism of action and evidence for the use of the most popular nutraceuticals for maintenance of skin health and anti-aging (16).

Aging Overview

Factors that contribute to aging are multifactorial and can broadly be categorized as intrinsic or extrinsic (17). Intrinsic aging is primarily genetic in nature but includes the ability of an individual to withstand and repair damage over time such that chronological aging may be rapid or slower depending upon innate responses to various insults (Figure 12.2). Extrinsic aging refers primarily to external injuries, primarily from environmental pollutants, chemical exposures, medications, and photoaging and nutrient intake or dietary factors (Figure 12.3) (18). An interplay between intrinsic and extrinsic factors exists such that we may also consider the process of aging through the prism of epigenetics, namely the ability of the environment to effect changes upon the individual's genome. In terms of nutrition, we know that diet in the context of intake of water, protein, trace elements, vitamins, fat, alcohol, and sugar or carbohydrates impact skin inflammation, autophagy, and the presence of advanced glycation end products or AGEs.

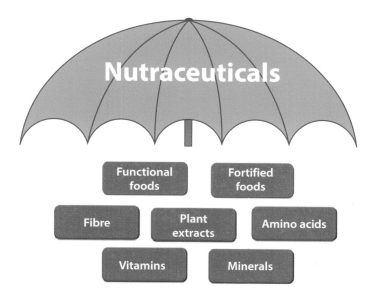

FIGURE 12.1 What are nutraceuticals?
(From Williamson EM, Liu X, Izzo AA. Trends in use, pharmacology, and clinical applications of emerging herbal nutraceuticals. Br J Pharmacol. 2020 Mar;177(6):1227–1240. Reprinted with permission.)

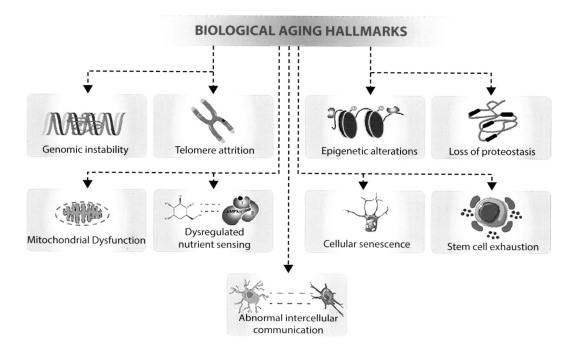

FIGURE 12.2 Biological aging hallmarks.
(From Chen Y, Hamidu S, Yang X, Yan Y, Wang Q, Li L, Oduro PK, Li Y. Dietary supplements and natural products: an update on their clinical effectiveness and molecular mechanisms of action during accelerated biological aging. Front Genet. 2022;1. Under Open Access.)

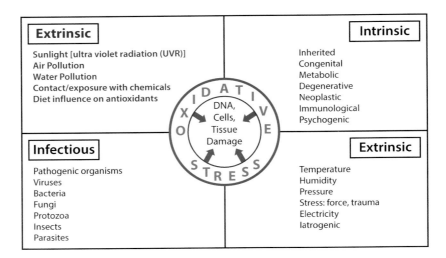

FIGURE 12.3 Extrinsic and intrinsic aging.
(From Lephart ED. Equol's anti-aging effects protect against environmental assaults by increasing skin antioxidant defense and ECM proteins while decreasing oxidative stress and inflammation. Cosmetics. 2018; 5(1):16. Under Open Access.)

Collagen

Collagen hydrolysates or peptides derived from bovine, porcine, or marine sources are increasingly used to improve skin and are primarily composed of Type 1 and III collagen. Type II collagen has been used to enhance joint health. These peptides are readily absorbed following ingestion as di- and tri-peptides (Figure 12.4). Their mechanism of action is based on in vitro studies showing an anti-inflammatory and antioxidant effect (19). There is also a chemotactic effect whereby the increased presence of these hydrolysates in the skin stimulates and attracts a fibroblastic activity. Stimulation of increased and thickened collagen fibers in vitro has been noted. Ingestion of collagen hydrolysates in irradiated hairless mice showed an increase in skin hydration, decreased wrinkle formation, stimulation of hyaluronic acid formation, downregulation of hyaluronidase, and a reduction of UVB-induced decrease in Type I collagen. Once absorbed, collagen peptides act as building blocks for fibroblasts, free radical scavengers, and inhibitors of AP-1, MMP-1, and MMP-3. Collagen peptides are noted to remain in the system for up to 96 hours after ingestion, suggesting that continued use is required for maintenance of effect (20–22).

A recent meta-analysis summarized the clinical effects on the skin in human subjects and noted wrinkle reduction, increased elasticity, and improved hydration. The amount and origin of collagen vary among studies. Dosing ranged from 2.5 to 12 g daily and was conducted over 90 days with the persistence of findings for an additional 30 days after supplementation ceased. While the origin of the peptides was agnostic (i.e., bovine, porcine, or marine) to the effect on the skin, the concentrations of proline-hydroxyproline and hydroxyproline-glycine in particular and at higher levels promoted a more rapid effect. Of note, some supplements contained other nutrients, including vitamins and coenzyme Q, which may have impacted results, although, in the studies supplementing with collagen peptides alone, the results were similar (23).

Probiotics

An adequate understanding of the role and potential promise of probiotic dietary supplementation in skin health and anti-aging requires consideration of the gut and skin microbiome and the gut-skin

Collagen

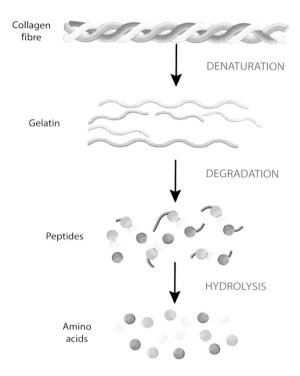

Collagen
fibre

DENATURATION

Gelatin

DEGRADATION

Peptides

HYDROLYSIS

Amino
acids

FIGURE 12.4 Collagen peptides.
(From iStock under license.)

axis. Both the gut and the skin play vital roles in the first exposure of the human body to the external environment, whether via oral intake on the one hand or external physical exposures on the other (Figure 12.5) (24–26).

Each system is comprised of a unique microbiome of trillions of organisms which requires an appropriate balance of commensal and pathogenic microorganisms to maintain intact barriers and homeostasis. Moreover, an imbalance or dysbiosis of the gut may disturb normal processes of cellular senescence, which may lead to both systemic and skin-specific aging and the promotion of various skin disorders. Identification and management of gut dysbiosis through pre- and probiotics may promote anti-senescence (27).

Longevity studies of the gut microbiota of centurions show the importance of the Firmicutes/ Bacterioidetes ratio, which decreases as we progress into old age, as a key finding with implications for the production of short-chain fatty acids (SCFAs), butyrate, and propionate, which are critical to an intact intestinal tract. Inadequate production of SCFAs promotes intestinal dysbiosis and cellular senescence. Cellular senescence is marked by a group of inflammatory markers, including pro-inflammatory cytokines, chemokines, proteases, lipids, growth factors, and extracellular matrix proteins. Interestingly, aging and diseased skin also exhibit microbial dysbiosis that results in elevated skin and serum inflammatory markers which are thought to contribute to systemic aging and disease. A skin-gut axis exists such that skin and gastrointestinal disorders may coexist and lead further to an association with other systemic disorders, thought to stem from dysbiosis, intestinal permeability, and increased systemic inflammation, such as cancer, diabetes, heart and kidney disease, as well as skin diseases. (28). Therefore, while anti-aging treatments and management of skin disease are critical, from a nutritional standpoint, dietary supplements targeting gut dsybiosis may also result in improved skin health (Figure 12.6). Prebiotics and

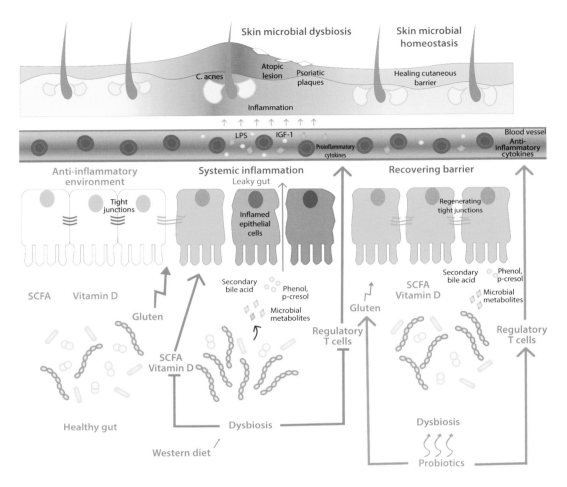

FIGURE 12.5 Gut-skin axis.
(From Szántó M, Dózsa A, Antal D, Szabó K, Kemény L, Bai P. Targeting the gut-skin axis-probiotics as new tools for skin disorder management? Exp Dermatol. 2019 Nov;28(11):1210–18. With permission.)

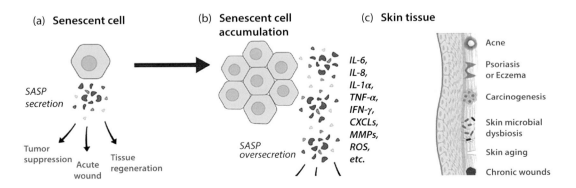

FIGURE 12.6 Senescent skin consequences.
(From Boyajian JL, Ghebretatios M, Schaly S, Islam P, Prakash S. Microbiome and human aging: probiotic and prebiotic potentials in longevity, skin health and cellular senescence. Nutrients. 2021 Dec 18;13(12):4550. (Under Open Access.)

TABLE 12.1

Uptake of Dietary Supplements

Category	Dermatologists Taking Supplements N = 225	Dermatologists Recommending Supplements N = 198
Overall health/wellness	42%	30%
Bone health	24%	25%
Skin, hair, and nails	16%	81%
Heart health	15%	12%
Anti-aging	14%	20%
Immune health	13%	12%

Source: Thompson KG, Kim N. Dietary supplements in dermatology: a review of the evidence for zinc, biotin, vitamin D, nicotinamide, and *Polypodium*. J Am Acad Dermatol. 2021 Apr;84(4):1042–50. With permission.

probiotics are used to treat intestinal dysbiosis and they have been shown to play an important role in the reversal of cellular senescence associated with an aging gut microbiome (29). *Lactococcus lactis* subsp. lactis strain Plasma (LC-Plasma) has a protective effect on cellular senescence and inflammation in mouse models which show a decrease in interferon-α. *Lacticaseibacillus rhamnosus*, *Lactococcus lactis*, *Lacticaseibacillus paracasei*, *Lactiplantibacillus plantarum*, *Bifidobacterium longum*, *Bifidobacterium adolescentis*, and *Brevibacillus brevis* have also been shown to play a similar role in reversing aging patterns. Synbiotics are a class of dietary supplements that combine probiotics with prebiotics. Prebiotics include substrates that promote bacterial metabolism and by-products that promote gut health (29). These include substrates such as plant phytochemicals or fiber or inulin. One study showed a significant increase in longevity of a synbiotic combination of a probiotic and an Ayurvedic herbal prebiotic known as triphala, over probiotics alone in aged Drosophila. Of note, the probiotic blend also improved longevity but with an increase in lifespan of 55% versus 60%. The increased longevity was correlated with improved metabolic biomarkers of reduced weight, glucose, and triglyceride levels (Table 12.1) (30).

Studies in mouse models and humans have shown anti-inflammatory and UV-protective effects as well as improvement of the skin barrier. A randomized, double-blind clinical trial of *L. plantarum* in a study of 110 patients showed statistically significant improvement in TEWL, skin hydration, wrinkles, and elasticity in the probiotic treated group compared to controls (31).

Metabolomics, the study of the by-products of the microbiome, may shed light on the status of an individual's gut and skin microbiome diversity and can allow for individualized treatment approaches for patients (32). Nevertheless, the ideal dosing, type of probiotic, and viability issues remain and ongoing studies are necessary to determine optimal treatment approaches. In addition, a balance must be achieved between the senescence-associated secretory phenotype (SASP), whereby its actions required in wound healing and regeneration are maintained while limiting its harmful effects on aging (Figure 12.7).

Vitamins and Minerals

Barring circumstances of malabsorption, malnutrition, chronic disease states, restrictive dietary choices, or the long-term use of certain pharmaceutical medications, a healthy individual should obtain adequate vitamins and minerals in their diet. Dietary supplements, including multi-vitamins or specific vitamins or minerals, have gained popularity as a general approach to optimizing health outcomes and performance and there is evidence to support supplementation of some vitamins and minerals based upon age-related changes that make a compelling argument for supplementation on an individual and case-by-case basis in a healthy individual (Table 12.2) (33).

Vitamin C or L-ascorbic acid is a potent antioxidant, is water-soluble, and must be acquired from the diet as it is not synthesized by the human body. Typically, a diet rich in fruits and vegetables provides adequate daily intake for biological processes and health (34).

Vitamin C is critical for collagen synthesis. Therefore, the absence of sufficient vitamin C intake can result in profound effects on the skin resulting in easy bruising, bleeding, delayed wound healing, and

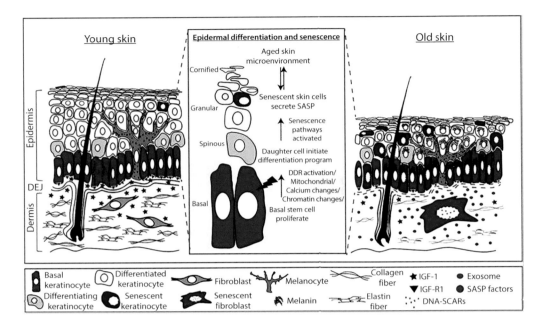

FIGURE 12.7   Cellular senescence in skin.
(From Ho CY, Dreesen O. Faces of cellular senescence in skin aging. Mech Ageing Dev. 2021 Sep;198:111525. Under Open Access.)

a condition known as scurvy. Specifically, vitamin C stabilizes the collagen triple helix by acting as a co-factor for lysyl and prolyl hydroxylase, has a role in cholesterol synthesis and iron absorption, and increases the bioavailability of selenium. Stable topical formulations of L-ascorbic acid are challenging to prepare and measures of effectiveness are not readily available. Studies suggest that the combination of vitamins C and E in combination provides photoprotection either orally or topically. Vitamin C helps to stabilize vitamin E, thus allowing an adequate formulation for the delivery of both vitamins (35).

Vitamin D is a fat-soluble vitamin that is synthesized by the body but requires sun exposure for its active form. With age, our ability to convert vitamin D into its active form reduces by 50% from ages 20 to 80. Therefore, oral supplementation is recommended particularly in older individuals, those who lack adequate sun exposure either because of sun protection for skin cancer prevention or because of innate skin type that prevents the penetration of sufficient amounts of UV light. Optimal serum levels of vitamin D should be maintained above 60 nmol/L, and in general, supplementation is recommended if the levels fall below 50 nmol/L (36).

Active vitamin D3 and its metabolites have anti-inflammatory, antimicrobial, anti-proliferative, pro-differentiating, anti-fibrotic, antioxidant, and photoprotective effects (Figure 12.8). A key mechanism of action includes increasing phosphorylation and expression of the p53 family of genes to exert photoprotection and repair and reduce skin aging and cancer. In general, vitamin D supplementation is recommended for general health based on age-specific recommendations and may, in this way, impact the overall health of the skin (37, 38).

Vitamin A

Vitamin A and its active metabolites have a long history of use in dermatology, both topically and orally, as isotretinoin. Acne, psoriasis, and certain refractory systemic skin conditions are treated with oral isotretinoin. In fact, therapeutic doses of non-pharmaceutical grade vitamin A have been used for medical treatment. In general, though, vitamin A supplementation, in the absence of a deficiency, is

TABLE 12.2

Effects of Dietary Supplements

Effect	Upregulated	Strains
Aging	MMPs TNF IL-6, −8, −1	Tyndallized *Lactobacillus acidophilus* was shown to suppress MMPs for wrinkle prevention in photoaged skin through inhibition of elastase activity An enrichment of *Cyanobacteria* can accompany a decrease in UV-induced damage and pigmentation, suggesting it to be a photoprotective species
Carcinogenesis	p38 MAPK IL-1 p16 INK4a	*Propionibacterium acnes* produces conjugated linoleic acid which was shown to inhibit carcinogenesis and modulate the immune system
Dyspigmentation	IL-1 TNF IL-6 HGF	Tyndallized *Lactobacillus acidophilus* exhibits antimelanogenesis effects by inhibiting the cAMP pathway and suppressing melanin secretion
Psoriasis and Atopic Dermatitis	IL-6, IL-1 TNF CXCL1, CXCL2, and CXCL8 T cells	*Lactobacillus pentosus* was shown to decrease levels of TNF and IL-6 among other cytokines in psoriasis-like skin
Acne Vulgaris	IL-1, −8, −12 p53 pathway	*Streptococcus salivarius* can inhibit the growth of *Propionibacterium acnes* and downregulate IL-8 in epithelial cells and keratinocytes
Chronic Wounds	CXCL1, CXCL2 p16INK4a, p53: MMPs	*Staphylococcus epidermis* can suppress skin inflammation during wound repair
Immunity Decline	*Dysregulated*: CD4+/CD8+ ratio *Upregulated*: TNF IFN IL-6	Colonization with *Staphylococcus epidermis* can enhance skin barrier and remodel skin immunity by inducing IL-17A+ CD8+ T cells

Source: Boyajian JL, Ghebretatios M, Schaly S, et al. Microbiome and human aging: probiotic and prebiotic potentials in longevity, skin health and cellular senescence. Nutrients. 2021;13(12):4550. Under Open Access.

Abbreviations: MMP = matrix metalloproteinase; TNF-α = tumor necrosis factor-alpha; IL = interleukin; UV = ultraviolet; MAPK = mitogen-activated protein kinases; p16INK4a = cyclin-dependent kinase inhibitor 2A; HGF = hepatocyte growth factor; CXCL = chemokine ligand; CD = cluster of differentiation; IFN-γ = interferon gamma.

not recommended for oral intake routinely and its positive anti-aging effects can be adequately harnessed through topical use. Provitamin A such as β-carotene, lycopene, and lutein are found naturally in plant products. The daily recommended doses for individual carotenoids are 2–4.8 mg/d for β-carotene, 10–20 mg/d for lutein, and 5.7–15 mg/d for lycopene (39). Interestingly, a reduction of UVA-inducing pigmentation was found to occur in a study comparing oral supplementation of an oral multi-carotenoid supplement to a placebo (40). Adequate amounts of provitamin A may be obtained simply through dietary habits, including even ingestion of tomato paste prior to spending time outdoors in the sun, so supplementation may be unnecessary in this author's opinion (41).

Vitamin B

Nicotinamide or vitamin B3 has shown promise as an oral supplement in the prevention and reduction of actinic keratoses and prevention of non-melanoma skin cancer (NMSC) in Phases II and III randomized clinical trials (42–44).

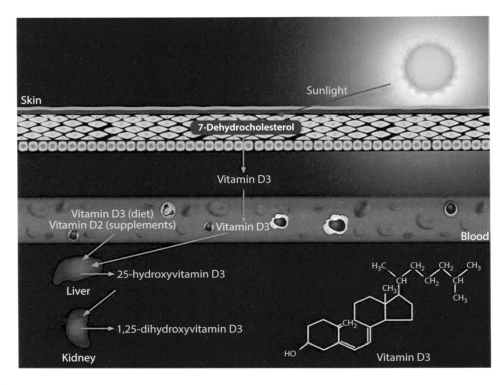

FIGURE 12.8 Effects of vitamin D3.
(From iStock under license.)

The role of B3 supplementation in the prevention of melanoma has not yet been determined. Ongoing treatment for chemoprevention and reduction of NMSCs is required as the effect, while rapid in onset, also dissipates quickly with cessation of supplementation (45).

Dosing is typically 500 mg twice a day. Niacinamide has been used as a non-primary treatment in inflammatory skin conditions such as acne and rosacea (46).

The role of B3 in anti-aging is complex and an understanding of the pathways involved and mechanism of action on the cellular level is important for the practicing dermatologist to make informed decisions about supplement recommendations. Nicotinamide (B3) is a precursor for Nicotinamide Mononucletide or NMH which is required for production of NAD+ biosynthesis. NAD+ is required to power a multitude of cellular enzymatic pathways metabolism relevant to cell death, aging, DNA repair, inflammation, and gene expression (Figure 12.9). In the prevention of skin cancer, the key roles of nicotinamide include one of modulating immunosuppression, inflammation, and DNA repair. The role of B3 or the precursor NMH in anti-aging has yet to be established. We know that with aging and age-related processes on the cellular level, there is increased utilization and subsequent depletion of NAD+ level. This, in turn, reduces mitochondrial energy production which increases oxidative stress and inflammation. The supplementation of NMN, as the precursor of NAD+, may reverse these age-related complications and slow down the rate of aging by enhancing NAD+ levels in the body. Nevertheless, studies supporting this hypothesis are derived primarily from in vitro or in vivo animal models. From the above review, it is shown that only very few pre-clinical and clinical studies have been conducted to investigate the safety of long-term administration of NMH. The safety profile of nicotinamide has been established in a few clinical trials, and that of NMH is ongoing. More data is necessary before recommending supplementation of B3 or NMH in healthy individuals without a history of numerous NMSCs, simply for the potential of a systemic or skin-specific anti-aging effect (Figure 12.9) (47).

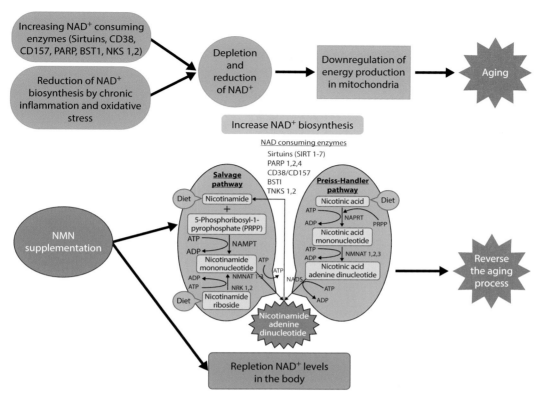

FIGURE 12.9 NAD metabolism and life cycle.
(From Nadeeshani H, Li J, Ying T, Zhang B, Lu J. Nicotinamide mononucleotide (NMN) as an anti-aging health product—promises and safety concerns. J Adv Res. 2021 Aug 11;37:267–78. With permission.)

Biologically Active Plant Polyphenols and Peptides

There are over 8,000 plant polyphenols which are broadly divided into flavanoid and non-flavanoid subtypes (Figure 12.10). Plant polyphenols as nutraceuticals may become increasingly relevant for their use as alternatives or adjunct treatments to topical sunscreens. Many of them show protection on a cellular level from the effects of up radiation (Table 12.3). Two polyphenols, resveratrol and equol, will be addressed here as they both have been prolifically studied for their effects on the skin and there is convincing evidence that supplementation can improve skin health (Figures 12.11 and 12.12). Equol has been the subject of fewer studies over the years as there has been a reluctance to tout estrogen-like hormonal treatment, either topical or oral, over concerns of tumorigenic potential (48). This is unlikely, as we know that diets high in soy are not associated with increased risks of gynecologic cancer in East and Southeast Asia, compared to women in the United States. The average daily consumption of soy in these regions is 20–50 mg/day versus 0.1–3 mg/day in the United States and even lower average consumption in Europe. Moreover, we know that plant isoflavones tend to be selective estrogen receptor modulators and preferentially hone to ER beta found in high amounts on the skin and scalp. A prospective study examined 29 women with visible signs of facial skin aging (36–76 years of age) that took two oral supplements daily for a total dose of 100 mg resveratrol plus 1000 mg of collagen. After six months, the subjects had significant improvements in facial pores, ultraviolet spots, wrinkles, and skin tone with no adverse events reported. The author's admission included not knowing which active ingredient (collagen, resveratrol, or both) resulted in the positive improvement of the skin parameters (49). Equol was examined in postmenopausal women in a pilot randomized placebo-controlled trial for 12 weeks in 101 Japanese women who were equol non-producers: 34 subjects in the placebo group, 34 subjects in the 10 mg dose, and 33 subjects

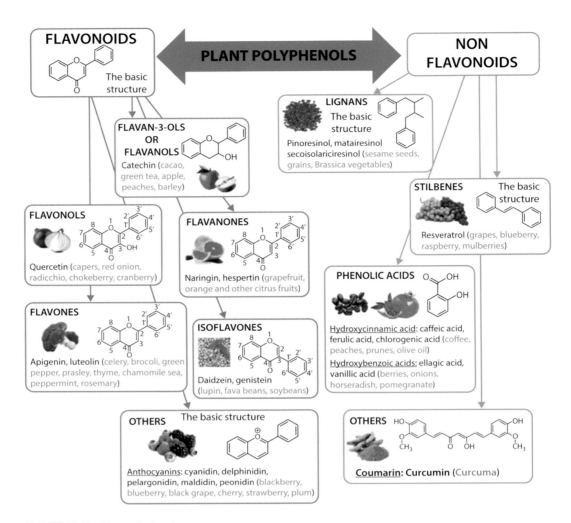

FIGURE 12.10   Plant polyphenols.
(Meccariello R, D'Angelo S. Impact of polyphenolic-food on longevity: an elixir of life. An overview. Antioxidants (Basel). 2021 Mar 24;10(4):507. doi: 10.3390/antiox10040507. PMID: 33805092; PMCID: PMC8064059.)

in the 30 mg dose of equol per day. The skin parameters measured included crow's feet wrinkles around the eyes, hydration, trans-epidermal water loss, and elasticity, which significantly improved for both equol dosing treatments (i.e., 10 mg and 30 mg per day) compared to the placebo-control group values and with no adverse events reported. Another randomized, placebo-controlled study showed that end glycation products in the skin were reduced in patients taking equol supplementation versus those on placebo (50). In this study, 57 women were randomized, with 27 receiving the supplement. Interestingly, a subset of women who were equol-producing showed a significant reduction in skin AGEs as measured by skin autofluorescence, suggesting a potentiating skin anti-aging effect with supplementation of equol in equol-producing women. Endogenous equol production status in women depends in large part on dietary factors and the use of antibiotics as equol is produced in the gut by specific bacteria microbiota from the precursor daidzein (51). These data suggest that S-equol oral supplementation may have beneficial effects on skin health in postmenopausal women with estrogen-deficient skin.

A prospective study examined 29 women with visible signs of facial skin aging (36–76 years of age) that took two oral supplements daily for a total dose of 100 mg resveratrol plus 1,000 mg of collagen. After six months, the subjects had significant improvements in facial pores, ultraviolet spots, wrinkles, and skin tone with no adverse events reported. The author's admission included not knowing which active

TABLE 12.3

Main Polyphenols: Their Origins and Effects on the Skin

Polyphenol	Source	Mechanism(s) of Action
Flavanols (catechin)	Tea leaves, grape seeds	• Inhibition of UVB-mediated phosphorylation of ERK1/2, JNK1/2 and p38 proteins. • Inhibition of UVB-mediated activation of NF-κB signaling and NF-κB DNA-binding activity. • Inhibition of UVB-induced AP-1 activity. • Reduction in UVB-mediated DNA damage through IL-12 dependent functional NER mechanism. • Inhibition of UVB-mediated phosphorylations of MAPKs and activation of NF-κB and NF-κB/p65 DNA-binding activity. • Reduction in UVB-mediated increase in protein expression of MMP-2, MMP-9, CD31, VEGF and PCNA. • Inhibition of UVB-mediated increase in infiltration of leukocytes, protein oxidation and lipid peroxidation. • Reduction in UVB-induced infiltration of CD11b+ cells and IL-10 production. • Induction in UVB-mediated decrease in IL-12 production. • Inhibition of UVB-mediated increase in COX-2, PGE2, cyclin D1, TNFα, IL-6, IL-1β. • Reduction in UVB-mediated increase in H_2O_2 producing cells, inducible nitric oxide synthase expressing cells, H_2O_2 and nitric oxide production. • Reduction in UVB-mediated DNA damage through IL-12 dependent functional NER mechanism. • Reduction in UVB-mediated formation of CPD+ cells. • Reduction in UVB-mediated DNA damage through IL-12 dependent induction of DNA repair. • Inhibition of UVB-mediated increase in H_2O_2 and nitric oxide production. • Inhibition of UVB-mediated increase in the production of PGE2, infiltration of leukocytes and myeloperoxidase activity.
Stilbenes (reservatrol)	Grapes	• Inhibition of UVB-mediated activation of IKKα and NF-κB, and phosphorylation and degradation of IκBα. • Reduction in the phosphorylation of Akt and pCREB, and downregulation of TGF-β2. • Inhibition in UVB-mediated infiltration of leukocytes, H_2O_2 production and PG metabolites, especially PGE2 and PGD2. • Reduction in UVB-mediated expression of TGF-β2.
Flavonoids (curcumin)	Vegetables, fruits, grains, roots, stems, leaves, bark (tree), flowers, tea, wine	• Inhibition of UVB-induced mitogenic and cell survival signaling involving AP-1 and NF-κB. • Inhibition of UVB-induced phosphorylation of MAPKs and AKT. • Induction of UVB-mediated E2F1 protein expression. • Suppression of UVB-mediated increase in inducible nitric oxide synthase and COX-2 protein expression, phosphorylation of STAT3 and NF-κB/p65. • Inhibition of UVB-induced infiltrating leukocytes, myeloperoxidase activity, IL-10 producing cells and its production. • Inhibition of UV-induced oxidative stress by targeting CD11b+ cell type in the skin.
Isoflavones (genistein)	Soy, legumes/legume seeds (peas, beans, lentils)	• Reduction in UVB-induced EGFR tyrosine phosphorylation and PGE2 synthesis. • Inhibition of UVB-mediated phosphorylated p66Shc at Ser36, and FKHRL1 at Thr32. • Reduction in UVB-mediated protein expression c-Fos and c-Jun. • Reduction in UVB-mediated formation of CPDs.

(Continued)

TABLE 12.3 (*Continued*)

Main Polyphenols: Their Origins and Effects on the Skin

Polyphenol	Source	Mechanism(s) of Action
Proanthocyanins	Red wine, pine bark, grape seeds	• Inhibition of UVB-mediated phosphorylation of MAPKs and activation of NF-κB signaling. • Reduction in UVB-mediated DNA damage through IL-12 dependent functional NER mechanism. • Inhibition of UVB-mediated phosphorylation of MAPKs, activation and nuclear translocation of NF-κB. • Inhibition of UVB-mediated infiltration and accumulation of activated macrophages and neutrophils, myeloperoxidase activity, COX-2, cyclin D1, PCNA, PGE2, TNF-α, IL-6, and IL-1β. • Reduction in the levels of CPD+ cells through IL-12 dependent induction of DNA repair. • Protection against UVB-mediated enhanced production of IL-10 by the epidermal and dermal cells of the skin, and in the draining lymph nodes. • Inhibition of UVB-induced immunosuppression by activating CD8+ effector T cells and inhibiting CD4+ T regulatory cells.
Ellagitannins and anthocyanins	Pomegranate, red wine, nuts, tea, fruits, vegetables	• Inhibition of UVB-mediated phosphorylation MAPKs, degradation and phosphorylation of IκBα, activation of IKKα, nuclear translocation and phosphorylation of NF-κB/p65 at Ser536. • Inhibition of UVB-mediated activation of NF-κB, downregulation of proapoptotic caspase-3, and accumulation of cells in G0/G1 phase of the cell cycle. • Inhibition of UVB-mediated phosphorylation of MAPKs, phosphorylation of STAT3 (Tyr705) and NF-κB/p65 (Ser536), activation of IKKα and phosphorylation and degradation of IκBα. • Inhibition of UVB-mediated expression of inducible nitric oxide synthase and COX-2. • Reduction in UVB-mediated formation of CPDs and 8-oxodG and H_2O_2. • Inhibition of UVB-mediated increase in protein expression of c-Fos and phosphorylation of c-Jun, 1), gelatinase (MMP-2, MMP-9), stromelysin (MMP-3), marilysin (MMP-7), and elastase (MMP-12). • Reduction in UVB-mediated formation of CPDs and 8-oxodG.
Phenolic acids (caffeic acids, pucinic acids, and ellagic acids)	Seeds, fruit skins, vegetable leaves	• Induction of endogenous protective enzymes leading to positive regulatory effects on signaling pathway. • Radical scavenging via hydrogen atom donation.

Source: Afaq F, Katiyar SK. Polyphenols: skin photoprotection and inhibition of photocarcinogenesis. Mini Rev Med Chem. 2011 Dec;11(14):1200–15; Panche AN, Diwan AD, Chandra SR. Flavonoids: an overview. J Nutr Sci. 2016 Dec 29;5:e47; Gacek M. Soy and legume seeds as sources of isoflavones: selected individual determinants of their consumption in a group of perimenopausal women. Prz Menopauzalny. 2014 Mar;13(1):27–31; Kumar N, Goel N. Phenolic acids: natural versatile molecules with promising therapeutic applications. Biotechnol Rep (Amst). 2019 Aug 20;24:e00370.

ingredient (collagen, resveratrol, or both) resulted in the positive improvement of the skin parameters (52). Finally, a placebo-control-led pilot study in men (37–56 years of age) showed that oral supplementation with 6 mg of racemic equol per day for 12 weeks significantly improved skin health parameters such as wrinkles, smoothness, and skin tone (discoloration) (53).

Another well-known Ayurvedic herbal supplement and flavonoid, Curcumin, is a highly biologically active polyphenol present in the plant whole herb Turmeric (Figure 12.13). Turmeric has been used for thousands of years as part of ancient medical traditions, both as a herbal medicine and to impact health as part of the diet. There is data supporting its use in the management of a variety of systemic medical

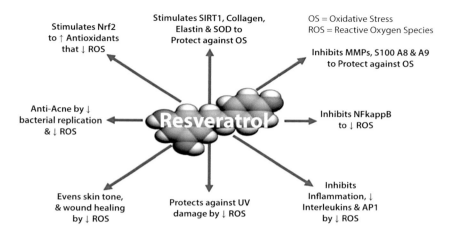

FIGURE 12.11 Resveratrol.
(From Lephart ED. Phytoestrogens [resveratrol and equol] for estrogen-deficient skin—controversies/misinformation versus anti-aging in vitro and clinical evidence via nutraceutical-cosmetics. Int J Mol Sci. 2021 Oct 18;22(20):11218. Under Open Access.)

conditions and more recent evidence suggestive of a role in a number of inflammatory skin conditions (54). Topical treatments of wounds, psoriasis, and atopic dermatitis have shown in vitro and in vivo improvement and a promising absorption profile. One drawback to topical administration can be the yellow discoloration that topical preparations impart. White curcumin can be sourced to counter this problem (personal comm). Oral bioavailability can be problematic and various methods have been used to counter this including the use of liposomes as well as coadministration with piperine which enhances bioavailability. In addition, the typical dosing parameters recommended in over-the-counter supplementation tend not to result in therapeutic effects for inflammatory dermatoses of the skin. Dosing of at least 4–8 g daily is typical for the treatment of systemic conditions. Nevertheless, even at doses of up to 12 g daily, side effects are minimal with the exception of mild gastrointestinal symptoms (55, 56).

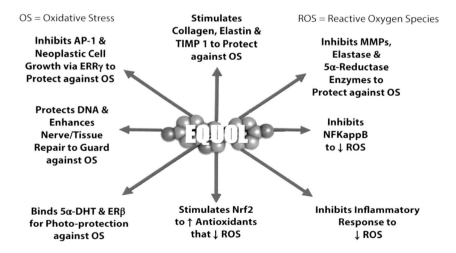

FIGURE 12.12 Equol.
(From Lephart ED. Phytoestrogens (resveratrol and equol) for estrogen-deficient skin—controversies/misinformation versus anti-aging in vitro and clinical evidence via nutraceutical-cosmetics. Int J Mol Sci. 2021 Oct 18;22(20):11218. (Under Open Access.)

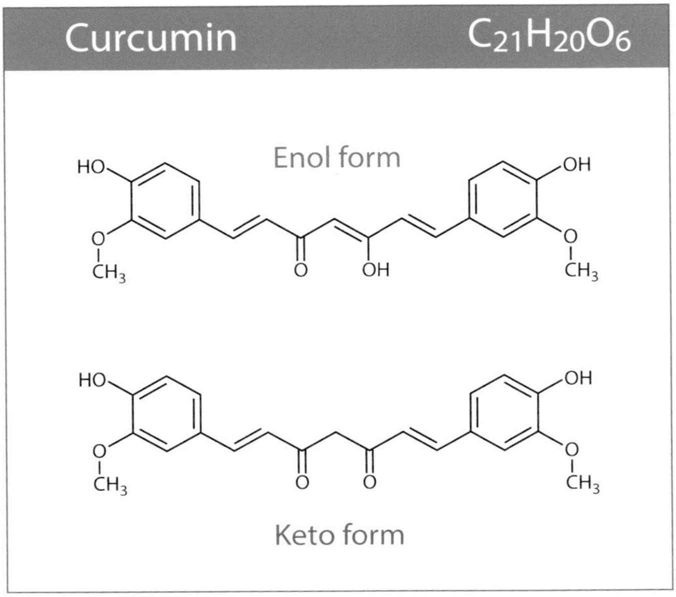

FIGURE 12.13 Curcumin.
(From iStock under license.)

Curcumin acts as an antioxidant and also as an anti-inflammatory, antimicrobial, and anti-prolifera-tive agent. It is thought to act in psoriasis by inhibition of TNF-α and subsequent reduction in inflam-matory cytokines such as IL-17 and IL-22 by blocking NF-κB. It also acts as a competitive inhibitor of phosphorylase kinase which is increased in psoriatic plaques. Curcumin's actions on wound healing are relevant to collagenesis and anti-aging as well as anti-inflammaging (57). Finally a number of phyto-chemicals, including curcumin, have photoprotective effects which are relevant both orally and topically and particularly in light of the search for alternative means to protect skin from sun damage by decreas-ing dependency on chemical sunscreens which may have unknown toxic effects on the skin and systemi-cally, as well as substituting for the cosmetic inelegance of physical blockers such as titanium and zinc with their well-known white discoloration upon application and difficult application (58).

Polyunsaturated Fatty Acids (PUFAs)

Omega-3 fatty acids are one of the most common dietary supplements recommended by dermatolo-gists (59). Omega-3 fatty acids are a type of PUFA which comprise two key fatty acids (Figure 12.14). These are eicosapentaenoic acid (EPA) and docosahexaenoic acid (DHA) which come mainly from fish (60–62).

Alpha linolenic acid (ALA), the most common omega-3 fatty acid in most Western diets, is found in vegetable oils and nuts (especially walnuts), flax seeds, flaxseed oil, leafy vegetables, and some animal fat, especially in grass-fed animals. These fatty acids cannot be synthesized by the human body and, therefore, must be obtained from food sources. There is much evidence from randomized clinical tri-als to suggest that they may improve cardiovascular outcomes. In some studies, fish oil supplementa-tion seems to help in improving acne, eczema, and psoriatic lesions due to a decrease in inflammation (63–65). The proposed mechanisms are via stimulation of anti-inflammatory prostaglandins; in addition, they upregulate the production of adiponectin, reduce reactive oxygen species, and suppress MAPKinase (66). In general, beneficial fats include alpha lipoic, oleic, and palmitoleic acid, omega-3 PUFAs, linoleic acid, trans-11 vaccenic acid, cis-9 and trans-11 conjugated linoleic acid, cholesterol, and phytosterol. Detrimental fats are palmitic, linoleic acid, and arachidonic acid (63, 67–68).

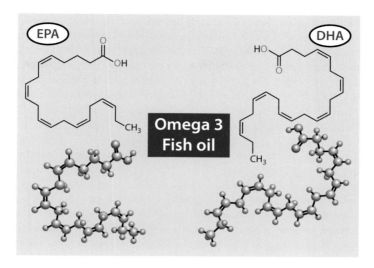

FIGURE 12.14 Omega-3 fatty acids.
(From iStock under license.)

Supplements and Safety

The significantly limited FDA oversight of supplements that are being used in many settings in pharmacologic doses for medicinal purposes, be it for weight loss, anti-aging, heart, and metabolic health, comes with risks that clinicians must understand. Their patients may be taking a number of supplements or they may recommend supplements on their behalf. Supplements can interact with other medications and each other. Drug interactions ought to be checked thoroughly prior to recommending specific supplements (69). Furthermore, some remedies result in increased bleeding risks or can cause liver toxicity in high doses; therefore, both dosing guidelines and precautions regarding side effects must be discussed with the patient, not dissimilar to counseling about prescription medications.

A number of studies have shown that supplementation of certain vitamins and minerals in excess of the recommended daily allowance obtained through diet can result in adverse outcomes and harm. For example, a study of β-carotene supplementation increased the risk of cancer in a study (70, 71).

Similarly, selenium supplementation may cause an increased risk of liver toxicity and cancer (70). Finally, we are well aware that high doses of vitamin A may result in teratogenicity in pregnant women. Another study shows an improvement in overall health that is linked to dietary supplementation of relevant bioactives obtained through food but no improvement with supplements. There are also risks of supplement to supplement interactions that may reduce bioavailability or result in increased side effects. Dosing parameters are murky for many supplements except the most widely used such as omega-3 fatty acids and vitamin D. Finally, the provenance of naturally derived versus synthetic supplements is relevant as local agricultural characteristics can influence the quality of the active supplement resulting in a less effective product or one that has increased contaminants, including arsenic or other compounds. Most supplements contain additives that may result in allergy, for example, and often the number of tablets required to be ingested for therapeutic dosing can be large and the risk of choking is significant (72).

Practical Perspectives and Testing

Approximately, one-third of Americans take supplements and also half of all cancer patients. Vitamins, C, D, and omega-3 fatty acids are the most commonly utilized supplements. Large-scale observational studies on cancer patients show equivocal results, neither benefit nor harm. Two RCTs in men showed a reduction in cancer incidence in men who took multi-vitamins, but it is unclear whether or not there was a deficiency in the relevant vitamins in these patients or not. A thorough history in patients with skin disorders and judicious testing for deficiencies may elucidate which individuals in our dermatology practices might benefit most from supplementation. As previously discussed, vitamin D supplementation is recommended if the serum levels fall below 60 mg/mL and if clinical findings and individual patient variation and circumstances prevent adequate sun exposure. Ferritin and iron levels can be evaluated and also corrected. Often, patients with refractory warts or eczematous dermatitis may warrant an evaluation of serum zinc levels and supplementation which if required long term, copper must also be given. Patients with malabsorption syndromes often require vitamin B12 supplementation and this can also be elucidated via testing. In general, it is a good idea to counsel patients regarding diet and nutrition so that obtaining adequate nutrients through dietary changes ought to be the first-line approach prior to testing and supplementation. In fact, Vedic traditions categorize patients into types and subtypes known as doshas and various foods and spices similarly. Depending upon an individual's type, subtype, and specific desires for wellness or symptoms of disease, food as medicine is often prescribed. Specific foods and herb combinations may improve or exacerbate diseases based on the complex interactions of individual variations and genetics, food, and herbal interactions. Supplements for anti-aging purposes to reduce wrinkles, increase elasticity, and even skin tone are best approached topically. Many topical antioxidant preparations such as vitamin A, resveratrol, and vitamins C and E have been studied and found to be useful in this regard, with limited systemic absorption. The use of nutraceuticals to support skin health as antioxidant sun protection may be of benefit particularly in patients at risk for skin cancer or suffering from pigmentary disorders that are exacerbated by sun exposure. The use of high doses of supplements with the potential to increase carcinogenesis or with known side effects or interactions with other medications, such as selenium, iron, or β-carotene is not recommended unless there is a proven deficiency and only until correction. Four hundred fifty-three people participated in a "Food Habits in Later Life" study conducted by the Union of Nutritional Sciences, and foods found to be protective were olive oil, legumes, fish, vegetables, and grains. Detrimental foods included meat, sugar, and dairy. The findings were based on dietary recall and cutaneous micro-topographic evaluation (73). The best diet for minimizing wrinkles included plentiful vegetables, fruits, and spices which are known to contain polyphenols, vitamins, and minerals. In addition, one that is low in sugar to avoid AGEs, low fat but high in omega-3 fatty acids and olive oils and obtaining polysaccharides from seaweed and mushrooms (74).

In fact, diets high in fats impair wound healing and increase inflammation through increased TNF and oxidative stress. Another recall study of 4,025 middle-aged women aged 40–74 had a 17-g increase in daily dietary fat and an increased appearance of wrinkled skin and atrophy (75, 76).

Conclusion

The future of nutraceuticals in the management of skin diseases, skin health, and anti-aging is promising, but significant resources need to be contributed to further study regarding safety, dosing, drug interactions, bioavailability, and sourcing. The author recommends that recommendations made to patients regarding the use of supplements be guided by practitioners familiar with their potential side effects, risks, and benefits. Moreover, specific brands and origins or supplements and nutraceuticals ought to be considered to ensure proper dosing, improve effectiveness, and allow for improved monitoring and moderation of side effects and interactions.

REFERENCES

1. Variant Market Research. Nutraceuticals Market. Food & Beverage. s.l.: Variant Market Research, 2017. p. 105.
2. Warriner S, Bryan K, Brown AM, Women's attitude towards the use of complementary and alternative medicines (CAM) in pregnancy. Midwifery 2014; 30: 138–43.
3. Fan D, Holistic integrative medicine: toward a new era of medical advancement. Front Med 2017; 11: 152–9.

4. Dwyer JT, Coates PM, Smith MJ, Dietary supplements: regulatory challenges and research resources. Nutrients 2018; 10(1): 41.

5. Brown AC, An overview of herb and dietary supplement efficacy, safety and government regulations in the United States with suggested improvements. Part 1 of 5 series. Food Chem Toxicol 2017; 107(Pt A): 449–71.

6. Wallace TC, Twenty years of Dietary Supplement Health and Education Act: How should dietary supplements be regulated? J Nutr 2015; 145: 1683–6.

7. Frankos VH, Street DA, O'Neill RK, FDA regulation of dietary supplements and requirements regarding adverse event reporting. Clin Pharmacol Ther 2010; 87: 239–44.

8. Kennett G, Time for change: stepping up the FDA's regulation of dietary supplements to promote consumer safety and awareness. J Law Health 2019; 1: 47–78.

9. Melethil S, Proposed rule: current good manufacturing practice in manufacturing, packing, or holding dietary ingredients and dietary supplements. Life Sci Mar 2006; 78: 2049–53.

10. Mukherjee PK, Harwansh RK, Bahadur S et al., Development of Ayurveda-tradition to trend. J Ethnopharmacol 2017; 2: 10–24.

11. Silverberg JI, Study designs in dermatology: a review for the clinical dermatologist. J Am Acad Dermatol 2015; 73: 721–31.

12. Dickinson A, Blatman J, El-Dash N et al., Consumer usage and reasons for using dietary supplements: report of a series of surveys. J Am Coll Nutr 2014; 33: 176–82.

13. Kantor ED, Trends in dietary supplement use among US adults from 1999-2012. JAMA 2016; 316: 1464–74.

14. Dickinson A, MacKay D, Wong A, Consumer attitudes about the role of multivitamins and other dietary supplements: report of a survey. Nutr J 2015; 14: 53–9.

15. Karla EK, Nutraceutical-definition and introduction. AAPS PharmSci 2003; 5: E25.

16. Williamson EM, Liu X, Izzo AA, Trends in US, pharmacology, and clinical applications of emerging herbal nutraceuticals. Br J Pharmacol 2020; 177: 1227–40.

17. Ho CY, Dressen O, Faces of cellular senescence in skin aging. Mech Ageing Dev 2021; 198: 111525.

18. Franco AC, Aveleira C, Cavadas C, Skin senescence: mechanisms and impact on whole-body aging. Trends Mol Med 2022; 28: 97–109.

19. Sato K, The presence of food-derived collagen peptides in human body-structure and biological activity. Food Funct 2017; 8: 4325–30.

20. Oesser S, Oral intake of specific bioactive collagen peptides reduces skin wrinkles and increases dermal matrix synthesis. Skin Pharmacol Physiol 2014; 27: 113–9.

21. Asserin J, The effect of oral collagen peptide supplementation on skin moisture and the dermal collagen network: evidence from an ex vivo model and randomized, placebo-controlled clinical trials. J Cosmet Dermatol 2015; 14: 291–301.

22. De Luca C, Skin antiageing and systemic redox effects of supplementation with collagen peptides and plant-derived antioxidants: a single-blind case-control clinical study. Oxid Med Cell Longev 2016; 2016: 4389410.

23. de Miranda RB, Weimer P, Rossi RC, Effects of hydrolyzed collagen supplementation on skin aging: a systematic review and meta-analysis. Int J Dermatol 2021; 60: 1449–61.

24. Salem I, The gut microbiome as a major regulator of the gut-skin axis. Front Microbiol 2018; 9: 1459.

25. De Pessemier B, Gut-skin axis: current knowledge of the interrelationship between microbial dysbiosis and skin conditions. Microorganisms 2021; 9: 353.

26. O'Neill CA, The gut-skin axis in health and disease: a paradigm with therapeutic implications. Bioessays 2016; 38: 1167–76.

27. Boyajian JL, Ghebretatios M, Schaly S et al., Microbiome and human aging: probiotic and prebiotic potentials in longevity, skin health and cellular senescence. Nutrients 2021; 13: 12.

28. Sinha S, Lin G, Ferenczi K, The skin microbiome and the gut-skin axis. Clin Dermatol 2021; 39: 829–39.

29. La Fata G, Weber P, Mohajeri MH, Probiotics and the gut immune system: indirect regulation. Probiotics Antimicrob Proteins 2018; 10: 11–21.

30. Westfall S, Lomis N, Prakash S, Longevity extension in Drosophila through gut-brain communication. Sci Rep 2018; 8: 8362.

31. Lee DE, Huh CS, Ra J, Choi ID et al., Clinical evidence of effects of *Lactobacillus plantarum* HY7714 on skin aging: a randomized, double blind, placebo-controlled study. J Microbiol Biotechnol 2015; 12: 2160–8.

32. Rinschen MM, Identification of boactive metabolites using activity metablomics. Nat Rev Mol Cell Biol 2019; 20: 353–67.
33. Shapiro SS, Saliou C, Role of vitamins in skin care. Nutrition 2001; 17: 839–40.
34. Grange M, Eck P, Dietary vitamin C in human health. Adv Food Nutr Res 2018; 83: 281–310.
35. Coerdt K. M., Goggins C. A., Khachemoune A, Vitamins A, B, and D: a short review for the dermatologist. Altern Ther Health Med 2021; 27: 41–8.
36. Pfotenhauer KM, Shubrook JH, Vitamin D deficiency, its role in health and disease, and current supplementation recommendations. J Am Osteopath Assoc 2017; 117: 301–5.
37. Williams SE, Vitamin D supplementation: pearls for practicing clinicians. Cleve Clin J Med 2022; 89: 154–60.
38. Thompson KG, Kim N, Dietary supplements in dermatology: a review of the evidence from zinc, biotin, vitamin D, nicotinamide, and *Polypodium*. J Am Acad Dermatol 2021; 84: 1042–50.
39. Toti E, Non-provitamin A and provitamin A carotenoids as immunomodulators: recommended dietary allowance, therapeutic index, or personalized nutrition? Oxid Med Cell Longev 2018; 2018: 4637861.
40. Baswan SM, Orally administered mixed carotenoids protect human skin against ultraviolet A-induced skin pigmentation: a double-blind, placebo-controlled, randomized clinical trial. Photodermatol Photoimmunol Photomed 2020; 46: 219–25.
41. Zinder R, et al., Vitamin A and wound healing. Nutr Clin Pract 2019; 34: 839–49.
42. Chen AC, A phase 3 randomized trial of nicotinamide for skin-cancer chemoprevention. N Engl J Med 2015; 373: 1618–26.
43. Martin AJ, Chen AC, Damian DL, Nicotinamide for skin-cancer chemoprevention. N Engl J Med 2016; 374: 790.
44. Snaidr VA, Damian DL, Halliday G, Nicotinamide for photoprotection and skin cancer chemoprevention: a review of efficacy and safety. Exp Dermatol 2019; 28(suppl 1): 15–22.
45. Giacalone S, Oral nicotinamide: the role in skin cancer chemoprevention. Dermatol Ther 2021; 34: e14892.
46. Kallis PJ, A biologically based approach to acne and rosacea. J Drugs Dermatol 2018; 17: 611–7.
47. Nadeeshani H, Nicotinamide mononucleotide (NMN) as an anti-aging health product—promises and safety concerns. J Adv. Res 2021; 37: 267–78.
48. Lephart ED, Phytoestrogens (resveratrol and equol) for estrogen-deficient skin-controversies/misinformation versus anti-aging in vitro and clinical evidence via nutraceutral-cosmetics. Int J Mol Sci 2021; 22: 11218.
49. Oyama A, The effects of natural S-equol supplementation on skin aging in postmenopausal women: a pilot randomized placebo-controlled trial. Int J Mol Sci 2021; 19: 202–10.
50. Yoshikata R, Effects of an equol-containing supplement on advanced glycation end products, visceral fat and climacteric symptoms in post-menopausal women: a randomized controlled trial. PLoS One 2021; 16: e0257332.
51. Mayo B, Vázquez L, Flórez AB, Equol: a bacterial metabolite from the Daidzein isoflavone and its presumed beneficial health effects. Nutrients 2019; 11: 2231.
52. Smoliga JM, Baur JA, Hausenblas HA, Resveratrol and health—a comprehensive review of human clinical trials. Mol Nutr Food Res 2011; 55: 1129–41.
53. Hausenblas H, Effects of resveratrol and collagen supplementation on facial aging. Nat Med J 2013; 5: 1–8.
54. Vaughn AR, Branum A, Sivamani R K, Effects of turmeric (*Curcuma longa*) on skin health: a systematic review of the clinical evidence. Phytother Res 2016; 30: 1243–64.
55. Gupta SC, Patchva S, Aggarwal BB, Therapeutic roles of curcumin: lessons learned from clinical trials. AAPS J 2013; 15: 195–218.
56. Nguyen TA, Friedman AJ, Curcumin: a novel treatment for skin-related disorders. J Drugs Dermatol 2013; 12: 1131–7.
57. Tundis R, Potential role of natural compounds against skin aging. Curr Med Chem 2015; 22: 1515–38.
58. Sharma RR, Deep A, Abdullah ST, Herbal products as skincare therapeutic agents against ultraviolet radiation-induced skin disorders. J Ayurveda Integr Med 2022; 13: 100500.
59. Dickinson A, Use of dietary supplements by cardiologists, dermatologists and orthopedists: report of a survey. Nutr J 2011; 10: 20.

60. Orengo IF, Wolf Jr JE, Black HS, Influence of fish oil supplementation on the minimal erythema dose in humans. Arch Dermatol Res 1992; 284: 219–21.
61. Rhodes LE, Dietary fish-oil supplementation in humans reduces UVB-erythemal sensitivity but increases epidermal lipid peroxidation. J Investig Dermatol 1994; 103: 151–4.
62. Ziboh VA, Miller CC, Cho Y, Metabolism of polyunsaturated fatty acids by skin epidermal enzymes: generation of anti-inflammatory and anti-proliferative metabolites. Am J Clin Nutr 2000; 71: 361s–6s.
63. Thomsen BJ, Chow EY, Sapijaszko MJ, The potential uses of omega-3 fatty acids in dermatology: a review. J Cutan Med Surg 2020; 24: 481–94.
64. Melnik BC, Linking diet to acne metabolomics, inflammation, and comedogenesis: an update. Clin Cosmet Investig Dermatol 2015; 8: 371–88.
65. Jung JY, Effect of dietary supplementation with omega-3 fatty acid and gamma-linolenic acid on acne vulgaris: a randomised, double-blind, controlled trial. Acta Derm Venereol 2014; 94: 521–5.
66. Latreille J, Association between dietary intake of n-3 polyunsaturated fatty acids and severity of skin photoaging in a middle-aged Caucasian population. J Dermatol Sci 2013; 72: 233–9.
67. Wang X, Wu J, Modulating effect of fatty acids and sterols on skin aging. J Functional Foods 2019; 57: 135–40.
68. Morse NL, Reid AJ, St-Onge M, An open-label clinical trial assessing the efficacy and safety of bend skincare anti-aging formula on minimal erythema dose in skin. Photodermatol Photoimmunol Photomed 2018; 34: 152–61.
69. Gurley BJ, Clinically relevant herb-micronutrient interactions: when botanicals, minerals, and vitamins collide. Adv Nutr 2018; 9: 524S–32S.
70. Buring JE, Hennekens CH, Beta-carotene and cancer chemoprevention. J Cell Biochem 1995; 22(suppl): 226–30.
71. Harvie M, Nutritional supplements and cancer: potential benefits and proven harms. Am Soc Clin Oncol Educ Book 2014; e476–86.
72. Burns EK, Perez-Sanchez A, Katta R, Risks of skin, hair, and nail supplements. Dermatol Pract Concept 2020; 10: e2020089.
73. Purba MB, Skin wrinkling: can food make a difference? J Am Coll Nutr 2001; 20: 71–80.
74. Muzumdar S, Ferenczi K, Nutrition and youthful skin. Clin Dermatol 2021; 39: 796–808.
75. Zhang Y, Oxidative stress-induced calreticulin expression and translocation: new insights into the destruction of melanocytes. J Invest Dermatol 2014; 134: 183–91.
76. Cosgrove MC, Dietary nutrient intakes and skin-aging appearance among middle-aged American women. Am J Clin Nutr 2007; 86: 1225–31.

13

New Delivery Systems for Novel Compounds

Zoe Diana Draelos

Introduction

The ability of cosmeceuticals to induce the desired change in the skin is primarily dependent on the delivery system. The delivery system is the carrier that takes an active ingredient from a formulation and places it in the proper location to achieve an effect. Delivery systems are customized to keep the active ingredient in a certain form for a specified length of time. For example, the delivery system for a sunscreen should not be designed for stratum corneum penetration. Sunscreens function on the skin surface to either absorb or reflect ultraviolet radiation. They create a protective coating over the skin surface. Delivery of a sunscreen beneath the stratum corneum would be counterproductive; however, this is not the case for antioxidants. Oxidation occurs in the viable epidermis and dermis where cellular lipid membranes are present. Thus, an antioxidant that remains on the skin surface, such as vitamin E or green tea, provides little protection from oxidative damage. This need to place cosmeceutical ingredients in a specified compartment is the primary goal of delivery systems.

Delivery systems are also designed to maintain the active ingredient in a target location for a specified duration. For example, a superior sunscreen should remain on the skin as long as possible. Since consumers are unlikely to reapply sunscreen thoroughly every two hours as directed, extended duration sunscreens offer superior photoprotection and the delivery system should resist rubbing, sweat, humidity, and water contact. Conversely, it would be unaesthetic for a therapeutic moisturizer rich in petrolatum to use a delivery system that kept the petrolatum on the skin surface all day. The skin would feel greasy, appear shiny, and stick to clothing. A better delivery system would allow small amounts of petrolatum to be released onto the skin surface avoiding the aesthetic drawbacks.

Unwanted side effects can also be minimized through careful delivery system selection. Retinoids are excellent agents for the treatment of acne, but exhibit unwanted dryness and irritation, especially when the concentration on the skin surface is high. A possible solution is the delivery of lower concentrations of retinoid for a prolonged time creating a time-released reservoir. This type of delivery increases efficacy by allowing skin retinoid exposure for more hours while minimizing side effects.

A variety of delivery systems have been developed to carry novel compounds to the skin. The simplest and oldest delivery systems are creams, lotions, and ointments. These represent delivery emulsions. Newer forms include liposomes, nanodelivery, microsponges, and patches. This chapter evaluates the ability of delivery systems to lend efficacy to cosmeceutical ingredients.

Emulsions

The most basic delivery system is the emulsion (1). An emulsion is formed from oil and water, which are mixed and held in solution by an emulsifier. Most emulsifiers are surfactants, or soaps, which dissolve the two nonmiscible ingredients. The most common emulsions are oil-in-water, where the oil is dissolved in the water (2). This emulsion is the most popular delivery system because the water evaporates leaving behind a thin film of oily ingredients. This is the basis for all moisturizers, the main method of transferring cosmeceuticals to the skin surface. If a large quantity of water is found in the emulsion, it is

DOI: 10.1201/9781315165905-13

considered a lotion, whereas a thicker emulsion with less water is considered a cream. Creams typically contain a higher concentration of oily ingredients than lotions accounting for the thicker film produced.

Creams and lotions are the main cosmeceutical delivery systems because they are inexpensive to produce. They also impart moisturizing qualities to the skin surface, one of the main methods used by cosmeceuticals to improve skin texture and appearance. Thus, carefully constructed emulsions can accomplish moisturization and delivery of an active agent simultaneously. For an emulsion to function as an effective cosmeceutical moisturizer, 1% or more transepidermal water loss must occur (3, 4). This is because transepidermal water loss is the signal for barrier repair, which must occur or the rehydration is temporary. Moisturizers do not rehydrate the skin, but rather form an environment optimal for barrier repair to occur, restoring the natural water balance in the skin. Water must be trapped in the skin that is drawn to the stratum corneum from the lower epidermal and dermal layers to achieve skin remoisturization (5).

The goal of all moisturizing emulsions is to accomplish skin remoisturization, which occurs in four steps: initiation of barrier repair, alteration of surface cutaneous moisture partition coefficient, onset of dermal–epidermal moisture diffusion, and synthesis of intercellular lipids (6). These steps must occur sequentially in order for proper skin barrier repair. Once the barrier has been repaired, there must be some substance that holds and regulates the skin water content. This substance has been termed the natural moisturizing factor (NMF). The constituents of the NMF have been theorized to consist of a mixture of amino acids, derivatives of amino acids, and salts. Artificially synthesized NMF has been constructed from amino acids, pyrrolidone carboxylic acid, lactate, urea, ammonia, uric acid, glucosamine, creatinine, citrate, sodium, potassium, calcium, magnesium, phosphate, chlorine, sugar, organic acids, and peptides (7). Ten percent of the dry weight of the stratum corneum cells is composed of NMF in well-hydrated skin (8). Cosmeceutical moisturizing emulsions try to duplicate the effect of the NMF.

Substances found in cosmeceutical oil-in-water emulsions include oily substances such as petrolatum, mineral oil, vegetable oils, and dimethicone. The water evaporates leaving the oil behind to place a water-impermeable barrier over the skin surface. Substances that attract water to the skin surface and function as humectants are found in the water portion of the emulsion. Naturally occurring humectants in the skin include dermal glycosaminoglycans, which function to maintain skin hydration. Glycosaminoglycans are the first substances to see a burst in production following barrier damage. Common cosmeceutical humectants include glycerin, sorbitol, propylene glycol, polyethylene glycol, lactic acid, urea, and gelatin (9, 10). Newer humectant substances include hyaluronic acid spheres, which hydrate on the skin surface to physically fill fine wrinkles on the face, especially around the eyes and on the lips. These spheres form the basis for the lip plumping and eye wrinkle minimizing cosmeceuticals; yet, they are specialized emulsions.

Water-in-oil emulsions, where the water-soluble substances are dissolved in the oil-soluble substances, are less popular due to their greasy aesthetics. Most ointments are water-in-oil emulsions, but they leave the skin feeling warm and sticky. Ointments deliver higher levels of moisturization because the water phase is small leaving behind a proportionately larger concentration of ingredients capable of retarding transepidermal water loss. Even though their efficacy is greater, cosmeceutical ointment moisturizers are uncommon. Newer triphasic emulsions, such as an oil-in-water emulsion in oil (O/W/O) or a water-in-oil emulsion in water (W/O/W), increasing in popularity. These emulsions are useful to isolate ingredients that are not necessarily compatible with one another.

A specialized form of emulsion is a serum. Serums are usually low viscosity oil-in-water emulsions that deliver a thin film of cosmeceuticals to the skin surface. This delivery system delivers minimal moisturizing benefits, but efficiently places cosmeceutical ingredients on the skin surface. Typically, a sera is placed on the skin immediately after cleansing to function as a skin "treatment" suitable for all skin types followed by an additional moisturizer, if necessary. Both water- and oil-soluble ingredients can be delivered in serum formulations.

Examples of substances that can be delivered in cosmeceutical emulsions include flavonoids, polyphenols, and carotenoids. These are all antioxidant substances that quench singlet oxygen and reactive oxygen species, such as superoxide anions, hydroxyl radicals, and hydroperoxides. Flavonoids possess a polyphenolic structure that accounts for their antioxidant, UV protectant, and metal chelation abilities. Polyphenols compose the largest category of botanical antioxidants. Carotenoids are chemically related to vitamin A. Cosmeceutical ingredients that fit into these categories include soy and silymarin as flavonoid-containing, curcumin and green tea as polyphenol-containing, and retinol as an example of a carotenoid.

Flavonoids

Soybeans and silymarin are examples of botanicals rich in flavonoids. Soy is a rich source of flavonoids called isoflavones, such as genistein and daidzein. These isoflavones function as phytoestrogens when orally consumed and have been credited with the decrease in cardiovascular disease and breast cancer seen in Asian women (11). Some of the cutaneous effects of soy have linked to its estrogenic effect in postmenopausal women. Topical estrogens have been shown to increase skin thickness and promote collagen synthesis (12). It is interesting to note that genistein increases collagen gene expression in cell culture; however, there are no published reports of this collagen-stimulating effect in topical human trials. This highlights the difference between cosmeceuticals and drugs.

Genestein has also been reported to function as a potent antioxidant scavenging peroxyl radicals and protecting against lipid peroxidation in vivo (13). The problem is that antioxidant protection prevents damage to the cell that is yet to occur, making measurement of its efficacy difficult. Furthermore, long-term protection from oxidation is necessary for any clinical benefit. Mix soy-derived genestein in a carefully constructed oil-in-water emulsion and you get moisturization benefits to decrease facial wrinkles of dehydration in the short-term and possible long-term benefits from antioxidant effects. It is this combination of delivery system and activeness that accounts for the success of the cosmeceutical category.

Another example of a flavonoid-rich botanical is silymarin. Silymarin is an extract of the milk thistle plant (*Silybum marianum*), which belongs to the aster family of plants, including daisies, thistles, and artichokes. The extract consists of three flavonoids derived from the fruit, seeds, and leaves of the plant. These flavonoids are silybin, silydianin, and silychristine. Homeopathically, silymarin is used to treat liver disease, but it is a strong antioxidant preventing lipid peroxidation by scavenging free radical species. Its antioxidant effects have been demonstrated topically in hairless mice by the 92% reduction in skin tumors following UVB exposure (14). The mechanism for this decrease in tumor production is unknown, but topical silymarin has been shown to decrease the formation of pyrimidine dimers in a mouse model, as well (15). Here again is a nice example of a cosmeceutical when silymarin is placed in a well-constructed emulsion. The emulsion repairs the barrier enhancing skin texture and appearance while delivering silymarin flavonoids to the skin surface. Is the silymarin improving skin appearance by decreasing pyrimidine dimers or by improving the skin barrier in an emulsion? Again, the cosmeceutical paradox is at work.

Polyphenols

Polyphenols are another category of botanicals popular in cosmeceutical moisturizer emulsions. Two currently popular examples include curcumin and green tea. Curcumin is a polyphenol antioxidant derived from the turmeric root, a popular natural yellow food coloring used in everything from pre-packaged snack foods to meats. It is sometimes used in cosmeceuticals as a natural yellow coloring in products that claim to be free of artificial ingredients. Curcumin is consumed orally as an Asian spice, frequently found in rice dishes to color the otherwise white rice yellow. However, this yellow color is undesirable in cosmetic preparations, since yellowing of products is typically associated with oxidative spoilage.

Tetrahydrocurcumin, a hydrogenated form of curcumin, is off-white in color and can be added to skin care products not only to function as a skin antioxidant, but also to prevent the lipids in the moisturizer from becoming rancid. The antioxidant effect of tetrahydrocurcumin is said to be greater than vitamin E, based on its food preservation effects. Many antioxidants are rated based on their ability to prevent the browning of foods, such as bananas, peaches, apples, and potatoes. Does this measure of antioxidant ability translate into cosmeceutical skin efficacy? It is unclear. Measuring the ability of a cosmeceutical to function as an antioxidant is difficult.

Probably the most accepted test to measure the ability of a product to prevent oxidative skin damage is the sunburn cell test. This test can be conducted with several experimental methods. One method is to apply the test product to one buttock and nothing to the opposite buttock for 8–12 weeks in subjects with Fitzpatrick skin type I who develop a consistent sunburn reaction to 2 MED of UVB and UVA radiation mimicking sunlight. The test is conducted on sun-protected skin to minimize the hardening effect of repeated solar exposure on the skin. Following radiation of both buttocks with 2 MED from a solar simulator, the skin is biopsied with a 3-mm punch to include the epidermis and superficial dermis. Following H&E staining, the specimen is sliced and the sunburn cells, which are apoptotic cells, are counted over several sections. Sunburn cell counts are compared between the untreated and treated sites to determine if the topical antioxidant reduced the number of apoptotic cells. Is this test medically relevant? Perhaps. However, it is the only standardized clinical test in human subjects that condenses years of oxidative damage into an 8- to 12-week realistic test period.

Are most topical antioxidants vetted with the sunburn cell test? Probably not. Most could not pass the test and this type of testing can only be performed by a clinician who can obtain and interpret the skin biopsies. This is the next challenge in cosmeceutical antioxidants, to demonstrate efficacy. In the meantime, skin benefits are achieved with the antioxidant in an emulsion that functions as a cosmeceutical vehicle.

Another topically applied food with antioxidant properties due to polyphenols is green tea. Green tea, also known as *Camellia sinensis*, is a botanical obtained from both the leaf and the bud of the plant. Orally, green tea is said to contain beneficial polyphenols, such as epicatechin, epicatechin-3-gallate, epigallocatechin, and eigallocatechin-3-gallate, which function as potent antioxidants (16). The term "green tea" refers to the manufacture of the botanical extract from fresh leaves of the tea plant by steaming and drying them at elevated temperatures, being careful to avoid oxidation and polymerization of the polyphenolic components. Green tea can be easily added to topical creams and lotions designed to combat the signs of photoaging, but it must be stabilized itself with an antioxidant, such as butylated hydroxytoluene.

A study by Katiyar et al. demonstrated the anti-inflammatory effects of topical green tea application on C3H mice. A topically applied green tea extract containing GTP ((–)-epigallocatechin-3-gallate) was found to reduce UVB-induced inflammation as measured by double skin-fold swelling (17). They also found protection against UV-induced edema, erythema, and antioxidant depletion in the epidermis. This work was further investigated by applying GTP to the back of humans 30 minutes prior to UV irradiation, which resulted in decreased myeloperoxidase activity and decreased infiltration of leukocytes as compared to untreated skin (18). This is a modified sunburn cell test previously described. The application of topical green tea polyphenols prior to UV exposure has also been shown to decrease the formation of cyclobutane pyrimidine dimers (19). These dimers are critical in initiating UV-induced mutagenesis and carcinogenesis, which represent the end stage of the aging process. Thus, green tea polyphenols can function topically as antioxidants, anti-inflammatories, and anti-carcinogens making them a popular botanical for inclusion in cosmeceutical emulsions.

Carotenoids

The final major category of cosmeceuticals discussed is carotenoids. The major carotenoid found in cosmeceuticals is retinol, the naturally occurring form of vitamin A found in fruits and vegetables with a red, orange, or yellow color (20, 21). Retinol and other carotenoids, such as lycopene, astaxanthin, and lutein, are found in tomatoes in high concentration and can be safely applied to the skin from these food sources. Topical retinol can function as an antioxidant, but exhibit a more profound biologic activity following cutaneous enzymatic conversion of retinol to retinoic acid, also known as tretinoin. It is this cutaneous conversion of retinol to retinoic acid that is responsible for the biologic activity of some of the new stabilized vitamin A preparations designed to improve the appearance of benign photodamaged skin (22). Unfortunately, only small amounts of retinol can be converted to tretinoin by the skin, accounting for the increased efficacy seen with prescription preparations. Yet, carotenoids can be placed in cosmeceutical emulsions for effective skin delivery.

This discussion has focused on the diverse use of emulsion technology to deliver cosmeceuticals to the skin surface, but emulsions have profound limitations. For example, creation of time-released delivery system is not possible with a simple emulsion. For this purpose, liposomes and multilamellar vesicles have been created, the next topic of discussion.

Liposomes

Liposomes are spherical vesicles with a diameter between 25 and 5,000 nm formed from membranes consisting of bilayer amphiphilic molecules, which possess both polar and nonpolar ends. The polar heads are directed toward the inside of the vesicle and toward its outer surface, whereas the nonpolar, or lipophilic tails, are directed toward the middle of the bilayer (Figure 13.1). This delivery system was discovered by AD Bangham who reported his work in the 1965 *Journal of Molecular Biology*. His discovery was based on the observation that phospholipids could be dispersed in an aqueous solution to spontaneously form hollow vesicles, known as liposomes.

Liposomes are based on the natural structure of the cell membrane, which has been highly conserved through evolutionary change. The name is derived from the Greek word "lipid" meaning fat and "soma" meaning body. Liposomes are primarily formed from phospholipids, such as phosphatidylcholine, but may also be composed of surfactants, such as dioleoylphosphatidylethanolamine. Their functionality may be influenced by chemical composition, vesicle size, shape, surface charge, lamellarity, and homogeneity.

The liposome is an extremely versatile structure. It can contain aqueous substances in its core, or nothing at all. Hydrophobic substances can dissolve in the phospholipid bilayer shell, which allows liposomes to deliver both oil-soluble and water-soluble substances. This characteristic is used in drug delivery where an oil-soluble drug can be dissolved in water if placed in the phospholipid shell. Similarly, water- and oil-soluble cosmeceutical ingredients can be dissolved in a stable solution without the use of an emulsifier with this technology.

It is unlikely that liposomes diffuse across the stratum corneum barrier intact. The corneocytes are embedded in intercellular lipids, composed of ceramides, glycosylceramides, cholesterol, and fatty acids, which are structurally different from the phospholipids of the liposome. It is postulated that liposomes penetrate through the appendageal structures. They may also fuse with other bilayers, such as cell membranes, to release their ingredients. This is the mechanism by which liposomes can function as moisturizers, supplementing deficient intercellular lipids.

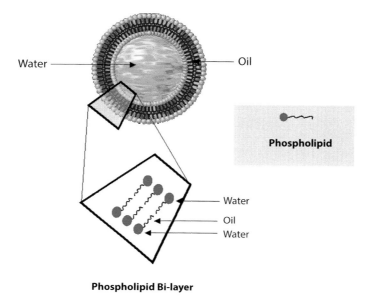

Phospholipid Bi-layer

FIGURE 13.1   The architecture of a liposome.

Liposomes can be specially devised to release their internal contents under certain conditions. For example, liposomes can release when a desired pH or temperature is present in the stratum corneum. Liposomes can be made of a certain size such that they are a natural target for macrophage phagocytosis, releasing their payload inside the macrophage phagosome and inducing a desired change. Liposomes can also be coated with opsonins and ligands to encourage endocytosis in other cell types, but this mechanism would be more appropriate for drug than cosmeceutical delivery, at present.

Niosomes are a specialized form of liposome composed of nonionic surfactants. These are detergents, such as ethoxylated fatty alcohols and synthetic polyglycerol ethers (polyoxyethylene alkylester, polyoxyethylene alkylether). These liposomes do not deliver the moisturizing phospholipids to the skin surface.

Another variant of the liposome is a multivesicular emulsion (MVE) (Figure 13.2). The MVE is created through a physical mixing technique, which makes them more stable, but also less expensive to produce. An MVE can be thought of as a liposome within a liposome. Thus, with the release of each liposome, additional moisturizing ingredients can be deposited on the skin surface. MVEs can deliver glycerin, dimethicone, sphingolipids, and ceramides to the skin surface simultaneously.

In summary, liposomes represent an important cosmeceutical delivery system. Their functionality is dependent on where the active ingredient is stored, which may be in the vesicle, in the lipid bilayer membrane, or on the vesicle surface, and the chemical nature of the active ingredient. However, liposomes are inherently unstable. They are readily deformed and possibly lysed by the weight of a cover slip when viewed under a microscope. They are subject to fusion, aggregation, and precipitation. Even vigorous shaking of a liposomal solution may lyse all of the lipid bilayers. The cosmeceutical strength of liposomes is in their ability to deliver time-released moisturizers and other active ingredients to the skin surface. Some of these drawbacks have been overcome with MVEs. However, the need remains for delivery systems that can reliably penetrate the stratum corneum enhancing the effect of cosmeceutical actives. Many cosmeceuticals could be more effective if penetration kinetics were better. One method of enhancing delivery is to make the particles of the active ingredient so small that they can penetrate through and around the corneocytes. This delivery system, known as nanodelivery, is the next topic for discussion.

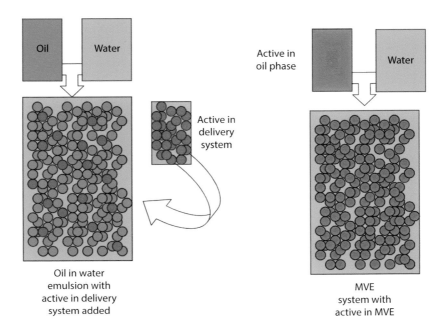

FIGURE 13.2 The left panel shows a traditional emulsion where the oil droplets are suspended in the water; the right panel depicts a multilamellar vesicular emulsion (MVE) where the oil droplets are suspended in specialized liposomes.

Nanodelivery

Nanodelivery is predicated on the use of very small particles, known as nanoparticles, of a cosmeceutical ingredient to enhance skin penetration. By definition, nano means smaller than 100 nm. The creation of nanoparticles is not new. Nanoparticles have been found on the ninth-century Mesopotamian pottery to create a glittery effect. Pottery from the Middle Ages and Renaissance with a copper metallic glitter contains copper nanoparticles dispersed homogenously within the ceramic glaze. Michael Faraday first explained the optics of this nanoparticle effect in 1857.

Nanoparticles are found in the environment as a byproduct of fire or combustion (Figure 13.3). Automobile exhaust, airplane exhaust, and air pollution in general contain nanoparticles. It is the nanoparticles inhaled in cigarette smoke that deposit in the alveoli creating the chronic inflammatory process leading to emphysema. Yet, life has evolved to deal with nanoparticle insults. The anatomy of the lung largely prevents nanoparticles from penetrating lung tissue and entering the body. Otherwise, salt nanoparticles from an ocean mist, dust nanoparticles from volcanic eruptions, or fuel aerosols would prove toxic. In nature, free nanoparticles tend to agglomerate, thus reducing their penetration abilities.

Yet, there is a growing concern over the presence of nanoparticles in the environment. These particles are invisible to the human eye and can penetrate the skin and lung tissues, gaining access to the lymphatics and blood circulation. From there, these particles can be widely distributed throughout the body.

Unfortunately, once these particles enter the body, they cannot be removed. Concern has been voiced in the medical community that nanoparticles of metals might be responsible for neurologic disease. Others have wondered if the chronic inflammation induced by nanoparticles might not cause other degenerative diseases.

At present, nanoparticles are being investigated for use in a variety of cosmeceutical products to include sunscreens, anti-aging moisturizers, and pigmented cosmetics. This discussion focuses on the use of nanotechnology as it relates to cosmeceuticals.

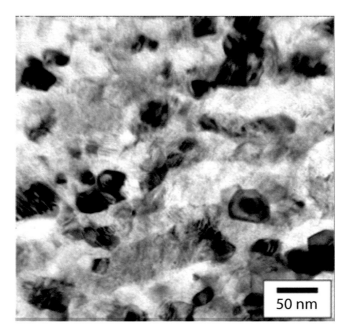

FIGURE 13.3   The appearance of impact diamond nanoparticles under transmission electron microscopy. (From Ohfuji H, Irifune T, Litasov KD, et al. Natural occurrence of pure nano-polycrystalline diamond from impact crater. Sci. Rep. 5, 14702. Under Creative Commons attribution.)

Nanoparticles

Nanoparticle technology has been applied to vitamins, sunscreens, fragrances, and essential oils (23). Since nanoparticles possess a high surface area to weight ratio, they can impart new characteristics to previously existing materials. For example, normally ductile copper becomes extremely hard when nanoparticles smaller than 50 nm are created. The melting temperature of many raw materials is raised when placed in nanoparticle form. Ten-nanometer nanoparticle ferroelectric materials can switch their direction of magnetization using room temperature thermal energy. This effect has been used to deliver multiple drugs into the body. Nanoparticles can be created that carry two different drugs with the first drug released by a small remotely generated electromagnetic pulse and the second drug released by a stronger pulse providing highly targeted delivery.

Nanoparticles also show promise as sunscreens. Nanoparticle zinc oxide and titanium dioxide are available to act as broad-spectrum inorganic filters by reflecting and to a lesser extent absorbing UVA and UVB radiation (24). Their concentration in sunscreen formulations is limited, however, by their white color. Nanoparticle zinc oxide and titanium dioxide are colorless conferring a large aesthetic advantage, but as of this writing, the cosmetics industry has voluntarily agreed to suspend the use of nanoparticle technology sunscreens. An expert panel was convened by the US FDA in 2007 to gather information on of the penetration of nanoparticles in the skin, but a final report is still forthcoming.

Nanoparticle sunscreens have health concerns of unwanted penetration, since sunscreen filters are intended to stay on the skin surface. Some experts believe that nanoparticle zinc oxide and titanium dioxide are unable to penetrate the stratum corneum; yet, others are concerned about the potential health consequences. Both titanium dioxide and zinc oxide are chemically inert. They are theorized to remain in the body indefinitely either forming a reservoir within the dermis or spreading throughout the body via the circulation. Concern arose over the possibility that sunscreen nanoparticles were capable of absorbing and reflecting UV radiation within the skin causing the generation of oxygen radicals within the dermis and initiating the inflammatory cascade. It is currently unknown if a dermal nanoparticle sunscreen reservoir might enhance the photoprotective abilities of the skin or prematurely age skin due to chronic low-grade inflammation characterized by unusually high levels of interleukins 8 and 12.

However, there are other cosmeceutical uses for nanoparticles where enhanced penetration may be desirable. Consider the ability of nanodelivered salicylic acid or benzoyl peroxide to enter the pilosebaceous unit. This would allow very small concentrations of OTC acne actives to reach the location of *Propionibacterium acnes* and more efficiently kill the organism eliminating unwanted epidermal irritation. Nanoparticle topical antibiotics would create similar opportunities to decrease the incidence of skin infection. Very small ingredient quantities with targeted delivery would increase efficacy while reducing toxicity and side effects.

Thus, the nanoparticle controversy continues regarding cosmeceuticals. It is unclear whether nanoparticles represent the next great formulation frontier creating huge therapeutic opportunities or a looming danger. Perhaps with better understanding, nanoparticles will become an important cosmeceutical delivery system.

Nanoemulsions

A variant on nanoparticles is nanoemulsions, similar in construction to the emulsions previously discussed at the beginning of this chapter as the oldest delivery system. Nanoemulsions, just like simple emulsions, are liquids with an oil-loving hydrophobic phase and a water-loving hydrophilic co-existing as a single phase with the aid of an emulsifier. The difference is that the droplets in these emulsions are on the nanoscale of 20–300 nm. If the nanodroplets are larger than 100 nm, the emulsion appears white, whereas nanoemulsions with droplets of 70 nm are transparent. Nanoemulsions offer the ability to deliver highly hydrophobic or lipophilic substances into the skin, which could not otherwise penetrate. The stratum corneum is an excellent barrier to lipophilic cosmeceuticals.

For example, new nanoemulsions of ubiquinone have been developed. Ubiquinone, also known as coenzyme Q10, is an important antioxidant manufactured by the body and found in all skin cells. It is found in both hydrophilic and hydrophobic cellular compartments, but topical delivery has been challenging.

Nanoemulsions have successfully delivered higher concentrations of ubiquinone into the skin with the goal of enhancing the skin's natural antioxidant capabilities. Nanodispersed organic sunscreen formulations containing benzophenone or octylmethoxycinnamate have also been created, but are not yet in widespread use. However, two other methods of enhanced delivery, microsponges and transdermal patches, are widely used for cosmeceutical delivery as of this writing.

Nanocarriers

Nanocarriers are useful for both drug and cosmeceutical deliveries. They include micelles, polymeric nanoparticles, solid lipid nanoparticles, and inorganic nanoparticle emulsions, to name a few. Emulsions that are fragmented to nanoparticle size have better aesthetics and superior penetration of the skin. Polymer-based nanoparticles, such as nanospheres and nanocapsules, are highly stable and can deliver the controlled release of actives due to the encapsulation of the active ingredient. This technology has been used to encapsulate small inhibitor ribonucleic acids that can modulate gene expressions. While this technique is currently used in the treatment of conditions such as pachyonychia congenital, it could be used to modulate aging in the future (25).

Microsponges

Microsponges are a delivery system designed for controlled time-extended release. They are macroporous beads 10–25 μm in diameter (26). Their active agent is released with temperature and rubbing as the sponge breaks down on the skin surface (27). Microsponges are presently used in prescription tretinoin formulations and OTC moisturizers and sunscreens. They are expensive to produce and leave a white residue on the skin. The main advantage of microsponges is to minimize irritation from active ingredients. For this reason, they can be effectively used to deliver cosmeceutical retinoids for anti-aging therapy (retinol, retinaldehyde), benzoyl peroxide for acne treatment, and hydroquinone for pigment lightening. The microsponge is useful for the delivery of ingredients that require constant contact with the skin to achieve efficacy.

Hydroquinone is an excellent example of a substance well suited for microsponge delivery since constant melanocyte pigment suppression is necessary for skin lightening. Hydroquinone, a phenolic compound chemically known as 1,4-dihydroxybenzene, functions by inhibiting the enzymatic oxidation of tyrosine and phenol oxidases. It covalently binds to histidine or interacts with copper at the active site of tyrosinase. It also inhibits RNA and DNA synthesis and may alter melanosome formation, thus selectively damaging melanocytes. These activities suppress the melanocyte metabolic processes inducing gradual decrease of melanin pigment production (28). The ability of the sponge to release hydroquinone over an extended period may increase the efficacy of 2% cosmeceutical preparations currently sold OTC. If extremely sustained delivery to a targeted area is desired, transdermal patches may offer additional efficacy, discussed next.

Transdermal Patches

Transdermal patches, also known as skin patches, were originally developed for pharmaceutical delivery and then adapted to cosmeceutical delivery of actives to a targeted area. The first commercialized patch was approved in 1979 for the delivery of scopolamine for motion sickness with subsequent approval of nicotine, estrogen, and nitroglycerin patches. The patch contains four components: liner, active agent, adhesive, membrane, and backing materials. The liner protects the patch and is removed before application. Removal of the liner exposes the drug, which is fixed to the skin with an adhesive. The membrane controls the release of drug onto the skin surface and the backing protects the patch from anything that rubs the skin.

This same patch technology has been adapted to cosmeceutical delivery. Patches containing vitamins C and E have been commercialized for application to wrinkles around the eyes, between the brows, and on the upper lip. These patches are an adaptation of an older product, known as frownies, which used adhesive to tape skin in place and minimize wrinkles overnight. The patch functions not only by immobilizing skin, but also by physically decreasing transepidermal water loss, delivering moisturizing ingredients, such as dimethicone to the skin surface, and placing vitamins or other cosmeceutical ingredients on the skin. The physical effect of the patch on the skin is just as important as the cosmeceutical delivered.

Transdermal patches are still a minor delivery method for cosmeceuticals. A variation of the transdermal patch is a film face mask. This delivery uses a polymer film to cover the face and deliver cosmeceutical moisturizers and other active ingredients without adhesive. The face is covered with the mask for 5–15 minutes, while reclining delivering vitamins and botanicals to the skin surface.

Paper Delivery Systems

Another form of face mask is a paper delivery system. Here, the paper is impregnated with a water-soluble ingredient. As the water evaporates, the active ingredient is left behind on the face. A variety of papers are available for this purpose to include nonwoven cellulose fiber, cotton fiber, and hydrogel. The nonwoven cellulose paper technology is used in inexpensive hand wipes with the paper being characteristically stiff with a low delivery capacity. The cotton fibers have a higher delivery capacity and are softer, making them more effective. However, the most effective and most expensive delivery system is the hydrogel. Here, the paper has two different parts, a top and bottom layer. The bottom layer is the cotton fiber, whereas the top layer contains water and active ingredient impregnated gel that is placed in contact with the face. The gel hyperhydrates the face resulting in a diminution of fine lines and wrinkles. The cosmetic effect is temporary, however, as removal of the paper will allow TEWL to return to normal levels with the extra water being lost to the environment.

The paper face masks are designed for single use and usually contain moisturizing ingredients, such as dimethicone and glycerin. The masks can be individualized for skin brightening, pore tightening, wrinkle minimization, and pigmentation improvement based on the ingredients in the mask. The delivery time is usually 20 minutes after which the paper mask is removed and disposed.

Mechanical Delivery Systems

Mechanical delivery systems rely on physical rather than chemical delivery mechanisms. Mechanical delivery systems physically remove the stratum corneum, which is the barrier to the penetration of all cosmeceutical actives. Several methods are employed to include skin poration and mircodermabrasion.

Skin Poration

Skin poration is a commonly used mechanical delivery system. This procedure is known as skin needling or derma-rolling. It requires a roller covered in plastic or stainless steel needles usually less than 0.3 mm. Longer needles are available on devices sold only to professionals. The poration can be used to deliver skin care products through two different methods. One method involves rolling the skin to create tiny holes and then immediately applying a skin serum with theoretically enhanced penetration through the newly created pores. The second method involves covering the face with the active ingredient following by poration to push the substance into the skin with the needles. The needle damage also is thought to initiate healing and collagen remodeling in addition to the effect of the active ingredient. Common ingredients that are rolled into the skin include hyaluronic acid, peptides, growth factors, hydroquinone, and retinoids. This delivery system must be used carefully because it is indiscriminate. Anything on the skin can be allowed to penetrate, including bacteria, soap residue, cosmetics, hydrocarbon pollution, etc.

Skin poration can also be achieved with laser microporation. Laser microporation applies light energy to the skin surface to excite water molecules resulting in explosive evaporation from the epidermis that leads to pore formation (29).

Microdermabrasion

Microdermabrasion enhances penetration of cosmeceutical actives by encouraging premature removal of the desquamating corneocytes. This can be facilitated by bombarding the skin surface with small particles, such as sand, and then vacuuming away the debris or by grinding the skin surface with a rotary drill apparatus. The same effect can also be achieved by running a sharp blade over the skin surface, a technique label microblading. All of these mechanical methods of removing the stratum corneum several cells at a time allow an easier access to the viable epidermis and facilitate delivery through penetration. Mechanical penetration enhancement is quite effective since both water-soluble and oil-soluble ingredient penetration can be increased. Care must be taken not to damage the dermis and create scarring. Further, overuse of this technique may result in the creation of sensitive skin (30).

Conclusion

This chapter has covered a variety of delivery systems for novel cosmeceuticals. As of this writing, cosmeceutical delivery is the biggest impediment to their efficacy. The stratum corneum is efficient at keeping substances out of the skin, a function consistent with life. Otherwise, hand washing could become a toxic event. Helping the skin maintain an intact barrier to prevent chemical entry and prevent disease is paramount; yet, allowing the entry of cosmeceutical actives designed to minimize oxidation, inflammation, and protein glycation might slow and possibly reverse the skin aging process. Liposomes, nanodelivery, microsponges, transdermal patches, paper delivery systems, and skin poration are a few of the currently available techniques to deliver novel cosmeceuticals.

REFERENCES

1. Chanchal D, Swarnlata S, Novel approaches in herbal cosmetics. J Cosmet Dermatol 2008; 7: 89–95.
2. Carlotti ME, Gallarate M, Rossatto V, O/W microemulsions as a vehicle for sunscreen. J Cosmet Sci 2003; 54: 451–62.
3. Jass HE, Elias PM, The living stratum corneum: Implications for cosmetic formulation. Cosmet Toilet 1991; 106: 47–53.
4. Holleran W, Feingold K, Man MQ, et al., Regulation of epidermal sphingolipid synthesis by permeability barrier function. J Lipid Res 1991; 32: 1151–8.
5. Wu MS, Yee DJ, Sullivan ME, Effect of a skin moisturizer on the water distribution in human stratum corneum. J Invest Dermatol 1983; 81: 446–8.
6. Jackson EM, Moisturizers: What's in them? How do they work? Am J Contact Dermatitis 1992; 3: 162–8.
7. Wehr RF, Krochmal L, Considerations in selecting a moisturizer. Cutis 1987; 39: 512–5.
8. Rawlings AV, Scott IR, Harding CR, Bowser PA, Stratum corneum moisturization at the molecular level. Prog Dermatol 1994; 28: 1–12.
9. De Groot AC, Weyland JW, Nater JP, Unwanted Effects of Cosmetics and Drugs Used in Dermatology, 3rd edn. Amsterdam: Elsevier, 1994: 498–500.
10. Spencer TS, Dry skin and skin moisturizers. Clin Dermatol 1988; 6: 24–8.
11. Glazier MG, Bowman MA, A review of the evidence for the use of phytoestrogens as a replacement for traditional estrogen replacement therapy. Arch Intern Med 2001; 161: 1161–72.
12. Maheux R, Naud F, Rioux M, et al., A randomized, double-blind, placebo-controlled study on the effect of conjugated estrogens on skin thickness. Am J Obset Gynecol 1994; 170: 642–9.
13. Wiseman H, O'Reilly JD, Adlercreutz H, et al., Isoflavone phytoestrogens consumed in soy decrease F-2-isoprostane concentrations and increase resistance of low-density lipoprotein to oxidation in humans. Am J Clin Nutr 2000; 72: 395–400.
14. Katiyar SK, Korman NJ, Mukhtar H, Agarwal R., Protective effects of silyarin against photocarcinogenesis in a mouse skin model. J Natl Cancer Inst 1997; 89: 556–66.
15. Chatterjee L, Agarwal R, Mukhtar H, Ultraviolet B radiation-induced DNA lesions in mouse epidermis: An assessment using a novel 32P-postlabeling technique. Biochem Biophys Res Commun 1996; 229: 590–5.

16. Katiyar SK, Elmets CA, Green tea and skin. Arch Dermatol 2000; 136: 989–94.
17. Katiyar SK, Elmets CA, Agarwal R, et al., Protection against ultraviolet-B radiation-induced local and systemic suppression of contact hypersensitivity and edema responses in C3H/HeN mice by green tea polyphenols. Photochem Photobiol 1995; 62: 855–61.
18. Elmets CA, Singh D, Tubesing K, et al., Green tea polyphenols as chemopreventive agents against cutaneous photodamage. J Am Acad Dermatol 2001; 44: 425–32.
19. Katiyar SK, Afaq F, Perez A, Mukhtar H, Green tea polyphenol treatment to human skin prevents formation of ultraviolet light B-induced pyrimidine dimers in DNA. Clin Cancer Res 2000; 6: 3864–9.
20. Goodman DS, Vitamin A and retinoids in health and disease. N Eng J Med 1984; 310: 1023–31.
21. Garmyn M, Ribaya-Mercado JD, Russel RM, Gilchrest BA, Effect of beta-carotene supplementation on the human sunburn reaction. Exp Dermatol 1995; 4: 104–11.
22. Duell EA, Derguini F, Kang S, Elder JT, Voorhees JJ, Extraction of human epidermis treated with retinol yields retro-retinoids in addition to free retinol and retinyl esters. J Invest Dermatol 1996; 107: 178–82.
23. Kaur IP, Agrawal R, Nanotechnology: A new paradigm in cosmeceuticals. Recent Patents Drug Deliv Formulat 2007; 1: 171–82.
24. Villalobos-Hernandez JR, Muller-Goymann CC, Sun protection enhancement of titanium dioxide crystals by the use of carnauba wax nanoparticles: The synergistic interaction between organic and inorganic sunscreens at a nanoscale. Int J Pharm 2006; 322: 161–70.
25. Nasir A, Nanodermatology: A bright glimpse just beyond the horizon. Skin Therapy Lett 2010; 15: 1–4.
26. Chadawar V, Shaji J, Microsponge delivery system. Curr Drug Deliv 2007; 4: 123–9.
27. Embil K, Nacht S, The microsponge delivery system (MDS): A topical delivery system with reduced irritancy incorporating multiple triggering mechanisms for the release of actives. J Microencapsul 1996; 13: 575–88.
28. Halder RM, Richards GM, Management of dischromias in ethnic skin. Dermatol Ther 2004; 17: 151–7.
29. Bachlav YG, Summer S, Heinrish A, Bragagna T, Bohler C, Kalia YN, Effect of controlled laser microporation on drug transport kinetics into and across the skin. J Control Release 2010; 146: 31–6.
30. Gill HS, Andrews SN, Sakthievel SK, et al., Selective removal of stratum corneum by microdermabrasion to increase skin permeability. Eur J Pharm Sci 2009; 38(2): 95–103.

14

Cosmeceuticals in Dermatologic Conditions

Mary P. Lupo and Skylar Souyoul

Introduction

All dermatologists make skin care recommendations to their patients. Whether you exclusively care for medical patients, are a Mohs surgeon, or have a practice heavily weighted in the aesthetic realm, we all recommend products to improve the medical or surgical condition we are treating or to complement and maintain our aesthetic results. All dermatologists, especially Mohs surgeons, recommend photoprotection and data verify the enhancing benefit of the addition of phytolase that can cleave damaged DNA as a chemo-preventative (1). Medical dermatologists must address the skin lipid barrier that is disrupted by the inflammatory disease process and dermatologist-designed skin care protocols can help reduce episodic flares in chronic skin diseases. In addition, new technology has been found effective in skin barrier repair for atopic dermatitis by human β defensin-3 via immune-modulating and antimicrobial actions (2). Finally, every aesthetic dermatologist understands the importance of pre-treatment skin preparation and post-treatment care to enhance and extend our results. Protocols including retinoids to speed re-epithelialization and pigment-reducing topical agents such as hydroquinone to decrease existing pigmentation are now standard for pre- and post-laser and light-based treatments (3, 4). More advanced protocols may add peptides, growth factors, and stem cell-activating products to enhance healing and stimulate new collagen.

For all these reasons, it is a natural extension of our professional, medical recommendations to include cosmeceuticals in the patient care discussions. Patients always will and should look to us for educated advice to navigate the many choices that can be confusing to a lay person. We must have a good understanding of the patient's unique needs and which product would best suit those needs. A good, ethical dermatologist lets science and medical professionalism always guide the suggestion, rather having this be a profit-only decision. Offering over-the-counter options is always a good way to ensure that patients do not feel overly pressured to make a purchase in your office. This entire textbook is about helping you as practicing dermatologists understand the science of cosmeceuticals to best serve your patient's needs and be offered in your practice for sale.

Global Considerations

Dermatologists recommend daily sun protection and emphasize the need for re-application during the day. When my patient says, "I don't go out in the sun," I point out that they live on planet earth and as such, they get sun when going to and from their car to get to my office as well as other brief exposures to ultraviolet radiation. I explain that sun exposure damage is cumulative (5). The first 10 minutes do count. Maybe there is no acute damage of erythema, but when it comes to cumulative solar damage, one needs to look no further than a clinical comparison of the left to the right cheek of trunk drivers over 40 years. In addition to SPF, the daytime use of antioxidants is often beneficial for pigment reduction and may help thwart malignant degeneration of cells and enhance the photoprotective effects of sunscreens (6). Nighttime, in contrast, is the best time for repair and restoration. Whether repairing the lipid barrier for aging, diseased, or inflamed skin, or regenerating collagen and dermal ground substance with the use of

DOI: 10.1201/9781315165905-14

fibroblast-stimulating cosmeceutical peptides and growth factors, or using retinoids for improved epidermal turnover, an evening product should be incorporated into the skin care protocol of each patient.

Product Selection

In order to make cosmeceutical recommendations to patients, it is important to understand the potential benefit that a product can deliver and which medical or cosmetic condition may respond to that product. Some of the clinical diagnoses that dermatologists treat which can be improved with the addition of appropriate complementary cosmeceuticals include skin cancer, photoaging, melasma, post-inflammatory hyperpigmentation (PIH), acne, rosacea, and any skin condition that results in lipid barrier disruption (i.e., atopy). Some topical prescription remedies, such as 5-fluoruracil, imiquimod, and aminolevulenic acid for actinic damage and adapalene, tretinoin, and tazarotene for acne or photoaging, all require complementary topical care to protect from ultraviolet light during the day and mitigate epidermal barrier disruption in the evening.

If a dermatologist wants to offer skin care products for sale out of their office, there are common categories of products that would likely be included. Photoprotective products, antioxidants, collagen-stimulating products, pigment-lightening, exfoliants, area-specific products (hands, neck, eye), cleansers, and barrier restorative would be good categories to offer. Many products do multi-tasking such as retinol, which is both pigment-lightening and collagen-stimulating, and alpha hydroxy acids which exfoliate, thereby improving acne as well as dyschromia.

Photoprotection creams, or sunscreens, are the most important recommendations that dermatologists can make to patients. Rosacea, skin cancers, melasma, photoaging, PIH, and light-sensitive dermatoses like polymorphic light eruption are just some of the medical conditions needing regular sunscreen use. It is critical that pulsed light, peel, and laser patients use sun protection before procedures to begin the process of correction, and immediately after the procedure to prevent PIH and consistently over time to maintain the benefit of these paid-out-of-pocket and costly cosmetic procedures. The benefits of using retinoids and hydroquinone both pre- and post-treatment have been proven to enhance results and these products can irritate the skin, so adequate sun protection enhances their tolerability (7). Much progress has been made recently in improvement of broad spectrum sunscreens, especially with improved protection from ultraviolet A rays and improvement in photo-stability of final product formulations.

Antioxidants purportedly complex free radicals that have various deleterious effects on the skin. Free radicals crosslink collagen and accelerate its breakdown (8). It would make sense to use this product class to protect from increases of matrix metalloproteinase I (MMP-1, collagenase) and sunburn cell formation that result from ultraviolet light exposure. UVR also causes NK-κβ activation and the production of pro-inflammatory mediators (9). Antioxidants have anti-inflammatory actions against these mediators and may protect against DNA damage. Table 14.1 lists some of the most popular antioxidant ingredients found in mainstream product lines. Since no sun protection cream can block all ultraviolet light, the use of antioxidants in the morning to complement the protective benefits of sunscreens would be a reasonable recommendation to patients.

Collagen-stimulating products are typically recommended for older skin in which wrinkles and fine lines are the primary concern. Table 14.2 lists some of the ingredients with cosmeceutical studies documenting in vitro or in vivo increases of collagen. These increases in collagen are the result of fibroblast stimulation (10). In addition to collagen, other components of the dermis, such as elastin and glycosoaminoglycans, are produced by fibroblasts. Aging skin and fine lines are the complaints for which these types of products are recommended (11). Exciting new advances in both stem cell-derived ingredients for direct cellular repair and ingredients that have been found to directly stimulate native adult skin cells show promise for both healing and cosmetic enhancements (12, 13). Improvement in skin texture is often the result of all of these fibroblast-stimulating effects.

Irregular pigmentation is a primary concern for many patients across all ethnic lines. Photoaging, PIH, and melasma are all medical conditions that may benefit from adjunctive use of skin care products (14). Primary recommendations include daily sun protection daytime and a hydroquinone plus retinoid prescription combination product at bedtime. Supplementing these agents with pigment-reducing

TABLE 14.1

Popular Antioxidants

Green tea extract
Grape seed extract
Genistein
CoffeeBerry
Co-enzyme Q10
Idebenone
Vitamin A
Vitamin C
Vitamin E
Pycnogenol
Alpha lipoic acid
Dimethylaminoethanol
Glutathione
Catalase
Selenium

TABLE 14.2

Collagen-Stimulating Ingredients

Stem cell-derived serums
Stem cell-stimulating serums
Peptides (copper peptide, pentapeptides)
Amino acids
Plant stem cell-derived serums
Human growth factors (transforming growth
  factor β epidermal growth factor)
Retinol
Niacinamide
CoffeeBerry

cosmeceuticals is a very popular protocol. Table 14.3 outlines ingredients that are prescribed for the lightening of pigment and reduction of sallow discoloration with regular use.

Products that facilitate keratinocyte turnover and maturation or act as keratolytics can improve the appearance of photoaged skin, discoloration, and acne (15). Regular exfoliation using certain exfoliation actives increases dermal matrix hyaluronic acid and glycosoaminoglycans, improving dermal thickness (16). Exfoliation can aid in the turnover of keratinocytes in the pilosebaceous unit and diminish micro-comedo formation, thus improving acne. Table 14.4 lists cosmeceutical ingredients that act as exfoliants. Products that produce a mechanical exfoliation rather than a chemical exfoliation using abrasive particles can also improve the appearance of aging or discolored skin and enhance penetration of prescription or dispensed topical skin lightening agents. Ingredients that work via enzymatic mechanisms are often the gentlest and are well-tolerated for those with sensitive skin. A new, natural enzyme sourced from salmon roe, for example, was recently found to have results similar to, but less irritating than creams containing glycolic acid (17).

TABLE 14.3

Pigment-Lightening Agents

Tetrahexyldecyl ascorbate
Magnesium ascorbyl phosphate
Ascorbyl phosphate
Ascorbic acid
Glycyrrhiza glabra
Ellagic acid
CoffeeBerry
Retinol
Soy extracts
Ferulic acid
Niacinamide
Acetyl glucosamine
Kojic acid
Azaleic acid
Glabridin
Arbutin
Aloesin
Hydroquinone

TABLE 14.4

Non-Physical Exfoliating Ingredients

Glycolic acid
Lactic acid
Malic acid
Polyhydroxy acids (gluconolactone,
  lactobionic acid)
Salicylic acid
Gluconic acid
Papain
Bromelain
Salmon roe protein

TABLE 14.5

Area-Specific Products

Eye creams/gels
Lip plumper/softener
Hand creams
Cuticle oils
Neck creams
Décolleté creams
Firming body lotions
Anti-cellulite creams
Foot creams

TABLE 14.6

Barrier Repair Ingredients

Lecithin
Triglycerides
Linoleic acid
Glycerin
Borage oil
Safflower oil
Shea butter
Ceramides
Omega oils
Argon oil
Allantoin
Fatty acids
Cholesterol
Squalene
Human β defensin-3

Sometimes, patient complaints are specific to a particular region of the skin. Table 14.5 lists common area-specific cosmeceuticals. Due to the very thin skin around the eyes, fine lines and discoloration can occur in even young patients. This area is often the first to concern a patient. Since lip augmentation is a very popular procedure performed in dermatologists' office, lip products to plump or smooth lips is another popular skin care product. The body may have areas of blotchy pigmentation and loss of elasticity, especially on the neck and décolleté. Finally, no area other than the face shows the ravages of cumulative ultraviolet light exposure over a lifetime more than the hands. For all these reasons, many patients are desirous of area-specific products to address such issues. Consumer demand results in the delivery of product when beauty is the issue, so neck creams, hands creams, and other treatments for the body (such as cellulite) are becoming more popular for sale to the public.

Dermatologists also make cleanser recommendations, especially for patients with eczema, contact dermatitis, and acne. Ingredients that hydrate and soothe, formulas that do not remove surface lipids and are pH-balanced, and those containing non-alkaline surfactants are typically offered by dermatologists. Procedures such as intense pulsed light, chemical peel, laser resurfacing, microdermabrasion, and aminolevulenic acid photodynamic therapy treatments all necessitate non-irritating cleansing to prevent redness, irritation, and flaking. One new trend is probiotic cleansers that claim to strengthen the immune system of the skin now being offered for patients undergoing peels and non-ablative laser resurfacing (18).

The stratum corneum is very important to the health and beauty of the skin. Simply hydrating this layer of the epidermis will improve the appearance of fine lines and improve skin's elasticity. The exfoliation of dead corneocytes and replenishing the lipids between the living keratinocytes gives the skin suppleness and a healthy glow. Barrier repair and protection is very important for many skin diseases as well as before and after procedures such as chemical peel and laser resurfacing. Emollients that replenish the lipid layer of the skin can be essential to the success and long-lasting improvement of several procedures and to complement prescription treatments of many diseases such as eczema and psoriasis. Aging skin often experiences dryness as a result of lipid barrier disruption. Barrier repair products are typically applied at bedtime since they can be heavier and do not contain necessary sun protection that is required for daytime products. Table 14.6 lists several effective ingredients known to repair and protect the epidermal lipid barrier.

Ethical Business Practices

The decision of whether to incorporate cosmeceutical suggestions into your patient treatment plan is usually easy and necessary. There are very good mass market products that, as cosmeceuticals, improve skin condition and make prescription remedies work even better. The decision of whether one should sell cosmeceuticals in the office can be more difficult. The ethical side of this issue has many opponents and proponents. Each physician must decide how best to handle product sales. The American Academy of Dermatology has a formal position on the subject (19). The decision to dispense must be in the best interest of the patient, with dermatologists never placing their personal financial interest above the welfare of patients. Patients should never be coerced into making a purchase. Listing of ingredients, advising the patient of less-expensive mass-marketed options, and fair pricing are also mandated. Products cannot be misrepresented as exclusive or unique unless it is true and all products should have valid claims of potential benefit. These recommendations are not only in line with the AAD, but also recommendations that will not diminish the reputation of dispensing dermatologists with patients, fellow physicians, and the general public. It is important to work with the patient so that they understand the product, use it as directed, and communicate reasonable expectations for what the cosmeceutical can realistically accomplish. It is just common sense and good business practice to conduct one's business practice in such an honorable way. Most dermatologists are comfortable dispensing cosmeceuticals because they feel that it improves compliance with skin care regimens and offers patients significant convenience. Products offered should be safe, effective, and able to be incorporated into the patient's lifestyle, so compliance can be achieved.

Once a decision to dispense is made, the dermatologist must choose a company that manufactures the desired products. Published data to support product claims are essential in offering products that will truly help the patients. Customer support issues such as brochures, credit for product returns, employee training, and volume purchase discounts are all important to financial success of adding cosmeceutical dispensing to the practice. Storage of products, purchase of correct amount to avoid expiring before sale as well as local and state regulations on sales tax collection and submission are all part of the internal logistics of retail sales. Employee training and data collection will take time from the medical part of the practice and must be efficiently managed. In general, the sale of physician dispensed cosmeceutical products is an ethical and practical way to increase income while providing a benefit to patients.

Conclusion

If accomplished in an ethical, knowledgeable, and responsible manner, the incorporation of cosmeceuticals into the practice of dermatology is good for both patients and doctors. Deciding if to dispense, what to dispense, and how to do it ethically and profitably are all necessary for success.

REFERENCES

1. Bhatia N, Berman B, Ceilley RI, Kircik LH. Understanding the role of photolyases: photoprotection and beyond. J Drugs Dermatol. 2017; 16(5 Suppl):61–66.
2. Kiatsurayanon C, Niyonsaba F, Smithrithee R, et al. Host defense (antimicrobial) peptide, human defensin-3 improves the function of the epithelial tight-junction barrier in human keratinocytes. J Invest Dermatol. 2014; 134.
3. Duke D, Grevelink JM. Care before and after laser skin resurfacing. Dermatol Surg. 1998; 24(2):201–206.
4. Ortonne JP. Retinoid therapy of pigmentary disorders. Dermatol Ther. 2006; 19(5):280–288.
5. Karagas MR, Zens MS, Nelson HH, et al. Measures of cumulative exposure from a standardized sun exposure history questionnaire: a comparison with histologic assessment of solar skin damage. Am J Epidem. 2007; 165(6):719–726.
6. Ebrahimzadeh MA, Enayatifard R, Khalili M, Ghaffarloo M, Saeedi M, Yazdani Charati J. Correlation between sun protection factor and antioxidant activity, phenol and flavonoid contents of some medicinal plants. Iranian J Pharm Research. 2014; 13(3):1041–1047.
7. Stanfield JW, Feldman SR, Levitt J. Sun protection strength of a hydroquinone 4%/retinol 0.3% preparation containing sunscreens. J Drugs Dermatol. 2006; 5(4):321–324.
8. Ryu A, Naru E, Arakane K, et al. Cross-linking of collagen by singlet oxygen generated with UV-A. Chem Pharm Bull. 1997; 45(8):1243–1247.
9. Larsson P, Ollinger K, Rosdahl I. Ultraviolet UVA- and UVB-induced redox alterations and activation of nuclear factor-kappa B in human melanocytes—protective effects of alpha-tocopherol. Br J Dermatol. 2006; 155(2):292–300.

10. Katayama K, Armendariz-Borunda J, Raghow R, et al. A pentapeptide from type I collagen promotes extracellular matrix production. J Biol Chem. 1993; 268:9941–9944.
11. Lupo MP. Peptides and proteins. In: Cosmeceuticals (Draelos ZD, Dover JS, Alam M eds). Philadelphia: Elsevier/Saunders, 2005: 119–124.
12. Nistor G, Poole AJ, Draelos Z, et al. Human stem cell-derived progenitors produce alpha 2 HS glyco-protein (fetuin): a revolutionary cosmetic ingredient. J Drugs Dermatol. 2016; 15(5):611–626.
13. Sundaram H. The mechanism and potential impact of stem cell activation in skin rejuvenation: an evidence-based analysis. J Drugs Dermatol. 2017; 16(4):378–384.
14. Rendon MI, Gaviria JI. Skin lightening agents. In: Cosmeceuticals (Draelos ZD, Dover JS, Alam M eds). Philadelphia: Elsevier/Saunders, 2005: 103–109.
15. Yu RJ, Van Scott EJ. Alpha-hydroxy-acids and carboxylic acids. J Cosmet Dermatol. 2004; 3(2):76–87.
16. Okana Y, Abe Y, Masaki H, et al. Biological effects of glycolic acid on dermal matrix metabolism medi-ated by dermal fibroblasts and epidermal keratinocytes. Experimental Dermatol. 2003; 12(Suppl 2): 57–63.
17. Mekas M, Chwalek J, MacGregor J, Chapas A. An evaluation of efficacy and tolerability of novel enzyme exfoliant versus glycolic acid in photodamage treatment. J Drugs Dermatol. 2015; 14(11):1306–1319.
18. Baldwin H, Bhatia ND, Friedman A, Eng RM, Seite S. The role of cutaneous microbiota harmony in maintaining a functional skin barrier. J Drugs Dermatol. 2017; 16(1):12–18.
19. https://www.aad.org/forms/policies/Uploads/AR/AR%20Code%20of%20Medical%20Ethics%20 for%20Dermatologists.pdf. Accessed 12/27/2017.

Index

Note: Locators in *italics* represent figures and **bold** indicate tables in the text.